T0073475

COMBATING PHYSICIAN BURNOUT

A Guide for Psychiatrists

COMBATING PHYSICIAN BURNOUT

A Guide for Psychiatrists

Edited by

Sheila LoboPrabhu, M.D.

Richard F. Summers, M.D.

H. Steven Moffic, M.D.

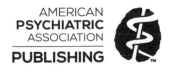

AMERICAN
PSYCHIATRIC
ASSOCIATION
PUBLISHING

If you wish to buy 50 or more copies of the same title, please go to www.appi.org/specialdiscounts for more information.

Copyright © 2020 American Psychiatric Association Publishing

ALL RIGHTS RESERVED

First Edition

Manufactured in the United States of America on acid-free paper
23   22   21   20   19   5   4   3   2   1

American Psychiatric Association Publishing
800 Maine Avenue SW
Suite 900
Washington, DC 20024-2812
www.appi.org

Library of Congress Cataloging-in-Publication Data
Names: LoboPrabhu, Sheila M., 1969– editor. | Summers, Richard F., editor. | Moffic, H. Steven, editor. | American Psychiatric Association, issuing body.
Title: Combating physician burnout : a guide for psychiatrists / edited by Sheila LoboPrabhu, Richard F. Summers, H. Steven Moffic.
Description: First edition. | Washington, D.C. : American Psychiatric Association Publishing, [2020] | Includes bibliographical references and index.
Identifiers: LCCN 2019027407 (print) | ISBN 9781615372270 (paperback ; alk. paper) | ISBN 9781615372720 (ebook)
Subjects: MESH: Burnout, Professional | Physicians—psychology | Compassion Fatigue | Psychiatry
Classification: LCC RC454 (print) | LCC RC454 (ebook) | NLM WA 495 | DDC 616.89—dc23
LC record available at https://lccn.loc.gov/2019027407
LC ebook record available at https://lccn.loc.gov/2019027408

British Library Cataloguing in Publication Data
A CIP record is available from the British Library.

Contents

PART I
Introduction

PART II
The Continuum of Stress, Burnout, and Impairment

PART III
Environmental Factors Leading to Burnout

PART IV
Addressing and Preventing Physician Burnout

PART V
Ethics and Burnout

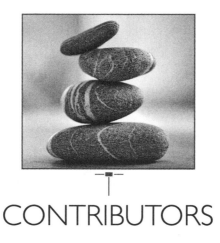

CONTRIBUTORS

Joan M. Anzia, M.D.
Professor of Psychiatry and Behavioral Sciences, Residency Program Director, and Vice Chair for Education, Northwestern University Feinberg School of Medicine; Physician Health Liaison, Northwestern Memorial Hospital, Chicago, Illinois

Stewart Babbott, M.D., FACP
Ward K. Ensminger Professor of Medicine and Associate Chair Ambulatory Services, Department of Medicine, University of Virginia, Charlottesville, Virginia

Lisa Boyars, M.D.
Assistant Professor, Department of Psychiatry and Behavioral Sciences, Medical University of South Carolina, Charleston, South Carolina

Julie Chilton, M.D.
Assistant Clinical Professor, Yale Child Study Center, Yale School of Medicine, New Haven, Connecticut

Gary Chinman, M.D.
Assistant Professor of Psychiatry, Harvard Medical School, Boston; Immediate Past President, Massachusetts Psychiatric Society, Wellesley, Massachusetts

Howard Dichter, M.D.
Private Practice, Bala Cynwyd, Pennsylvania

Anita Everett, M.D., DFAPA
Past President American Psychiatric Association; Director, Center for Mental Health Services, U.S. Department of Health and Human Services, SAMHSA, Rockville, Maryland

Constance Guille, M.D., MSCR
Associate Professor, Departments of Psychiatry and Behavioral Sciences and Obstetrics and Gynecology, Medical University of South Carolina, Charleston, South Carolina

Philip J. Kroth, M.D., M.Sc.
Director, Biomedical Informatics Research, Training and Scholarship, Health Sciences Library and Informatics Center, and Professor and Section Chief for Clinical Informatics Division of Translational Informatics and General Internal Medicine, Department of Internal Medicine, University of New Mexico School of Medicine, Albuquerque, New Mexico

Rishi Kumar
Student, MBChB course, University of Auckland, Auckland, New Zealand

Shailesh Kumar, M.D., FRANZCP, FRCPsych, Diploma in Psychological Medicine, MPhil
Consultant Psychiatrist, Department of Forensic Psychiatry, and Honorary Clinical Associate Professor, University of Auckland, Auckland, New Zealand

Randall M. Levin, M.D., FACEP-Life
Chair, Wellness Section, 2018–2020, American College of Emergency Physicians, Milwaukee, Wisconsin

Sheila LoboPrabhu, M.D.
Associate Professor of Psychiatry, Menninger Department of Psychiatry and Behavioral Sciences, Baylor College of Medicine; Staff Psychiatrist, Michael E. DeBakey Veterans Affairs Medical Center and South Central Mental Illness Research Education Clinical Center, Houston, Texas

Andrés Martin, M.D., M.P.H.
Riva Ariella Ritvo Professor, Child Study Center, Yale School of Medicine, New Haven, Connecticut

Laurel E.S. Mayer, M.D.
Associate Professor of Psychiatry, Vagelos College of Physicians and Surgeons, Columbia University; Associate Professor, New York State Psychiatric Institute; Director, House Staff Mental Health Service–Columbia Campus, NewYork-Presbyterian Hospital, New York, New York

H. Steven Moffic, M.D.
Member, the American Psychiatric Association Board of Trustees Ad Hoc Work Group on Psychiatrist Well-being and Burnout, 2016–2018; Retired Tenured Professor of Psychiatry, Medical College of Wisconsin, Milwaukee, Wisconsin

Victor Molinari, Ph.D.
Professor, School of Aging Studies, University of South Florida, Tampa, Florida

Nidal Moukaddam, M.D., Ph.D.
Associate Professor, Menninger Department of Psychiatry and Behavioral Sciences, Baylor College of Medicine; Adult Outpatient Services Director, Ben Taub Hospital; Medical Director, Stabilization, Treatment and Rehabilitation (STAR) Program for Psychosis, Houston, Texas

David Pollack, M.D.
Professor Emeritus for Public Policy, Oregon Health and Science University, Portland, Oregon

Anthony L. Rostain, M.D., M.A.
Professor, Psychiatry and Pediatrics, Department of Psychiatry, University of Pennsylvania Perelman School of Medicine, Philadelphia, Pennsylvania

Hillary Rouse, M.A.
Doctoral Student, School of Aging Studies, University of South Florida, Tampa, Florida

Luis T. Sanchez, M.D.
Chair, Committee on Senior Physicians, Massachusetts Medical Society and Director Emeritus, Physician Health Services, subsidiary of Massachusetts Medical Society, Waltham; Alternate Delegate, Senior Physician Section, American Medical Association, Chicago, Illinois

Eva Schernhammer, M.D., Dr.P.H., M.Phil.
Professor of Epidemiology and Head, Department of Epidemiology, Medical University of Vienna, Vienna, Austria

Asim Shah, M.D.
Professor and Executive Vice Chair for Psychiatry and Behavioral Sciences, Baylor College of Medicine; Chief of Psychiatry, Ben Taub Hospital, Houston, Texas

Cynthia M. Stonnington, M.D.
Consultant and Chair, Department of Psychiatry and Psychology, Mayo Clinic Arizona; Associate Professor of Psychiatry and Wellness Director, Mayo Clinic College of Medicine and Science, Arizona Campus, Phoenix/Scottsdale, Arizona

Richard F. Summers, M.D.
Clinical Professor of Psychiatry and Senior Residency Advisor, Perelman School of Medicine of the University of Pennsylvania, Bryn Mawr, Pennsylvania

Kenneth Thau, M.D.
Professor of Psychiatry, Department of Psychiatry and Psychotherapy, Medical University of Vienna, Vienna, Austria

Linda L. M. Worley, M.D.
Associate Regional Dean, University of Arkansas for Medical Sciences Northwest College of Medicine, Fayetteville; Professor of Psychiatry and Behavioral Sciences and Professor of Obstetrics and Gynecology, UAMS; Adjunct Professor of Medicine, Vanderbilt University Medical Center, Center for Professional Health, Nashville, Tennessee

Claudia Zimmermann, M.A., M.Sc. (Oxon)
Doctoral Student, Department of Epidemiology, Medical University of Vienna, Vienna, Austria

Disclosure of Competing Interests

The following contributors to this book have indicated a financial interest in or other affiliation with a commercial supporter, a manufacturer of a commercial product, a provider of a commercial service, a nongovernmental organization, and /or a government agency, as listed below:

Philip J. Kroth, M.D., M.Sc.—*Royalties*: Jones & Bartlett

Sheila LoboPrabhu, M.D.—*Coauthor*: 1–2 hour Ethics CME live, internet, and home study courses on physician burnout, wellness and professionalism in my capacity as a volunteer Regional Education team member of the Physician Health and Wellness Committee of the Texas Medical Association, available at www.texmed.org, no income received for authoring these courses, travel expenses incurred, if any, to write courses reimbursed by TMA

Richard F. Summers, M.D.—*Royalties:* Guilford Press, Inc.

The following contributors to this book have indicated no competing interests to disclose:

> Stewart Babbott, M.D., FACP
> Lisa Boyars, M.D.
> Gary Chinman, M.D.
> Julie Chilton, M.D.
> Randall M. Levin, M.D., FACEP-Life
> Andrés Martin, M.D., M.P.H.
> Laurel E. S. Mayer, M.D.
> H. Steven Moffic, M.D.
> Victor Molinari, Ph.D.
> David Pollack, M.D.
> Hillary Rouse, M.A.
> Luis T. Sanchez, M.D.
> Eva Schernhammer, M.D., Dr.P.H., M.Phil.
> Asim Shah, M.D.
> Cynthia M. Stonnington, M.D.
> Kenneth Thau, M.D.
> Linda L. M. Worley, M.D.
> Claudia Zimmermann, M.A., M.Sc. (Oxon)

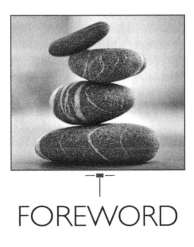

FOREWORD

Are you well? This is a multilayered question with a myriad of possible meanings and answers. I invite you to ponder this question relative to yourself and the profession of medicine—and psychiatry in particular—as you read this book. Broadly, we know that a sense of wellness varies in amplitude throughout a day, a week, and years. The widely accepted paradigm of occupation-related wellness or its opposite, burnout, that was developed by Christina Maslach and Susan E. Jackson in 1981 includes three parameters: emotional exhaustion, lack of a sense of personal accomplishment, and depersonalization. I invite you, as you read this foreword and this book, to make a few notes regarding your own professional wellness status, both now and during periods of time in your past. Reflect on your own wellness and also on that of your professional colleagues.

In preparing this work, we anticipate that readers will predominantly be psychiatrists; some will be physicians from other specialties and other health professionals. Other readers may be stakeholders with an interest in the well-being and burnout phenomenon of modern-day physicians. Stakeholders may include various family members, teachers, other professionals, or individuals. Are you well in the moment as you read these words ("well" in the immediate context and balance of satisfiers and dissatisfiers in your day-to-day life)? Are you well in the overall life trajectory of past accomplishments and losses as well as the opportunities that you anticipate will be in your future? There are many layers to physician wellness.

only increase your wellness but also that of your patients because burnout is correlated with quality of care.

I am honored to have been selected to serve as the APA president and to have had the privilege during that year to have collaborated with the APA Work Group on Psychiatrist Well-being and Burnout. This work will serve to improve the health and well-being of our profession so that we are, in fact, able to better serve our patients.

Anita Everett, M.D., DFAPA
Past President (2017–2018), American Psychiatric Association
Director, Center for Mental Health Services, U.S. HHS, SAMHSA

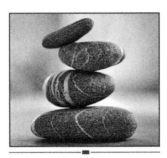

PART I

INTRODUCTION

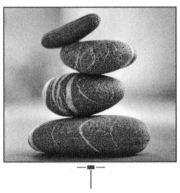

CHAPTER I

THE HISTORY OF BURNOUT IN SOCIETY, MEDICINE, AND PSYCHIATRY

H. Steven Moffic, M.D.

Randall M. Levin, M.D., FACEP-Life

Hillary Rouse, M.A.

What is burnout? Given that it is a colloquial term, does something spiritual fit best, such as, burnout is the process that blocks you from being connected to your inner strengths and sense of purpose, along with the subsequent symptoms that follow. Or, as it has been researched, is there a more academic definition that is widely accepted, such as, burnout is a psychological syndrome that is the direct response to prolonged stressors on the job (Leiter and Maslach 2016)? Perhaps we still need more research and analysis to settle on a definition and conception of what burnout and the process of burning out mean. It will take an historical examination of how burnout became a concern in society, medicine, and psychiatry to try to provide the answers to these questions.

Burnout in many workplaces in the United States first began to receive attention in the 1970s. In 1980, the American Medical Association first began to pay attention to the issue of burnout as it applies to physicians by adding secondary priorities on colleagues and self in the preamble to its update on ethical principles (Riddick 2003). In medical workplaces specifically, such concern started later. Around 1990, among the first specialties to pay attention to the issue of physician burnout was emergency medicine. Surveys showed that burnout rates in medicine had reached epidemic levels over the last decade, with rates that actually greatly exceeded those reported in other workplaces (Shanafelt et al. 2015; The Physicians Foundation 2018). Psychiatry, in particular, became concerned more recently, and in response, the American Psychiatric Association (APA) established the Board of Trustees Ad Hoc Work Group on Psychiatrist Well-being and Burnout in 2017; this became an ongoing committee in 2018. New data in the Medscape National Physician Burnout and Depression Report 2018 indicate that the endeavors of emergency medicine may be resulting in a striking reduction in burnout prevalence in that specialty (Peckman 2018), while at the same time the findings of the APA Board of Trustees Ad Hoc Work Group were promising and indicated that the knowledge and skills of psychiatrists may play a unique role in additional solutions. Emergency medicine and psychiatry have now been joined by other medical specialties—for example, the National Academy of Medicine (NAM) created the Action Collaborative on Physician Well-Being and Resilience in 2017 in a collective effort to enhance the mental health of physicians and the consequent quality of care of their patients.

Recognizing Burnout in Society

Burnout began to receive more attention in the 1970s (Schaufeli et al. 2009; Weber and Jaekel-Reinhard 2000). Around that time, the phenomenon received a comprehensive analysis by the psychologist and psychoanalyst Herbert Freudenberger, Ph.D. (Freudenberger 1980). He seemed to connect the term *burn-out* (as he spelled it) with the burning out of the substance abusers that he encountered during his mental health care work on the streets. He also felt that those who tried to help such substance abusers were also burning out. In extrapolating from his specific circumstances, he came to feel that a change from an industrial society to a service economy was causing more widespread burnout. Industry was no longer promising lifetime jobs or loyalty to employees. He correctly predicted that as time went on, burnout was also likely to increase in workers in the service economy, including those in healthcare, as healthcare workplaces would begin to be characterized by less loyalty to employees.

Around the late 1970s, a Job Demands-Control Model, labeled *job strain*, also emerged and became particularly popular in the occupational medical world (Karasek 1979). When high-demand jobs are paired with a low degree of being able to control one's work, workers seem to be at higher risk for adverse psychological and physical effects.

Around the same time, and apparently independently, the social psychologist Dr. Christina Maslach became interested in a related work phenomenon (Maslach and Leiter 2016). The genesis of Dr. Maslach's concern emerged with the Stanford Prison Experiment of 1971 (Zimbardo 2008). In this experiment, students who were divided into prison guards and inmates in a mock prison went on to exhibit brutal behavior as "guards" and expressed submissive behavior as "inmates." The experiment was cut short after 5 days when Dr. Maslach, having just received her Ph.D., witnessed the experiment and told Dr. Philip Zimbardo, who led the research group conducting the experiment, that it was unacceptable to her professionally and personally. After a heated argument, he agreed and ended the experiment.

Forty years later, when interviewed (Ratnesar 2011) about what came to be considered a heroic ethical effort, Dr. Maslach was asked if the prison study experience had something to do with her eminent research on burnout, and she thought it did. She interviewed real prison guards in a real prison and then healthcare workers, including those who worked in hospitals and emergency departments. She and colleagues at Stanford University learned that the workers felt emotionally exhausted, with a loss of idealism when they felt overly controlled (Maslach 1976). They thought that burnout occurred when workers were dealing with a social environment involving certain kinds of stressors and constraints and generally not because they were weak, had poor coping skills, or had mental problems.

To Dr. Maslach's surprise, her 1976 publication received much attention in the popular press. Even more intrigued, Dr. Maslach developed a method for assessing burnout as a multidimensional construct (Maslach and Jackson 1981). As part of this initial work, burnout was redefined as a response to constant emotional pressure that leads to exhaustion, cynicism, and work stress. It had become apparent at that time that some sort of psychometric tool was needed in order to assess burnout. Using the qualitative research on burnout, Maslach and Jackson (1981) created the Maslach Burnout Inventory (MBI). This scale is composed of three subsections for a total of 22 questions. These sections include nine questions on emotional exhaustion, eight questions on personal accomplishment, and five questions on depersonalization. These questions are answered using a seven-point Likert scale, with higher scores indicating feelings occurring every day or feelings that are very strong.

The MBI has been found to be a relatively reliable, valid tool. One of its major strengths is that it can, and has been, easily adapted to different occupations. It has also been translated into many languages for worldwide use. In addition, in a study investigating the clinical validity of the MBI, researchers tested patients on this scale and then compared the results with a psychiatrist's assessment of individuals using the criteria of "work-related neurasthenia" as a guideline for burnout. The study concluded that the MBI had strong clinical validity, with results from both assessments being very similar (Schaufeli et al. 2001).

Although the MBI is an excellent tool, it has some limitations. First, it is proprietary and thus has a cost. This has contributed to the use of particular items from the inventory, such as emotional exhaustion, in lieu of the entire MBI. A total score can be derived with the MBI; however, there is no set cutoff score that signifies burnout. In addition, what constitutes burnout in different occupations has been found to vary, in terms of both the overall score and the scores in each subscale of the MBI. Finally, the Likert-style nature of the MBI does not allow researchers to obtain an in-depth understanding of what individuals are feeling (Doulougeri et al. 2016), which is an important concern for psychiatry.

Over the years, the MBI has become the most well-known and most often used proprietary survey tool (Maslach et al. 1996). However, there have been more modifications on how to conceptualize and understand burnout. In 1983, Meir defined burnout as a state that occurs in individuals who expect little reward, in addition to considerable punishment, from their work because of a lack of reinforcement, controllable outcomes, and/or personal competence. Maslach and Jackson (1986) subsequently expanded their prior definition of burnout to include specifically emotional exhaustion, depersonalization instead of cynicism, and a reduced sense of personal accomplishment rather than work stress. Further, in 1988, Pines and Aronson defined burnout as a state of physical, emotional, and mental exhaustion caused by long-term involvement in emotionally demanding situations. This became a popular definition for current research because it described burnout as a condition that could occur regardless of the nature of the job. Pines and Aronson used their definition to create a psychometric tool, called the Burnout Measure, to assess burnout in individuals. This scale has 21 questions that assess burnout according to their definition—according to the three components of exhaustion. These questions also are answered using a seven-point Likert scale, with higher scores indicating more significant feelings (Pines and Aronson 1988). This assessment is administered not only in occupational contexts; the assessment is also implemented in nonoccupational areas, for example, the marriage relationship and political conflict (Pines 1994, 1996). Although this tool has also been established as reliable and valid, it should be noted that the Burnout Measure is used in only about 5% of research on burnout, whereas the MBI is used in more than 90% of studies (Schaufeli et al. 2001).

In 1990, the concept of burnout was further developed by Lee and Ashforth (1990), who recognized burnout as a syndrome encompassing the three dimensions of the Maslach and Jackson (1986) model. In 2001, Maslach et al. further expanded upon this by defining burnout as a psychological syndrome relating to chronic interpersonal stressors; and in 2002, Winstanley and Whittington identified burnout as a dynamic process caused by high workload and low coping resources. Two additional revisions were done in 2005. One revision was by Gil-Monte (2005), who believed that there should be a fourth dimension to Maslach's conception of burnout. Gil-Monte's definition of burnout included dividing the personal accomplishment dimension into enthusiasm toward the job and feelings of guilt. The other revision, by Kristensen et al. (2005), proposed that Maslach's definition of burnout was flawed because only fatigue and exhaustion are identified as the core features of burnout. Kristensen et al. argued that depersonalization is a coping strategy for burnout and that reduced personal accomplishment is a consequence of burnout. The definitions of burnout have changed throughout time. However, the most consistently used definition is the one coined by Maslach and Jackson (1981); this is the definition that helped to quantitatively conceptualize burnout through the MBI, the most widely used burnout scale.

There have also been other survey instruments to measure burnout (Louie et al. 2017). In terms of physicians and other healthcare personnel specifically, the Research, Data, and Metrics Working Group of NAM recently concluded that there were several validated instruments available to assess work-related dimensions of well-being. For burnout, they are the MBI–Human Services Survey for Medical Personnel; the Oldenburg Inventory; Physician Work-Life Study's Single-Item; and the Copenhagen Burnout Inventory. For composite well-being, instruments are the Stanford Professional Fulfillment Index and the Composite Global Well-Being Index.

The term *burnout* caught on more generally and has continued to be used, even though it is more of a colloquial term than a scientific one. Why hasn't another term emerged? Perhaps it is because *burnout* has a metaphoric power in conveying the dying down of worker passion to be like the dying down of a fire's embers.

Beyond the switching from an industrial to a service society, what other factors seemed to contribute to more burnout? First of all, the "cultural revolution" of the 1960s seemed to weaken the authority of helping paternalistic professionals such as teachers, social workers, police officers, nurses, and physicians. With the development of bioethics around that same time, the importance of the principle of patient autonomy came to rival that of paternalism. Empowered patients began to feel more entitled to ask for what they thought they needed. Even so, as long as the work setting supported the idealism of those professionals adequately, as it did in settings like monasteries, Montessori schools, and religious sectors, burnout was virtually absent (Cherniss and Kranz 1983).

Physicians and dentists generally had only a reported 10% rate of burnout around the year 2000 (Schaufeli et al. 2011). Actually, this 10% rate of burnout was an increase from virtually nothing and was caused by the rise in patient autonomy and the new demands that patients placed on physicians. Thus, some physicians felt blocked and disconnected from their ability to heal when patients demanded something that the physician would not recommend (Tauber 2005).

However, in the mid-1990s, other external forces were emerging along the lines of Freudenberger's prediction, causing exceptional increases in burnout even among pockets of healthcare professionals that foreshadowed the more general increase of physician burnout as for-profit managed care developed. A study of two staff model health maintenance organizations (HMOs) found that more than half of the physicians reported high emotional exhaustion, a key indicator of burnout (Deckard et al. 1994). Staff models involved physicians being employed and paid a salary. At the same time in community psychiatry, there was a concern that clinical and administrative psychiatrists were losing their authority, while they continued to have ethical and legal responsibility for patient care (Vaccaro and Clark 1996). All these warning signs were apparently ignored in medicine. More generally, the rates of burnout in most physicians, which were relatively low, began rising dramatically at the beginning of the twenty-first century and came to exceed that of other sectors of the economy (Shanafelt et al. 2012).

Although first researched in the United States, by the new millennium the general concern with burnout had spread to countries as diverse as the Philippines and Israel, to Western Europe, and then to Asia, Latin America, Africa, and India (Schaufeli et al. 2009). The interest in the rise of perceived burnout seemed to correspond to the degree of economic development in the countries studied.

Probably because parenting was often not thought of as being work and because of the original focus on the workplace, researching burnout in parents is a more recent phenomenon. It turns out that *parental burnout* seems to also be on the rise. One study from Belgium reported a high level of burnout of up to 12% for both working women and men who take on more parenting, according to a new parental burnout inventory (Roskam et al. 2017). "So exhausted" was described as the primary symptom. There are more similarities than differences between parental burnout and workplace burnout. Parental obstacles include work obligations and two parents working. Moreover, parental burnout seems even more serious and worrisome to parents than workplace burnout because of how their children are adversely affected. Of course, parental and workplace burnout can coexist and worsen the overall impact of being burned out, which can become crucial for work and home life stress and balance.

Definition of Burnout

The definition of *burnout* is elusive, despite being studied for almost 50 years. In the early work of Drs. Freudenberger and Maslach, burnout seemed like some sort of syndrome, somewhere between what was considered as normality and a mental disorder. Because it was connected to the workplace and not home life, burnout was regarded as a social problem. One challenge was defining a cutoff for severity in the surveys used. On the MBI, the key subscales measure exhaustion, cynicism, and a sense of being ineffective, with the various kinds of exhaustion receiving the most attention. The question is this: What meaning do the cutoff scores for designating burnout on such scales have (Balon 2017)? Indeed, at least when applied to physicians, there is concern that cutoff scores that result in more than 50% prevalence do not have much clinical or theoretical meaning (Brisson and Bianchi 2017).

A different thread of thought considers burnout to possibly be a medical disorder. Historically, this can be traced back to the emergence of neurasthenia (Schaufeli et al. 2009). *Neurasthenia* emerged in the early 1800s as a concept to describe a "weakness of the nerves." Most likely to occur in isolated farm workers or overworked businessmen, the symptoms of neurasthenia included fatigue, anxiety, depressed mood, and headaches. In the United states, this psychopathological diagnosis was included in the *Diagnostic and Statistical Manual of Mental Disorders* (DSM) until 1987 (American Psychiatric Association 1987); it continues to be included in the *International Classification of Diseases*, 10th Revision (ICD-10) as F48: "Other nonpsychotic mental disorders." Some physicians equate neurasthenia with severe burnout, as long as the symptoms are work related and the individual is receiving professional treatment. According to this description, it is a culturally accepted diagnosis in some countries, for example, in China (Schwartz 2002).

Although the term *burnout* as related to job satisfaction is not mentioned in DSM-5 (American Psychiatric Association 2013), it is coded in ICD-10 as Z73, in the category of "problems related to life management difficulty." This problem is loosely described as "a state of vital exhaustion" (Van Diest and Appels 1991), harkening back to the most emphasized component in the MBI. In Sweden, "exhaustion disorder" was added to their national version of ICD-10 as a medical diagnosis. Criteria included 2 weeks of daily mental exhaustion, difficulty in concentration, decreased ability to cope with stress, irritability, sleep problems, muscle pains, dizziness, or palpitations, along with subjective suffering, impaired work capacity, and not being related to other medical diagnoses. Similarly, the Netherlands has included burnout as a psychiatric illness, characterized by work-related neurasthenia and long-term loss of the occupational role (van der Klink and van Dijk 2003). Thus, in America and Europe, burnout is a popular term for different reasons. In America, it is a nonmedical label that is thus not stigmatized like other psychiatric disorders tend to be. In contrast, in Europe it is a nonstigmatized medical diagnosis that in some welfare states comes with compensation claims and reimbursed treatment programs. Whether burnout is considered a problem or a diagnosis of an illness, it can coexist with other mental disorders. When such coexistence is present, being burned out can inhibit getting help for major psychiatric disorders, or, in turn, having psychiatric disorders can make it harder to recognize coexisting burnout.

Another medical point of view connects burnout with depression. This point of view considers whether burnout leads to clinical depression or, perhaps, whether burnout is a subcategory of depression (Maslach and Leiter 2016). However, the limited neuropsychiatric studies suggest brain changes more similar to those of major trauma in childhood, and physicians have described thousands of everyday microtraumas as the cause of burnout (Michel 2016). That would suggest that burnout could be a subclinical variety of posttraumatic stress disorder (PTSD). As in the description of microtraumas associated with exposure to racism, such everyday microtraumas for physicians would include unrealistic scheduling, system limitations in resources, patient complaints, and administrative criticism or bullying. Cortisol levels that do not return to normal after repeated trauma can lead to a cascade of health problems, including low-grade inflammation and coronary heart disease (Toker et al. 2012). One physician concerned with physician suicide says that physician burnout is actually physician abuse and that the term *abuse* should be used instead (Wible 2016). That recommendation has not caught on widely, but the physician suicides reported have evoked much concern.

As with soldiers returning from Iraq and Afghanistan, an alternative and overlapping way of describing PTSD is that of a moral injury (Shay 1995). From this perspective, the problem in treating veterans as if they had usual PTSD is that it ignores the moral and ethical dilemmas of committing violence in combat for what may have been questionable reasons.

In healthcare, *moral distress* has also been discussed in the nursing literature for decades as "the experience of knowing the right thing to do while being in a situation in which it is nearly impossible to do it" (Jameton 1984). Moral distress has more recently been deliberated by veterinarians, especially concerning euthanasia (Moses et al. 2018). For physicians, the moral injury might be the perception that making money for the organization is more important than providing quality care for patients. Similar to burnout, they can sense, or know, that they can potentially provide better care if these system obstacles did not exist, especially if the obstacles are perceived to be unnecessary. If, on the other hand, a physician lowers expectations to accommodate the organization, guilt related to doing so could accumulate over time. Indeed, research is beginning to show a correlation of burnout with mistakes, reduced patient satisfaction, and other quality-of-care problems that could haunt physicians (Shanafelt et al. 2010). Another perspective on moral distress is the finding that enabling physicians to adequately devote 20% or more of their work time to what is most meaningful to and valued by them helps to prevent burnout (Rothenberger 2017).

A psychiatrist, in an excerpt from a poem he wrote, "Numbers Game," describes his personal guilt and anguish regarding working with for-profit managed care companies (Berlin 2017, available at https://www.psychiatrictimes.com/poetry/numbers-game). Burnout can be an existential crisis in which specific aspects of the work environment make peak, or even adequate, performance impossible (Pines and Aronson 1988).

With the recent emergence of what is termed *positive psychology* in the United States, burnout can also be considered to be an erosion of work engagement, with engagement being the positive and burnout the negative pole on a continuum of employee well-being (Bakker and Schaufeli 2008). When burnout is viewed this way, burnout prevention turns into the promotion of work engagement.

What burnout is not is compassion fatigue (Carpenter-Song and Torrey 2015). *Compassion fatigue* comes from a short-term, emotionally draining experience, such as in disaster medicine, or from many years of treating emotionally needy and draining people, including patients (Figley 1995). Burnout, to the contrary, is not a response to long hours on a challenging job, nor does it emerge quickly. In years gone by, medical residents worked much longer hours, as did many physicians in practice. Yet the burnout rate was low, likely because in those work hours, although physicians may have been physically tired at times, the physicians felt that their healing self was being called on and not thwarted. However, there are some data to suggest that physicians with higher degrees of compassion, and possibly empathy, are more vulnerable to burning out (Gleichgerrcht and Decety 2013; Kumar 2016). The reason may be that physicians with high compassion and empathy feel worse when the system thwarts their ability to connect with the patient emotionally. Similarly, feeling that one's career is a calling, which is so common among physicians, puts one at higher risk for burning out because of being more emotionally taxed and vulnerable to administrative demands and to sacrificing one's personal life to work demands (Shell 2018).

Recent review studies on the nature and prevalence of burnout clearly indicate that it needs further clarification (Schwenk and Gold 2018). Many physicians suggest that psychiatry, with its experience in classifying mental disorders, is most able to meet this challenge.

Reducing Burnout

The diversity in the definitions of burnout seems to be reflected in the diversity of approaches to prevent, reduce, or treat it (Bahrer-Kohler 2013). Relevant to the presumed causative factors, these approaches to reduce burnout in the general workplace focus on both the individual and the workplace.

It is assumed that there must be some individual variation in vulnerability. This focus is reflected in wellness programs. Such programs may, or may not, be provided in the workplace. Some of the more common recommendations focus on the following:

- Exercise and leisure activities
- Balance between work and personal life
- Emotional intelligence
- Conflict resolution
- Meditation of various types, including mindfulness and the therapeutic use of musical sounds in sound healing
- Social networks of support
- Process groups on burnout, including Balint groups (educational small-group case discussions about the clinician-patient relationship) that focus on clinician challenges (Kjeldmand and Holmström 2008)

Similarly, the organization can establish various measures to prevent or reduce burnout, including the following:

- Empowerment of workers
- Appreciation of workers
- Better communication
- Job resources
- Trustworthy monitoring of burnout by colleagues and administration
- Prevention of bullying and abuse
- Coaching and mentorship
- Discussion of the moral concerns and conflicts in the work setting
- Wellness programs and/or appointment of a chief wellness officer

In essence, the key is the fit between the worker and the workplace. Therefore, it is a dynamic process of trying to ensure that both the worker's and the organization's basic needs are met as best as possible.

There have been some evaluations of the effectiveness of such intervention programs. In a study of 25 primary intervention studies, of which 17 were person directed, 2 were organization directed, and 6 were a combination, 80% of all programs led to some reduction in burnout (Awa et al. 2010). The person-directed interventions modestly reduced burnout in the short term of 6 months or less, whereas the combination interventions had longer-lasting positive effects of 12 months or more. However, in all of these studies, the positive intervention effects diminished over time. There are also natural fluctuations of the degree of burnout because it is a process that reflects various situational and personal factors. The tentative conclusion for the general workplace is that systemwide interventions are best, but intermittent reassessment and refresher programs are necessary for the benefits to continue. However, because burnout in the healthcare workplace is of more recent concern, it is uncertain whether the same conclusion will hold there, although recent research does suggest similar results (Panagioti et al. 2017).

Given the importance of the system, then, the best "treatment" (which would be a cure for burnout) would be to leave the system. Of course, that is not always a practical or desired option. More models and studies are needed before we can develop the kind of expert guidelines we have for DSM disorders.

Burnout in Emergency Medicine

In medicine, compared with other societal workplaces, concern about reducing burnout was delayed until medicine became more business oriented with the development of for-profit managed care in the 1980s (Moffic 1997). Over time, both patients and physicians became frustrated with the emphasis on cost savings and profit over patient care. Within psychiatry, that frustration was illustrated in the dramatic play *Good for Otto* by David Rabe. A

New York Times review of the play depicted some of those business impera-
tives in the following excerpt about a patient and therapist (Isherwood 2015):

> As Frannie's condition deteriorates…Dr. Michaels attempts with increasing
> frustration to get approval from her insurance company for more-intensive
> care…. We witness phones calls with a functionary from the insurance
> company…whose calm recitations of the strict procedures required for any
> change in care—endless paperwork, no guarantees of reimbursement for
> anything not preapproved, etc.—push the doctor to lash out at her. (While
> no polemic, the play presents a persuasive indictment of the power insurers
> have over both doctors and their patients.) (Isherwood 2015, p. C1)

Although it is beyond the scope of this book focusing on psychiatrists to
review burnout in all medical specialties, it may be particularly instructive
to focus on a specialty that was one of the first to respond to the repercus-
sions of such business and organizational changes. This specialty is emergency medicine. The endeavors of emergency medicine practitioners can be
viewed as an example of a long-term, committed attempt to increase wellness and reduce burnout. The impact of their efforts may have significant
meaning for future endeavors in the rest of medicine, including psychiatry.

The premier organization of emergency medicine is the American College of Emergency Physicians (ACEP), which was first established in 1968. In
1989, in response to the concerns of members, ACEP put together a Personal
and Professional Well-Being Task Force, with the mission of finding solutions to the barriers and obstacles to having a sense of well-being along with
a long, fulfilling career. From this agenda, the group produced a 128-page
booklet that has been updated over the years (Manfredi and Huber 2019;
available at https://www.acep.org/globalassets/sites/acep/media/wellness/
acepwellnessguide.pdf). An Aging Physician Task Force was established
around 2005–2006 as an offshoot of this general approach to address concerns related to the experienced emergency physician, including not only the
need to continue to provide optimal patient care but also the need to maintain
perceived well-being while doing so. Once again, an organizational self-
published booklet was issued in 2009 and was reaffirmed in 2015 (American
College of Emergency Physicians 2015; available at https://www.acep.org/
patient-care/policy-statements/considerations-for-emergency-physicians-in-
pre-retirement-years/.

In 1992, ACEP's Well-Being Committee began offering a "wellness booth"
at their scientific assemblies. This consisted mostly of medical testing and the
opportunity to take the MBI, with the goal of understanding personal health
status and the risk of becoming burned out. In 2004, a Wellness Section was
established separately from the Well-Being Committee. This Wellness Section
was designed to encourage the development of a community of like-minded
practitioners in a psychologically safe environment where discussion related to
career journeys could take place, as well as to support the Well-Being Committee's strategic goals.

Early in these ACEP endeavors, the focus was on what was described as the "self-prong"—personal wellness and resiliency. In other words, the assumption was that "if only I was stronger and better, then everything would be fine." However, over the ensuing years, this approach seemed to have limited benefits, and some regarded it as blaming the victim. Discussion evolved, and the likelihood that other factors were at play, especially organizational factors in the system in which one works, was recognized.

This perspective was consistent with the burgeoning research studies being conducted simultaneously on the burnout of physicians across specialties. A supportive home life, spirituality, meditation, mindfulness, and embracing positive psychology could all support well-being and resilience, but a disempowering and toxic organizational system could tear all that down (Taylor 2008). A pivotal document was the Rand Report sponsored by the American Medical Association and The Rand Corporation (Friedberg et al. 2013), as it became clearer that the "Triple Aim" of enhancing patient experience, improving population health, and reducing costs was insufficient. Systems need healthy physicians, and the "Quadruple Aim"—with the added fourth aim of improving the work lives of physicians—became an alternative system goal (Bodenheimer and Sinsky 2014). Not only is it now thought that up to 80% of the variance in causing physician burnout is coming from the system, but it is also acknowledged that it is financially sound for organizations to invest in physician well-being (Shanafelt and Noseworthy 2017).

In recognizing the importance of the workplace environment in the process of burning out physicians, the ACEP Well-Being Committee in 2016 internally released *Wellness in the Workplace: An Information Paper* (available at www.acep.org/globalassets/uploads/uploaded-files/acep/clinical-and-practice-management/resources/wellness/wellness-in-the-workplace.pdf), highlighting the importance of redesigning workplaces at the institutional level generally and specifically in the emergency department. Also in 2016, the ACEP Wellness Section sponsored a speaker with expertise as a human factors and systems engineer for their section meeting at the annual ACEP17 Scientific Assembly to help physicians develop the leadership skills to become engaged and empowered partners at the table. Identifying the need to bring onboard a human factors and systems engineer, a unique psychological approach that we often do not see in clinical psychology, was also noted to be relevant in the July 2017 Collaborative Symposia organized by NAM. Indeed, the collaborative work of NAM is viewed as having great potential to comprehensively address the forces primarily causing burnout (Dzau et al. 2018).

Medscape (an online medical information resource) has been conducting surveys of physician burnout for many years using a one-question item. Although there is much criticism over the validity of the survey results, it is the only survey that has been monitoring burnout in physicians year by year. The survey found that the prevalence of burnout among emergency physicians increased over many years and that the rates were among the highest of any specialty. In the 2017 Medscape Lifestyle Report, emergency physicians ranked first among all specialties, at 59%, in having the emergency physicians who participated acknowledge a symptom related to burnout (Peckman 2017). However, in 2018, their ranking dropped to eighth place at 45% (Peckman 2018). If this first-time and unprecedented degree of drop in burnout prevalence in emergency physicians has validity, it suggests that perhaps interventions to reduce burnout in emergency medicine have finally begun to pay off. Those interventions included the following:

- A complete organizational involvement, from the board of directors down to individual committees and sections of ACEP
- Consistent publication of substantial self-produced literature
- A newsletter that invited participation from other related professions, including psychiatry
- A persistent but fluid approach that changed as peer-reviewed literature emerged with new data and/or the needs of the membership evolved
- A reflection of wellness and burnout concerns in their mission statement, vision statement, and policies on impaired physicians

Emergency physicians have successfully recognized that to care for the communities that they serve, they need to be supported in focusing on their own well-being. In that light, ACEP's inaugural wellness conference and retreat took place in February 2019, with the rationale that quality of patient care goes hand in hand with the well-being of physicians (Shanafelt 2009).

Burnout and Psychiatrists

The earlier section "Recognizing Burnout in Society" indicated that the study of burnout in general workplaces has spread internationally; burnout has also been studied in psychiatrists in particular. Rates for burnout in psychiatrists seemed to hover around 20% in Milan, Italy (Bressi et al. 2009), and Canada (Kealy et al. 2016). Given that healthcare systems are different in other countries, such studies indicate that there are other significant causes of psychiatrist burnout in addition to factors specific to our systems in the United States.

In contrast to these other countries and the ACEP, organized psychiatry in the United States has been relatively late to join in the concern about wellness and burnout (Moffic 2015). This is despite the fact that psychiatry was an early target of for-profit managed care systems. Scholarly consideration seemed to gain traction in 2016, when a textbook on psychiatric ethics (Roberts 2016) included a chapter on clinician well-being and impairment (Trockel et al. 2016). Recently, an issue of *Academic Psychiatry* focused on psychiatrist wellness (Gengoux and Roberts 2018). As was the case with emergency medicine, this focus on wellness has been followed by a focus on burnout and on how psychiatrists can contribute our particular expertise and knowledge.

One explanation for this delay is that our rate of burnout seems to be less than that of many other specialties. However, in the annual Medscape surveys, it had climbed above 40% by 2017. Moreover, an early warning sign occurred in community psychiatrists in the mid-1980s, when a small study suggested that about half of community psychiatrists might be burning out (Clark and Vaccaro 1987). This survey followed the dismantling of the federally funded Community Mental Health Act, with a consequent loss of resources, during the administration of President Reagan.

Another explanation is that there are so many everyday practice concerns in our field that we do not "see the forest for the trees." Ironically, we psychiatrists among all physicians may have been using the defense mechanism of denial even more than other specialists to prevent the painful recognition that we, of all physicians, are burning out. On the other hand, because of our expertise about such defense mechanisms and other psychological processes, we may be able to play a special role in reducing the epidemic increase of burnout in physicians in general (Moffic 2018).

Consider another psychological coping mechanism that has been touted to be an antidote to burnout: resilience. The development of resilience in anyone has been viewed as a positive development—coming back stronger after encountering trauma or other severe stress. Certainly, the inevitable challenges in just becoming a physician lead to increased resilience in most of us. These stressors include the need to master large amounts of relevant knowledge and to cope with patients who die despite our best efforts. Nevertheless, any helpful psychological mechanism can become a problem when used or experienced in excess (Brody et al. 2016; Kumar 2016). In the case of physicians, if the potential of burning out is not kept in mind, more resilience can allow the burning-out physician to plow ahead at work and still claim job satisfaction (Coleman et al. 2015). Such relentless willpower can endanger the physician's own health, including premature aging of immune cells (DeSteno 2018). To counter that, physicians (if the system in which they work does not) can periodically measure their own burnout, resilience, and job satisfaction with any of the major assessment tools available.

Given that about half of all physicians do not seem to be burning out, it is interesting to consider what the predictors are for well-being. Are the non-burned-out physicians just in a better system, or are they treated better in a disempowering system? In psychiatry, is the still common solo practice—a system of one—a protective factor (Morse et al. 2012)? Or does the development of burnout also have something to do with personal histories and personality? If there is a relationship between burnout and trauma, as suggested earlier (see the section "Definition of Burnout"), those physicians with more of a history of unresolved trauma could be at greater risk (Dunne 2015). For an individual physician, exploring the personal history and meaning of choosing a career in medicine can reveal important psychodynamic issues that might need to be addressed (Pines 2000). For instance, a history of being traumatized by an authority figure would likely increase the psychiatrist's vulnerability to bullying administrators of disempowering systems.

All medical specialties have their own unique characteristics and stressors. For instance, emergency physicians are routinely first responders to crises and disasters. The unique stressors that may affect a psychiatrist include the following (Maslach and Leiter 2016):

• Being part of a stigmatized medical specialty
• Being thought of as not a "real" doctor
• Experiencing secondary trauma from working with traumatized patients
• Being at risk from angry and violent patients
• Facing potential suicides of patients
• Being an early and primary target of for-profit managed care
• Working with limited resources
• Experiencing role diffusion

Before psychiatry became more biologically oriented, psychiatrists were expected to have their own psychotherapy when they were in training to better understand themselves and how their personal issues affected patient care. *Countertransference*—that is, the transferring of one's personal issues onto the patient—is always looming. Has the disappearance of the expectation of psychiatrists undertaking personal psychotherapy contributed to a lack of collective introspection about a psychological problem like burnout?

Historically, we psychiatrists have also tended not to share publicly much about ourselves. This started with the "blank screen" of classical Freudian psychoanalysts and continues to permeate our concern about personal disclosure. Jung seemed ambivalent about sharing his own self-analytic journal, not sharing it with others during his lifetime (Corbett 2009). This may help explain why we have very few personal disclosures about our own burnout compared with other medical specialists and other mental health care disciplines (Moffic 2017). However, without enough of those narratives, empathy and concern for collegial burnout may be insufficient (Hankir and Zaman 2013).

Given that the rate of burnout continues to increase among most physicians despite many years of trying to reduce it, perhaps psychiatry is the missing therapeutic ingredient (Everett 2017). Time will perhaps tell if we can provide some unique help. In an effort to do so, the APA Board of Trustees Ad Hoc Work Group on Psychiatrist Well-being and Burnout established a portal on the APA website with information on burnout, brief educational videos by members of the work group, and survey tools for burnout and depression (available at www.psychiatry.org/psychiatrists/practice/well-being-and-burnout). Instead of the MBI, because of considerations of cost and concerns about whether the MBI is the best tool to use for psychiatrists, the Oldenburg Burnout Inventory was used (Reis et al. 2015), and a tentative cutoff point of 35 for burnout was established. Those who filled out the survey over the first year had a prevalence rate that was hovering around 74%, with the highest levels among women and early-career psychiatrists.

The work group also developed tools for knowledgeable psychiatrists to be ambassadors to educational systems and organizations to help them in assess-

ing and addressing wellness and burnout. Although tools like the MBI and Oldenburg Burnout Inventory can be used to periodically assess the degree of
burnout and the result of interventions in individuals and groups, there are significant pros and cons, as well as ethical concerns, in measuring physician
burnout. Administrators could use high scores either to help or to harm given
individuals. Therefore, as in patient care (Roberts and Dyer 2004), informed
consent might be a minimal requirement for use in those being assessed so that
the tools do not add to the sense of disempowerment that contributes to burnout. For psychiatric residents in training, such assessments of burnout could
potentially be used during each year of training to monitor their well-being.

Already, the APA has begun to engage other psychiatrists via town hall
meetings at the annual APA meeting. Knowing you are not alone in struggling with burnout can be reassuring. Better understanding can be helpful
by itself, but this must also lead to better therapeutic tools to be of the most
use. The usual therapeutic tools we have for disorders, such as the variety of
psychotherapies and medications, are unlikely to be of similar use for burnout if it is different qualitatively from DSM-5 disorders. Perhaps positive
psychology and psychiatry approaches would work better as burnout prevention and reduction strategies (Jeste and Palmer 2015). This is already
suggested by the popularity of meditation. If burnout results from thousands of microtraumas during the day, then would thousands of moments of
joy and awe be an antidote? For instance, pediatric residents seem energized,
less cynical, and more confident when attending physicians brought them
flowers of gratitude at the end of a rotation, when fellow residents high-fived
each other for good bedside manner, and when they embraced each other after some sort of perceived or real failure (Bayer and Capucilli 2018). Gratitude, compassion, and pride seem to provide some relief from the harm of
trying to use too much willpower (DeSteno 2018). Humor is a time-tested
positive coping mechanism for stress. Some physicians and psychiatrists
have incorporated the use of clowning in healing activities for health and
mental health problems (Hammerschlag 2011).

Like administrators in all medical specialties, psychiatrist administrators
are the conduit for workplace management, at the fulcrum between the financial resources of an organization and the organization's clinicians; their
approach to burnout may well be the key to success in their workplaces (Carpenter-Song and Torrey 2015). The particular psychological attitude and
skills of these psychiatrists may make them adept managers, and as psychiatrists, they have unique knowledge, including how to manage regressive
group processes that threaten the functioning of the work group (Kernberg
1998). From the perspective of classic psychoanalytic group theory, one
helpful strategy for psychiatric administrators is to have a "slight paranoia,"
exercising vigilance to protect against envious attacks by members of the organization on the leader. Another is to have an ethical kind of love (Moffic
2016), a sublimated love (Kernberg 1998), for the staff and clinicians. This is
the conditional love that will help to empower the clinicians to grow and

thrive, along with realistic expectations, akin to what a parent needs to do with children. Of course, although there are no surveys about their specific degree of burning out, psychiatrist administrators must also be aware of their own mental health if they are not empowered and valued by those who are the financial decision makers in their system.

Projecting into the future from our past knowledge, here are some of the ways that the APA can address the challenges of defining and addressing burnout:

- Educate psychiatrists about the problem and how to enhance our own well-being.
- Bring in our diagnostic research experts to seek more clarification of the nature of so-called burnout.
- Focus particularly on any subgroups that have the highest rates of psychiatrist burnout.
- Recognize that there seem to be many counterintuitive processes in burnout that need to be better understood and addressed, for example, whether more resilience is helpful or harmful, the counterphobic denial of burning out as it is occurring, vulnerability of the most compassionate to burning out, dissociation from microtraumas, and learned helplessness, all of which seem to call for experts in group and individual psychodynamics.
- Encourage the sharing of more carefully considered psychiatrist self-reports of their own burnout processes.
- Understand what unique psychological "treatments" help burnout.
- Integrate psychiatrists more into medical settings, where they seem to have lower rates of burnout and where they can help to ensure that wellness checkups include mental health in addition to physical health.
- Connect with other medical specialties in the United States, as well as internationally, such as national medical and veterinary organizations, given that burnout seems to be a problem in healthcare across many different organized systems of care.

Conclusion

> Those who cannot remember the past are condemned to repeat it.
>
> George Santayana
> *The Life of Reason*

The genesis of trying to understand burnout seems to reside more in the social component of psychiatry's biopsychosocial model (Engel 1980). Historically, the study of clinical practice in prison systems, hospitals, and substance abuse treatment programs led to the scholarly examination of burnout.

It is now more evident that the social system generally has a stronger influence on burnout than individual vulnerability. The development of the current epidemic rate of physician burnout can be traced from the loss of authority in some HMO and community psychiatry systems in the mid-1990s; this loss of authority later spread more widely as the dominance of for-profit health systems increased (Tracer 2018). However, uncertainty exists about whether it is possible to simultaneously improve quality, lower costs, and achieve better medical outcomes, let alone add the fourth component of clinician wellness (Burns and Pauly 2018). Ironically, perhaps, the business orientation that helped to cause physician burnout may be an important part of its solution because it is becoming clearer that physician burnout is costly to the organization (West et al. 2018). Even malpractice insurance companies are beginning to support wellness programs, at least in part because they may reduce physician mistakes and the consequent successful lawsuits.

Although psychologists have long been involved in studying and addressing burnout, psychiatrists have not. Perhaps the delayed concern of psychiatrists and psychiatric organizations about burnout will prove to be more beneficial than harmful if we continue to follow the pace and pathways established by the APA Board of Trustees Ad Hoc Work Group on Psychiatrist Well-being and Burnout as it moves forward as a standing APA committee. Ongoing efforts and attention directed to the issue of burnout (as emergency medicine has done) are key because this is not an acute crisis but a chronic one. Our expertise and skills can supplement what has already been learned and done in emergency medicine as well as other medical and mental health care specialties. The NAM is trying to develop a comprehensive model of how to consider burnout in physicians, and psychiatrists can play an important role in this.

To try to summarize a complex challenge, here is a prototype for preventing or reducing burnout, however it is defined, in any workplace:

1. Process any personal psychological wounds as well as possible.
2. Engage in wellness activities for your body and mind.
3. Work in a system that best fits and supports your abilities and potential.
4. Seek out leadership that has the interest and power to enhance well-being.

KEY POINTS

- Burnout is an important mental health problem in America and around the globe.

- Physicians, including psychiatrists, apparently now have the highest rate of burnout of any profession or work group.

- Those physicians and psychiatrists who view their career as a calling, and who are the most compassionate, seem to be at higher risk for burning out.

- Psychiatrists have paid relatively less attention to this challenge until the past couple of years; however, they may have the special skills and knowledge to provide heretofore missing solutions.

- Although measurement tools are available, whether burnout is a syndrome, problem, moral distress, a variation of a psychiatric disorder, or an example of the Jungian "wounded healer" is still uncertain at this time, and clarification is needed.

- The key to wellness and preventing burnout is having a good and ethical fit and relationship between the clinician and the system, which at a minimum should include 20% of work time devoted to activities that the physician values the most.

- Even if a disempowering system is the major causative factor, there are wellness-oriented activities that can be helpful, including hobbies, meditation, laughter, and feelings of awe.

- Individual "treatments" for burnout are under further investigation.

- The psychiatrist administrator, conveying ethical love and realistic expectations, is the essential cog in the wheel of the healthcare system.

- Burnout is the rare issue that touches on all the responsibilities noted in the preamble of the American Medical Association's Code of Medical Ethics—from quality of patient care to the needs of society, colleagues, and oneself.

References

American College of Emergency Physicians: Considerations for Emergency Physicians in Pre-retirement Years, 2015. Available at https://www.acep.org/patient-care/policy-statements/considerations-for-emergency-physicians-in-pre-retirement-years/. Accessed June 17, 2019.

American Psychiatric Association: Diagnostic and Statistical Manual of Mental Disorders, 3rd Edition, Revised. Washington, DC, American Psychiatric Association, 1987

American Psychiatric Association: Diagnostic and Statistical Manual of Mental Disorders, 5th Edition. Arlington, VA, American Psychiatric Association, 2013

Awa WL, Plaumann M, Walter U: Burnout prevention: a review of intervention programs. Patient Educ Couns 78(2):184–190, 2010 19467822

Bahrer-Kohler S (ed): Burnout for Experts: Prevention in the Context of Living and Working. New York, Springer, 2013

Bakker A, Schaufeli WB: Positive organizational behavior: engaged employees in flourishing organizations. J Organ Behav 29:147–154, 2008

Balon R: What about burnout? Ann Clin Psychiatry 29(2):81–82, 2017 28463342

Bayer N, Capucilli P: Small steps to address medical resident burnout. JAMA Pediatr 172(2):113–114, 2018 29279902

Berlin R: Numbers game. Psychiatr Times 34(5):28, 2017. Available at: https://www.psychiatrictimes.com/poetry/numbers-game. Accessed June 17, 2019.

Bodenheimer T, Sinsky C: From triple to quadruple aim: care of the patient requires care of the provider. Ann Fam Med 12(6):573–576, 2014 25384822

Bressi C, Porcellana M, Gambini O, et al: Burnout among psychiatrists in Milan: a multicenter survey. Psychiatr Serv 60(7):985–988, 2009 19564233

Brisson R, Bianchi R: Stranger things: on the upside down world of burnout research. Acad Psychiatry 41(2):200–201, 2017 27815715

Brody GH, Yu T, Miller GE, Chen E: Resilience in adolescence, health, and psychosocial outcomes. Pediatrics 138(6):e20161042, 2016 27940681

Burns L, Pauly M: Transformation of the health care industry: curb your enthusiasm? Milbank Q 96(1):57–109, 2018 29504199

Carpenter-Song E, Torrey WC: "I always viewed this as the real psychiatry": provider perspectives on community psychiatry as a career of first choice. Community Ment Health J 51(3):258–266, 2015 24989962

Cherniss C, Kranz D: The ideological community as an antidote to burnout in the human services, in Stress and Burnout in the Human Services Professions. Edited by Farber D. New York, Pergamon, 1983, pp 198–212

Clark GH Jr, Vaccaro JV: Burnout among CMHC psychiatrists and the struggle to survive. Hosp Community Psychiatry 38(8):843–847, 1987 3610084

Coleman M, Dexter D, Nankivil N: Factors affecting physician satisfaction and Wisconsin Medical Society strategies to drive change. WMJ 114(4):135–142, 2015 26436181

Corbett S: The holy grail of the unconscious. The New York Times Magazine, Sept 16, 2009

Deckard G, Meterko M, Field D: Physician burnout: an examination of personal, professional, and organizational relationships. Med Care 32(7):745–754, 1994 8028408

DeSteno D: Emotional Success: The Power of Gratitude, Compassion, and Pride. Boston, MA, Houghton Mifflin Harcourt, 2018

Doulougeri K, Georganta K, Montgomery A: "Diagnosing" burnout among healthcare professionals: can we find consensus? Cogent Med 3(1):1–10 2016

Dunne C: Carl Jung: Wounded Healer of the Soul (Reprint Edition). London, Watkins Publishing, 2015

Dzau VJ, Kirch DG, Nasca TJ: To care is human—collectively confronting the clinician-burnout crisis. N Engl J Med 378(4):312–314, 2018 29365296

Engel GL: The clinical application of the biopsychosocial model. Am J Psychiatry 137(5):535–544, 1980 7369396

Everett A: Response to the presidential address. Am J Psychiatry 174(8):734–736, 2017 28760017

Figley C: Compassion Fatigue. New York, Taylor and Francis Group, 1995

Freudenberger H: Burnout: The High Cost of High Achievement. Norwell, MA, Anchor Press, 1980

Friedberg M, Chen PG, Van Busum KR, et al: Factors Affecting Physician Professional Satisfaction and Their Implications for Patient Care, Health Systems, and Health Policy. Santa Monica, CA, RAND Corporation, 2013. Available at: https://www.rand.org/pubs/research_reports/RR439.html. Accessed July 24, 2018.

Gengoux GW, Roberts LW: Enhancing wellness and engagement among healthcare professionals. Acad Psychiatry 42(1):1–4, 2018 29297148

Gil-Monte PR: El Síndrome de Quemarse por el Trabajo (Burnout): Una enfermedad laboral en la sociedad del bienestar. Madrid, Pirámide, 2005

Gleichgerrcht E, Decety J: Empathy in clinical practice: how individual dispositions, gender, and experience moderate empathic concern, burnout, and emotional distress in physicians. PLoS One 8(4):e61526, 2013 23620760

Hammerschlag C: Kindling Spirit—Healing From Within. Seattle, WA, Turtle Island Press, 2011

Hankir A, Zaman R: Jung's archetype, 'The Wounded Healer', mental illness in the medical profession and the role of the humanities in psychiatry. BMJ Case Rep Jul 2013 Epub

Isherwood C: Review: David Rabe's "Good for Otto" introduces a world of pain. New York Times, November 16, 2015, p C1

Jameton A: Nursing Practice: The Ethical Issues. Englewood Cliffs, NJ, Prentice Hall, 1984, p 6

Jeste D, Palmer B (eds): Positive Psychiatry: A Clinical Handbook. Washington, DC, American Psychiatric Publishing, 2015

Karasek RA: Job demands, job decision latitude and mental strain: implications for job redesign. Adm Sci Q 24:285–308, 1979

Kealy D, Halli P, Ogrodniczuk JS, et al: Burnout among Canadian psychiatry residents: a national survey. Can J Psychiatry 61(11):732–736, 2016 27310237

Kernberg O: Ideology, Conflict, and Leadership in Groups and Organizations. New Haven, CT, Yale University Press, 1998

Kjeldmand D, Holmström I: Balint groups as a means to increase job satisfaction and prevent burnout among general practitioners. Ann Fam Med 6(2):138–145, 2008 18332406

Kristensen TS, Borritz M, Villadsen B, Christensen KB: The Copenhagen Burnout Inventory: a new tool for the assessment of burnout. Work Stress 19(3):192–207, 2005

Kumar S: Burnout and doctors: prevalence, prevention and intervention. Healthcare (Basel) 4(3):37, 2016 27417625

Lee RT, Ashforth BE: On the meaning of Maslach's three dimensions of burnout. J Appl Psychol 75(6):743–747, 1990 1981064

Leiter MP, Maslach C: Latent burnout profiles: a new approach to understanding the burnout experience. Burn Res 3(4):89–100, 2016

Louie AK, Trockel MT, Balon R, et al: "Physician Wellness" as published in Academic Psychiatry. Acad Psychiatry 41(2):155–158, 2017 28213884

Manfredi RA, Huber JM: Being Well in Emergency Medicine: ACEP's Guide to Investing in Yourself, 2019. Available at https://www.acep.org/globalassets/sites/acep/media/wellness/acepwellnessguide.pdf. Accessed June 17, 2019.

Maslach C: Burned-out. Hum Behav 9:16–22, 1976

Maslach C, Jackson SE: The measurement of experienced burnout. Journal of Occupational Behaviour 2:99–113, 1981

Maslach C, Jackson SE: Maslach Burnout Inventory Manual, 2nd Edition. Palo Alto, CA, Consulting Psychologists Press, 1986

Maslach C, Leiter MP: Understanding the burnout experience: recent research and its implications for psychiatry. World Psychiatry 15(2):103–111, 2016 27265691

Maslach C, Jackson S, Leiter M: MBI: The Maslach Burnout Inventory Manual, 3rd Edition. Palo Alto, CA, Consulting Psychologists Press, 1996

Maslach C, Schaufeli WB, Leiter MP: Job burnout. Annu Rev Psychol 2:397–422 2001 11148311

Meir ST: Toward a theory of burnout. Hum Relat 36(10):899–910, 1983

Michel A: Burnout and the brain. Observer, February 2016

Moffic HS: The Ethical Way: Challenges and Solutions for Managed Behavioral Healthcare. San Francisco, CA, Jossey-Bass, 1997

Moffic HS: Is our profession breaking our hearts? A Valentine's Day concern. Psychiatr Times, Feb 11, 2015. Available at: http://www.psychiatrictimes.com/blogs/our-profession-breaking-our-hearts-valentine-day-concern. Accessed December 25, 2017.

Moffic HS: Ethics column: ethical love and the prevention of burn-out by psychiatric leadership. Journal of Psychiatric Administration and Management 5(2):45–54, 2016

Moffic HS: A psychiatrist burns out. Psychiatr Times, March 30, 2017. Available at: http://psychiatrictimes.com/blogs/couch-crisis/psychiatrist-burns-out. Accessed December 25, 2017.

Moffic HS: Some aspects of burnout are natural for psychiatry to address. Psychiatric News 53(7):3, 21, 2018

Morse G, Salyers MP, Rollins AL, et al: Burnout in mental health services: a review of the problem and its remediation. Adm Policy Ment Health 39(5):341–352, 2012 21533847

Moses L, Malowney M, Boyd J: Ethical conflict and moral distress in veterinary practice: a survey of North American veterinarians. Journal of Veterinary Internal Medicine 32(6):2115–2122, 2018

Panagioti M, Panagopoulou E, Bower P, et al: Controlled interventions to reduce burnout in physicians: a systematic review and meta-analysis. JAMA Intern Med 177(2):195–205, 2017 27918798

Peckman C: Medscape lifestyle report 2017: race and ethnicity, bias and burnout. Medscape, Jan 11, 2017

Peckman C: Medscape national physician burnout and depression report 2018. Medscape, Jan 17, 2018

Pines A, Aronson E: Career Burnout: Causes and Cures. New York, The Free Press, 1988

Pines AM: The Palestinian intifada and Israelis' burnout. J Cross Cult Psychcol 25(4):438–451, 1994

Pines AM: Couple Burnout: Causes and Cures. New York, Routledge, 1996

Pines AM: Treating career burnout: a psychodynamic existential perspective. J Clin Psychol 56(5):633–642, 2000 10852150

Ratnesar R: The menace within. Stanford Magazine, July/August, 2011

Reis D, Xanthopoulou D, Tsaousis I: Measuring job and academic burnout with the Oldenburg Inventory (OLBI): factorial invariance across samples and countries. Burn Res 2(1):8–18, 2015

Riddick FA Jr: The code of medical ethics of the American Medical Association. Ochsner J 5(2):6–10, 2003 22826677

Roberts LW: A Clinical Guide to Psychiatric Ethics. Washington, DC, American Psychiatric Association Publishing, 2016

Roberts LW, Dyer AR (eds): Ethics in Mental Health Care (Concise Guides Series; Hales, RE, series ed). Arlington, VA, American Psychiatric Publishing 2004

Roskam I, Raes M-E, Mikolajczak M: Exhausted parents: development and preliminary validation of the parental burnout inventory. Front Psychol 8:163, 2017 28232811

Rothenberger DA: Physician burnout and well-being: a systematic review and framework for action. Dis Colon Rectum 60(6):567–576, 2017 28481850

Schaufeli WB, Baker AB, Hoogduin K, et al: On the clinical validity of the Maslach Burnout Inventory and the Burnout Measure. Psychol Health 16(5):565–582, 2001 22804499

Schaufeli WB, Leiter MP, Maslach C: Burnout: 35 years of research and practice. Career Development International 14(3):204–220, 2009

Schaufeli WB, Maassen GH, Bakker AB, et al: Stability and change in burnout: a 10-year follow-up study among primary care physicians. J Occup Organ Psychol 84(2):248–267, 2011

Schwartz PY: Why is neurasthenia important in Asian cultures? West J Med 176(4):257–258, 2002 12208833

Schwenk TL, Gold KJ: Physician burnout—a serious symptom, but of what? JAMA 320(11):1109–1110, 2018 30422283

Shanafelt TD: Enhancing meaning in work: a prescription for preventing physician burnout and promoting patient-centered care. JAMA 302(12):1338–1340, 2009 19773573

Shanafelt TD, Noseworthy JH: Executive leadership and physician well-being: nine organizational strategies to promote engagement and reduce burnout. Mayo Clin Proc 92(1):129–146, 2017 27871627

Shanafelt TD, Balch CM, Bechamps G, et al: Burnout and medical errors among American surgeons. Ann Surg 251(6):995–1000, 2010 19934755

Shanafelt TD, Boone S, Tan L, et al: Burnout and satisfaction with work-life balance among US physicians relative to the general US population. Arch Intern Med 172(18):1377–1385, 2012 22911330

Shanafelt TD, Hasan O, Dyrbye LN, et al: Changes in burnout and satisfaction with work-life balance in physicians and the general US working population between 2011 and 2014. Mayo Clin Proc 90(12):1600–1613, 2015 26653297

Shay J: Achilles in Vietnam: Combat Trauma and the Undoing of Character. New York, Simon & Schuster, 1995

Shell E: The Job: Work and Its Future in a Time of Radical Change. New York, Penguin Random House, 2018

Tauber A: Patient Autonomy and the Ethics of Responsibility. Cambridge, MA, MIT Press, 2005

Taylor S: Fostering a supportive environment at work. The Psychologist-Manager Journal 11:265–283, 2008

The Physicians Foundation: 2018 Survey of America's Physicians: Practice Patterns and Perspectives. 2018. Available at: https://physiciansfoundation.org/research-insights/the-physicians-foundation-2018-physician-survey/. Accessed June 10, 2019.

Toker S, Melamed S, Berliner S, et al: Burnout and risk of coronary heart disease: a prospective study of 8838 employees. Psychosom Med 74(8):840–847, 2012 23006431

Tracer Z: Health insurance startups bet it's time for a nineties revival. Bloomberg, July 24, 2018

Trockel M, Miller M, Roberts LW: Clinician well-being and impairment, in A Clinical Guide to Psychiatric Ethics. Edited by Roberts LW. Washington, DC, American Psychiatric Association Publishing, 2016

Vaccaro J, Clark G (eds): Practicing Psychiatry in the Community: A Manual. Washington, DC, American Psychiatric Publishing, 1996

van der Klink JJ, van Dijk FJ: Dutch practice guidelines for managing adjustment disorders in occupational and primary health care. Scand J Work Environ Health 29(6):478–487, 2003 14712856

van Diest R, Appels A: Vital exhaustion and depression: a conceptual study. J Psychosom Res 35(4):535–544, 1991 1681098

Weber A, Jaekel-Reinhard A: Burnout syndrome: a disease of modern societies? Occup Med (Lond) 50(7):512–517, 2000 11198677

West CP, Dyrbye LN, Shanafelt TD: Physician burnout: contributors, consequences and solutions. J Intern Med 283(6):516–529, 2018 29505159

Wible P: Physician Suicide Letters Answered. Eugene, OR, Pamela Wible, MD, 2016

Winstanley S, Whittington R: Anxiety, burnout and coping styles in general hospital staff exposed to workplace aggression: a cyclical model of burnout and vulnerability to aggression. Work Stress 16(4):302–315, 2002

Zimbardo P: The Lucifer Effect: Understanding How Good People Turn Evil. New York, Random House, 2008

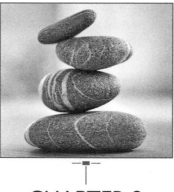

CHAPTER 2

THE SOCIAL CONTEXT OF PHYSICIAN BURNOUT

Richard F. Summers, M.D.

"Institutions are where the human heart either gets welcomed or thwarted or broken."

Parker J. Palmer
Living the Questions (Intrator 2005)

Several years ago, psychiatry residency directors discussed their professional identities and values regarding work-life balance in a workshop at a national meeting. One gray-haired participant spoke eloquently about the wonderful long-term relationships he had developed with patients and how this was such a source of professional satisfaction and meaning. He reminisced about a patient with whom he had worked for many years, at whose funeral he had received tremendous appreciation and gratitude from family members for the compassionate care he had provided. The residency director talked about the feeling of satisfaction and validation he felt and how this gave him a sense of meaning in his work. However, a younger psychiatrist in the group quickly spoke up with some alarm. Smart, successful, creative, warm, and humanistic, this man passionately explained that he did not want to become one of those doctors whose practice life overran his time at home with his family. He would never attend the funeral of a patient and saw this as above and beyond the call of our work. Such behavior was over the line.

Needless to say, a controversy ensued, with some participants expressing shock and disappointment at the erosion of the culture of medicine, the devaluing of a deep doctor-patient relationship. Yet others agreed with the younger psychiatrist's viewpoint and noted that the first speaker's level of personal involvement and the porosity of his work-life boundaries was inimical to a healthy personal life for physicians. Some politely decried the "millennial values," whereas others complained about the "dinosaurs."

Leaving aside the merits of the moral and lifestyle choices involved here, what was clear to many in the discussion was that this difference in perspective said everything about how medicine was changing and that the experience of doctors—their identities, values, and behavior—was in transition. In this chapter, I aim to explore this transition, identify the crucial elements of the social context of the practice of medicine, and connect this context to the evolving epidemic of physician burnout. My background for working on this topic includes 30 years as a practicing psychiatrist and educator, a knowledge of the literature in this area, and my role as chair of the American Psychiatric Association (APA) Board of Trustees Ad Hoc Work Group on Psychiatrist Well-being and Burnout.

From Marcus Welby, M.D., to Randolph Bell

The traditional medical career was regarded by physicians and nonphysicians alike as a privilege, both in terms of the satisfaction and meaning of the work and the prestige and economic reward. Physicians have gone from this now nostalgic view, which was always somewhat romantic, to the opposite, where many regard burnout and dissatisfaction as an inevitable part of a career in medicine. The kindly, gentle general practitioner has been replaced as an exemplar by Meredith Grey, the miserable house officer on *Grey's Anatomy,* and more recently by the selfish and manipulative Randolph Bell on the cynical new television series *The Resident.*

Burnout is defined by Maslach and Leiter (2016) as a syndrome of emotional exhaustion, depersonalization, and decreased sense of personal efficacy. This conceptualization, which remains a core notion as the discussion about physician burnout has spread and becomes more complex and nuanced, seeks to distinguish burnout from other conditions such as depression, anxiety disorders, posttraumatic states, and neuropsychological impairment. A competing viewpoint looks at physician well-being, holding that this desirable state reflects a combination of positive factors such as thriving and vigor as well as negative factors such as exhaustion and dysphoria. Indeed, Brady et al. (2018) proposed a comprehensive definition:

> Physician wellness (well-being) is defined by quality of life, which includes the absence of ill-being and the presence of positive physical, mental, social, and integrated well-being experienced in connection with activities and environments that allow physicians to develop their full potentials across personal and work-life domains. (p. 103)

This chapter identifies three major social and economic trends that have shaped the profession of medicine over recent decades—the social transformation of the profession of medicine, the corporatization of healthcare, and the Triple Aim of healthcare—and discusses how these trends affect the important domains of work-related risk factors that have been identified in the occupational literature as relevant to burnout: workload, control, reward, community, fairness, and values (Maslach et al. 2001; Schaufeli and Enzmann 1998). Next, the major changes in practice of medicine over the twentieth and twenty-first century are discussed as they impact the satisfaction and dissatisfaction of physicians in general and psychiatrists in particular. Finally, the chapter concludes by looking toward the future and explores those forces that may help to mitigate burnout and promote well-being.

Other chapters in this volume discuss the phenomenology of burnout and its epidemiology in more detail, along with the associated physician mental health problems. Specific drivers of burnout and depression, and the interventions for them, are also covered elsewhere in the volume.

Three Social and Economic Forces Shaping Physician Experience

The social transformation of the profession of medicine over the twentieth century, corporatization of healthcare, and the adoption of the Triple Aim of healthcare (Berwick et al. 2008) are three interrelated trends that have had profound effects on the lived experience of physicians working in diverse clinical settings.

THE SOCIAL TRANSFORMATION OF MEDICINE

Paul Starr (1982), the sociologist and author of the definitive work on the sociology of medicine in the twentieth century, took on the first of these major trends. He noted as follows:

From a relatively weak, traditional profession of minor economic significance, medicine has become a sprawling system of hospitals, clinics, health
plans, insurance companies, and myriad other organizations employing a
vast labor force. This transformation has not been propelled solely by the advance of science and the satisfaction of human needs. The history of medicine has been written as an epic of progress, but it is also a tale of social and
economic conflict over the emergence of new hierarchies, of power and authority, new markets, and new conditions of belief and experience. (p. 4)

Starr's narrative reminds us that physicians emerged from their relatively low status role, unremarkable economic circumstances, and delimited
professional identity and became the high-status and high-earning drivers
of an explosively expanding healthcare industry by riding the coattails of science and harnessing a uniquely American marketplace. We physicians developed not only economic and social status but also political strength and
power. Our profession's increasing reliance on science provided a basis for
this transformation, but it required economic and political strength to implement. The economic and political structures ultimately determined its
new position.

Physicians reached a peak of autonomy, professionalism, and affluence
somewhere in the 1970s or 1980s. This was when physicians were frequently
the leaders of healthcare organizations, and government and insurance
companies paid the bills and exerted a modicum of control. Yet the same
economic and political forces that brought physicians this power have
driven further transformation of the healthcare system, which has resulted
in deprofessionalization, commoditization, and a new role for physicians as
service providers in a complex corporate marketplace. As the share of gross
domestic product spent on medicine increased (Centers for Medicare and
Medicaid Services 2018) and the needs of the population became clearer, the
economic mechanisms for driving improvements in healthcare clearly lie
beyond the economics of physicians' practices. Insurers, employers, and
federal and state governments stepped in to manage healthcare. This included increasing restrictions but also selective deregulation, such as allowing for-profit health maintenance organizations (HMOs). With these
changes, the role of physicians morphed from decider to provider.

Psychiatry has participated in its own unique version of this arc. As medicine rode the wave up through the mid-twentieth century, psychiatry shared
the fruits of the new power and prosperity. Bolstered by its contribution to
the recognition of posttraumatic stress disorder (PTSD) in World War II, its
robust role in popular culture, and the excitement of psychoanalytic insights,
many flocked to psychiatry training programs, and practice flourished in hospitals, Veterans Affairs programs, community systems, and cottage-industry
private practices. As the broader economic and political forces drove consol-
idation of healthcare institutions in general, mental healthcare institutions responded to the same pressures. This meant aggregation of physicians into
group practices, provider panels, and salaried positions in larger organizations.

The need for population-based care, accountability, and standardization—and more recently the electronic health record (EHR)—accelerated these trends.

Psychiatry yielded to many of these general pressures earlier than many other specialties, probably because of its relatively low profitability, inherent community focus, and stigmatization, which rendered it more vulnerable to aggressive cost cutting by insurance companies and government. Lack of parity in insurance coverage contributed to the squeeze on resources. Applications to psychiatry residency programs peaked in the 1950s and 1960s (Neff et al. 1987) and then began to decline until their nadir in the late 1990s. This trend probably follows psychiatry's transformation. Thankfully, since that time, there has been a marked upward trend in U.S. medical graduates applying to psychiatry residencies as the transformation of the rest of medicine has caught up, and the students now see that psychiatry offers practitioners a unique combination of personal connection, engagement with important social issues, and cutting-edge science.

CORPORATIZATION OF MEDICINE

The relentless pressure for financial performance, spread of for-profit medicine, and rise of new healthcare start-ups reflect an extension of the path predicted by Starr (1982). Nonprofit entities now function like corporations, employing management strategies and accountability used in the business world. The corporatization of medicine has resulted in a loss of physician autonomy, change in the doctor-patient contract, and new pressures on physician behavior.

Some physicians have adapted by becoming businessmen. Arnold Relman (1992; available at www.theatlantic.com/past/docs/politics/healthca/relman.htm) lamented the impact of this trend, noting that "at every turn in the road physicians both in practice and in academic institutions are being attracted by financial arrangements that can compromise their professional independence." Most have become employees.

Physicians as employees experience their work differently. On the positive side, they are freed from the pressure to provide more units of service to generate income, have clearer lines between work and personal life, and have more structured collegial relationships to share the burden of patient care. However, they are more likely to experience conflict between their values and those of the organization for whom they work and more likely to chafe under the requirements and accountability expected from those organizations. They experience a loosening of the very personal doctor-patient relationship, diffusion of responsibility, and the sense of having to serve too many masters—patients, employers, and their internalized ideals about patient care.

As corporate entities, for-profit and not-for-profit, respond to the demands of the marketplace, they make decisions accordingly, and the norms of many healthcare organizations begin to shift toward those more typical of businesses. The culture of medicine, and of medicine as a profession, begins to erode and physicians are treated as valuable employees.

THE TRIPLE AIM

The Triple Aim of the healthcare system, as defined by Berwick et al. (2008, p. 759; available at www.healthaffairs.org/doi/pdf/10.1377/hlthaff.27.3.759), involves a focus on three simultaneous goals: "improving the experience of care, improving the health of populations, and reducing per capita costs of health care." This elegantly articulated vision has been highly influential and is reflected in the increased attention now paid to data collected on patient satisfaction, health outcomes, and transparency in the cost of care. The streams of data on these indicators influence managers making decisions on physician staffing, patient flow, pathways of care, service delivery design, capital investment, and other fundamental organizational priorities.

The Affordable Care Act attempted to incentivize attention to these system parameters, based on the notion that the effective pursuit of the Triple Aim requires a reorganization of healthcare into defined populations, a commitment to universality among its members, and an integrator—that is, an entity with responsibility for the population and the ability to control the important parameters in providing care to that population.

The transformation driven by the Triple Aim, which has successfully shifted attention to populations, has been limited. There is persistence of care provided based on fee-for-service incentives side by side with many programs designed to meet these new parameters. In psychiatry, the integrated care approach is responsive to the demands of the Triple Aim, as are many innovative programs designed to address the needs of high utilizers of care, chronically ill patients, and those with comorbid psychiatric illness and medical illness.

Mediators of Burnout

The result of these three trends—the longer-term historical transformation of the profession of medicine, corporatization of healthcare, and most recently the pursuit of the Triple Aim—is a very different system of care from several decades ago. The question for this discussion of burnout is what is the impact of those trends on the six domains of activity regarded as mediators of workplace-based stress. Maslach et al. (2001) conceptualized burnout as a problem with person-job fit and identified workload, control, reward, community, fairness, and values as the occupational dimensions most relevant to satisfaction and burnout.

A review of these six psychiatric job domains suggests that at least four may present challenges for psychiatrists. There is a perception that *workload* is greater with the increased prevalence of psychiatric illness, greater patient complexity and acuity, more effective patient scheduling systems, and greater productivity demands or incentives to produce more. Increased time spent on documenting in the EHR (Arndt et al. 2017) cuts into time spent with patients. It is a generally accepted notion that physicians have decreased autonomy and *control* (this is addressed in greater detail in Chapter 14, "Establishing and Maintaining Proportional Authority, Responsibility, and Expertise to Prevent Burnout"). It is difficult to assess the impact of these social trends on the *rewards* of providing care. Current salaries are increasing with the psychiatrist workforce shortage, which represents an increase in reward. Many regard the *community* of physicians to be weaker than in the past, a reflection of less time for bonding and more workplace conflict regarding values and management. Ethical conflicts over limiting resources for individual patients or between a physician's recommendation and the available resources often show themselves in concerns about *fairness* and *values*. This includes conflict between the mission to care for patients and the need to maintain the financial health of the organization.

Satisfiers and Dissatisfiers: Herzberg's Two-Factor Theory

Frederick Herzberg's two-factor or motivation-hygiene theory takes this discussion of mediators of burnout further (Herzberg et al. 1959). The two-factor theory posits that some workplace factors result in job satisfaction and others cause dissatisfaction and that these are separate and distinct factors. Some workplace factors lead to an intrinsic sense of meaning and satisfaction— motivators, and enough of these experiences must be present for job satisfaction. Other factors, those that cause dissatisfaction, must be kept in check, such as through proper "hygiene" in the workplace. Job satisfaction is only achieved through adequate opportunities for satisfaction and a relative absence of dissatisfactions. This model has achieved validity and acceptance and is a useful framework for thinking about the social context of burnout.

Taking into account the three broad forces shaping the physician experience, the discussion in this chapter details more specific factors in the social context, dividing them into those that contribute to physician satisfaction, those affecting dissatisfaction, and those that seem to have effects in both areas.

SATISFIERS

Reminding us of the intrinsic rewards of practicing medicine, Sir James Paget, the great nineteenth-century pathologist, said, "Being a doctor offers the most complete and constant union of those three qualities which have the greatest charm for pure and active minds—novelty, utility, and charity" (Bryan 1997, p. 35). Despite the changes in the structure of healthcare and the workflow in many clinical settings, the doctor-patient relationship remains an experience that inspires and nurtures a sense of *medicine as a calling*. Indeed, in a study of physicians at the Mayo Clinic, those who self-reported experiencing their careers in medicine as a calling had a lower rate of burnout (Jager et al. 2017).

It is not clear how much this sense of a calling expresses itself among current medical students, house staff, and younger psychiatrists. Medical students, residents, and younger physicians are at increased risk of burnout (Dyrbye et al. 2014), and some have raised the question of whether this is related to seeing medicine as a job rather than a calling. The account of the younger psychiatrist earlier in this chapter who would never attend a patient's funeral may represent that less-engaged perspective.

Traditionally, the deepest satisfaction for psychiatrists was thought to be the long-term psychotherapy relationship, with its opportunity for intimacy, reflectiveness, and nurturance. Many do regard these relationships as the most satisfying of their work mix, but new practice models are providing other engaging alternatives. Psychiatrists working in assertive community treatment teams often enthusiastically describe the flexibility of that role, the activity and variety of meeting patients where they live, and the closeness of the treatment team. The sense of providing an urgently needed service is profoundly meaningful and satisfying. Psychiatrists engaged in collaborative practice using the integrated care model frequently report this as well. There are interesting data suggesting that physicians who provide telemedicine services are a more satisfied group (Whitten and Love 2005), although it is not clear yet whether this is the case for psychiatrists, too.

Second, the *advance of knowledge in psychiatry*, limited as it is, does provide for increased satisfaction for practitioners. This refers to both knowledge about the mechanisms of psychopathology and treatment as well as outcome data. The experience of knowledge and mastery is an essential part of the intrinsic satisfaction of being a physician. As psychiatry develops more data to guide treatment, an awareness of what constitutes evidence-based practice and an increased range of treatment options will provide additional satisfaction for psychiatrists. Although the imperative for evidence-based practice has certainly resulted in some distortions in determining appropriate treatment, such as economically driven insurance company protocols that merely reference evidence-based practice, overall this development in the field has likely led to increased attention to the effectiveness of treatments offered.

Third, the increased *aspiration* of our field to meet the needs of the population has resulted in an activation of idealism and altruism that has affected many psychiatrists. Not long ago, applicants to psychiatry residency programs aspired to be department chairs, or researchers, or well-balanced clinicians versed in psychotherapy and psychopharmacology. Now, the most frequent residency application essay is about the aspiration to take care of diverse populations and provide service to underserved communities. The increased attention to population-based care, with the awareness of scarce resources, the disturbing disparities in care among racial and ethnic groups and between those with and without mental illness, and the importance of interprofessional collaboration, are new themes in psychiatric practice that support these aspirations and are a consequence of them.

Fourth, awareness of the centrality of mental health and mental illness in *public discourse* is a satisfier. There is increased recognition that mental health is central to physical health and effective functioning, and this has become a widely agreed-upon topic in public policy and media (New York Times Editorial Board 2018). Public figures who discuss their personal struggles with mental illness, the exploding opioid epidemic, and the public debate about the relationship between gun violence and mental health are specific manifestations of this greater awareness and openness. Mental health policy is increasingly recognized as an essential part of human services policy because of the interconnection of social services systems—education, justice, welfare, and healthcare. Although some use these conversations to support stigma and exclusion, clearly the predominant effect of increased public discussion of mental health and illness has been to place psychiatry in a more favorable light and thus increase the satisfaction and status of the profession. Psychiatrists are increasingly seen as experts in this crucial societal domain, and this sense of inclusion in broader social concerns and the value of that role add to the intrinsic satisfactions of being a psychiatrist.

Thus, the positive side of the work satisfaction ledger is fairly full in the context of the broader social forces shaping medicine. The experience of medicine as a calling, better scientific knowledge, increased aspirations of the profession, and our greater centrality in public discourse are all intrinsic satisfactions of being a psychiatrist, and they have found new forms and new expressions as the overall healthcare system and public discourse evolves and changes.

SATISFIERS OR DISSATISFIERS?

Some would suggest that the most profound shift in the experience of being a doctor has to do with the change in the *business practice of medicine.* Small business has given way to corporate structure, and individual private practice has yielded to employed positions. These changes reflect the increased administrative complexity and cost of practicing medicine and the need to share overhead, increased participation by for-profit corporations, concentration of ever larger for-profit and nonprofit entities, and the need to organize physicians into entities that can care for populations. These changes create new opportunities for satisfaction but also for dissatisfaction.

On one hand, physicians can be freed of the administrative tasks and focus on providing the best care to their patients. They can work with clearer boundaries in terms of hours and responsibilities because they are part of a larger organization, and they may experience increased financial stability and less uncertainty related to illness and disability. On the other hand, they lose a meaningful sense of ownership over their workplace procedures and the more personal commitment to patients that can come from a more direct business relationship with patients. They may experience more dissonance between their personal values and view of medical care and the broader culture of the large organization they are part of. Indeed, smaller practices are less associated with physician burnout among primary care doctors (Blechter et al. 2018).

Second, the *consumer movement* flattens the power and knowledge gradient between physician and patient. The leads to increased patient knowledge and empowerment regarding the management of their illnesses and all of the benefits attendant to that—increased access to care, better matching between treatments and patient preferences, improved communication between patient and provider, improved compliance with treatments, decreased stigma and shame, and hopefully improved outcome. Psychiatrists benefit from all of these factors, and this adds to the intrinsic satisfaction of the work. It also creates opportunities for new kinds of partnerships and the incorporation of technology to enhance communication and sharing of data that can further enhance physician satisfaction. However, struggles regarding control, time spent undoing misinformation from the internet and pharmaceutical company advertisements, the favoring of media impression over science, unreasonable patient expectations, unfair and inaccurate online evaluations, and an atmosphere of contention in the doctor-patient relationship are all potential side effects of the consumer movement that may constitute significant dissatisfiers.

Third, the long history of the *stigma of psychiatric illness* profoundly affects those with mental illness, and psychiatrists are secondarily affected. We have been frequently stigmatized along with our patients, and there are many stereotypes and biases against psychiatrists because we have served as advocates and representatives of those with mental illness and have served to remind people of the prevalence and seriousness of these problems when there is often a strong urge to deny, ignore, and marginalize them. The decrease in stigma goes hand in hand with the centrality of mental health concerns in public policy discourse and the rise of the consumer movement. This development is mostly a satisfier for psychiatrists, but many have observed that a historical adaptation to our stigmatized status has been a particular "clannishness" among psychiatrists and a paradoxical feeling of specialness. To become more like doctors in the rest of medicine will involve some loss of that specialness.

Fourth, there has been a change in the *culture of medicine.* Associated with the three broad social forces shaping modern medicine—social transformation, corporatization, and pursuit of the Triple Aim—physicians have changed how they view themselves and relate to one another differently. The old "boys' club" culture is thankfully substantially reduced, but the traditional values of collegiality, mutual respect, autonomy, effacement of self-interest, and commitment to individual patients may also be eroding. Although it may be helpful in the new systemic context, this cultural shift can result in role strain and discontent at the same time that it is largely adaptive. Fulfilling the requirements of a medical job is different from caring for specific individuals. Functioning as an employed physician requires loyalty to the system and commitment to a job description as opposed to a commitment to specific individual patients.

Connected to this issue is the *generational shift* in culture among physicians. Younger doctors are frequently focused on appropriate limits and structures in the practice environment and the development of effective systems of care; this conflicts with older doctors who tend to focus more on individual relationships and responsibilities. Although generalizations about the generations of physicians—silent generation, baby boomers, Generation X, Generation Y—risk simplifying our understanding, they do hold some currency and help to identify potential areas of friction and discontent (Evans et al. 2016). Younger doctors can be pushed to function in ways that are uncomfortable and seem excessively burdensome, and older physicians feel they are pressured to abandon important values about caring for individuals, which can be disheartening.

Fifth, the crucial goal of *residency training* is to prepare the psychiatrists of the future for the needs and demands of their patients and the system of care. This includes knowledge, skills, and attitudes and thus a set of expectations about the practice environment. The American Association of Directors of Psychiatry Residency Training and other psychiatry education organizations, as well as the APA, have taken on the challenge of prognosticating about the needs of the future and strategizing about how to meet them (American Psychiatric Association 2015). The recent APA work group on this topic identified four critical educational goals (American Psychiatric Association 2015, p. 2):

- Ensuring a robust pipeline of psychiatrists to meet the public health needs now and in the future
- Aligning residency structure with current educational demands
- Preparing faculty to meet the educational needs of trainees
- Training residents for effective integration of behavioral healthcare with primary care

To the extent that the training experiences, both in content and expectations, are aligned with the system that psychiatrists will practice in, we can expect professional satisfaction. Inevitably, however, there is a disparity between those expectations and the reality. Residencies exist within academic settings that may differ in important ways from the employment setting of psychiatrists, and their educational priorities may reflect educational leaders' attempts to influence the field as opposed to adapt to it. Finally, residents' choices in training experiences may reflect their wishes about the kind of work they will do without recognizing the actual opportunities that are available.

The question of how much and what kind of emphasis should be placed on psychotherapy training in residency is an example of this potential mismatch. Because relatively few psychiatrists are incentivized by the current system to practice psychotherapy as a specific billable procedure, the emphasis on learning psychotherapy in residency may enhance some intrinsic satisfactions of the work but also result in dissatisfaction because of the lack of demand for these specific skills.

Sixth, with the increasing cost of and increased demands on our healthcare system, whether we pursue the Triple Aim or the Quadruple Aim that includes physician well-being as a desired outcome, it is clear that continued *innovation* will be necessary to meet our goals. New psychopharmacological approaches have been increasingly scarce, new psychotherapy outcome data add only incrementally to our capacity, and little is new in the combination of psychotherapy and psychopharmacology. Neurostimulation is a new avenue for intervention, but its promise for widespread impact is uncertain. Thus, in psychiatry, innovation mostly refers to new care delivery models such as integrated care, telepsychiatry, and the use of technology.

At its best, innovation provides interesting and exciting new activities for psychiatrists that can add to their intrinsic satisfaction. Assertive community treatment, integrated care systems, and telepsychiatry are examples of this. Technological innovation, including activity monitoring, social media monitoring, and other forms of enhanced communication between patients and providers can improve outcomes and offer improved efficiency in the use of psychiatrists' time, but there is also a concern that a new role of monitoring data flows and implementing protocolized decision making can be alienating and isolating. Thus, system innovation offers the possibility of increased satisfaction but may inadvertently lead to increase in dissatisfaction as well.

DISSATISFIERS

The single most common complaint of physicians about their work is the intrusion of the EHR (see Chapter 8, "Electronic Health Records and Physician Burnout"). The EHR is clearly a necessity and holds great promise as the systems are improved and made more user-friendly, efficient, and unobtrusive. They provide valuable clinical decision support. Yet the day-to-day reality of EHR use leads to profound dissatisfaction. Attention to screens and time spent completing lengthy templates, along with the higher bar for documenting every care interaction, has led to a deeply frustrating diversion of time and attention away from the experience of providing care to "feeding the beast." Documenting the day's work later in the evening at home, time spent typing while patients are sitting in the office, and "checking boxes" about patient history and necessary screenings often lead to a feeling of wasted time and decreased compassion and clinical creativity. The advantages of the EHR, including coordination of care and reduction of waste and error, does provide some satisfaction, but virtually everyone in the healthcare system regards the EHR at this early point in its evolution as a major dissatisfier.

The longstanding trend toward the practice of *defensive medicine* in order to minimize medical-legal liability adds to the alienation from the intrinsic satisfactions of patient care. Although psychiatrists are at lesser risk than many other specialties, there are special situations of particular concern for us. Suicide and violence represent high-stakes clinical situations associated with particular anxiety about liability. Suicide prevention programs are critically important and have shown to be effective, but some extensions of this approach, such as the Zero Suicide Initiative (Coffey et al. 2015) may confer additional anxiety, and therefore dissatisfaction, because the aspiration is greater than the clinician's reach.

The impact on a clinician of committing a *medical error* may be quite significant and long-lasting. Some suggest the term *second victim* to refer to the effect on the doctor who is responsible for the medical error (Marmon and Heiss 2015). The experience of shaming that may result from root cause analyses and morbidity and mortality committee discussions can exacerbate ongoing dissatisfactions and fan the flames of discontent for the clinician involved. Indeed, if a doctor feels he or she has been unfairly blamed or castigated for an error, this can be the basis for a grudge that is hard to get over.

The *economic status of doctors* is less favorable in recent decades (Moawad 2017), although it remains high. However, even among an extraordinarily privileged group, downward economic pressure leads to discontent. Sometimes this is manifested directly with dissatisfaction about compensation, but it may also become attached to the prevailing problems and irritations of the work and result in an increased intensity about many of the factors listed here under "dissatisfiers."

Finally, the *physician community* has weakened and thus provides less vital support to physicians in finding and engaging in their intrinsic satisfaction with the work as well as supporting those who are struggling with the dissatisfactions. Increased productivity demands with less downtime, documentation demands, adherence to job descriptions rather than commitment to relationships, and the creep of corporate culture have all contributed to the weakening of the traditionally strong bonds among physicians. Indeed, one of the interventions thought to increase physician satisfaction and combat burnout is the creation of physician groups that aim to promote sharing and communication among doctors in the workplace about their experiences.

Conclusion

We physicians can surely anticipate that the three broad trends shaping medicine—transformation of medicine, corporatization, and the system transformation driven by the Triple Aim—will continue. Although America is engaged in a polarized debate on the merits of health system reform, there is little to suggest a significant departure from the current path. In this chapter, I describe the forces leading to greater satisfaction and those resulting in decreased satisfaction for physicians. The last task is to prognosticate about the future and those trends that may impact physician well-being and burnout.

The use of artificial intelligence to develop decision-making systems, analyze data, and automate healthcare will surely result in significant change. It is hard to estimate the speed and nature of this impact. Medicine is considered one of the professions least likely to be automated, but components of the work surely will be. Artificial intelligence has the potential to be a profound satisfier, freeing the clinician from the demands of the EHR and allowing for better use of time to interact with patients and their families to support, educate, and care for patients. Yet there is also the potential for physicians to become implementers of software-driven treatment plans, and this could be the greatest dissatisfier of all. Much will depend on the way that artificial intelligence is used and how much healthcare systems prioritize physician well-being and the importance of the physician-patient relationship.

Advocacy and awareness about the problem of physician burnout has been startlingly effective. From a problem discussed infrequently, and at the margins, to a topic that figures prominently in the professional meetings and journals of many specialties, the increase in awareness about well-being and burnout has been dramatic. There is increased attention by national organizations, including the National Academy of Medicine and its Action Collaborative on Clinical Well-Being and Resilience (National Academy of Medicine 2018), the Accreditation Council for Graduate Medical Education, and the American Association of Medical Colleges. Many healthcare systems and departments are forming well-being committees and task forces, and training programs are mobilizing their resources as well. In psychiatry, the APA Board of Trustees Ad Hoc Work Group on Psychiatrist Well-being and Burnout (American Psychiatric Association 2018) has collected data on psychiatrist well-being, and numerous other organizations have convened task forces to study and disseminate resources to combat this problem.

The proposal of the Quadruple Aim, including physician work experience as a desired outcome, has tremendous promise as a mechanism to promote a healthy physician workforce (Bodenheimer and Sinsky 2014). The Institute for Healthcare Improvement has not formally embraced this concept, pointing out that the Triple Aim is focused on the patient experience and not the physician's, but they note that physician well-being and prevention of burnout are essential and implied in the need to have an effective workforce to implement the Triple Aim (Feeley 2017). Measurement of physician well-being will surely cause leaders to focus on this area more and attend to this problem in organizational decision making and resource allocation. Indeed, the Accreditation Council on Graduate Medical Education has begun to survey faculty well-being on a regular basis as a potential indicator related to accreditation.

In conclusion, the trends that have shaped modern healthcare have been the context for the current problem of physician burnout. Burnout, experienced as emotional exhaustion, depersonalization and cynicism, and a decreased sense of personal effectiveness, is not the inevitable price of progress but its unfortunate byproduct. In this chapter, I describe the social context for the problem, and subsequent chapters address specific aspects of burnout and how to combat it.

KEY POINTS

————————■————————

- The experience of practicing medicine has been profoundly affected by three major trends over the past century—the social transformation of medicine, corporatization of healthcare organizations, and pursuit of the Triple Aim.

- The changes in the practice of medicine are the context for the current epidemic of burnout among physicians and psychiatrists.

- Multiple factors in the medical workplace impact the physician's experience of satisfaction and dissatisfaction with practicing medicine.

- Artificial intelligence, advocacy, and awareness about physician burnout and the advent of the Quadruple Aim (including physician work experience as a goal in system transformation) are three factors that will affect physician well-being and burnout in the future.

————————■————————

References

American Psychiatric Association: Training the Psychiatrist of the Future: A Report by the Board of Trustees Work Group on Education and Training. Arlington, VA, 2015

American Psychiatric Association: Well-Being and Burnout: Take Charge of Your Well-Being. An Urgent Issue for Psychiatrists and Medicine. Washington, DC, American Psychiatric Association, 2018. Available at: https://www.psychiatry.org/psychiatrists/practice/well-being-and-burnout. Accessed June 1, 2018.

Arndt BG, Beasley JW, Watkinson MD, et al: Tethered to the EHR: primary care physician workload assessment using EHR event log data and time-motion observations. Ann Fam Med 15(5):419–426, 2017 28893811

Bodenheimer T, Sinsky C: From triple to quadruple aim: care of the patient requires care of the provider. Ann Fam Med 12(6):573–576, 2014 25384822

Berwick DM, Nolan TW, Whittington J: The triple aim: care, health, and cost. Health Aff (Millwood) 27(3):759–769, 2008 18474969. Available at: www.healthaffairs.org/doi/pdf/10.1377/hlthaff.27.3.759. Accessed June 1, 2018.

Blechter B, Jiang N, Cleland C, et al: Correlates of burnout in small independent primary care practices in an urban setting. J Am Board Fam Med 31(4):529–536, 2018 29986978

Brady KJS, Trockel MT, Khan CT, et al: What do we mean by physician wellness? A systematic review of its definition and measurement. Acad Psychiatry 42(1):94–108, 2018 28913621

Bryan CS: Osler: Inspirations from a Great Physician. New York, Oxford University Press, 1997

Centers for Medicare and Medicaid Services: National Health and Expenditure Data: Historical. Baltimore, MD, Centers for Medicare and Medicaid Services, 2018. Available at: https://www.cms.gov/Research-Statistics-Data-and-Systems/Statistics-Trends-and-Reports/NationalHealthExpendData/NationalHealthAccountsHistorical.html. Accessed June 1, 2018.

Coffey MJ, Coffey CE, Ahmedani BK: Suicide in a health maintenance organization population. JAMA Psychiatry 72(3):294–296, 2015 25607598

Dyrbye LN, West CP, Satele D, et al: Burnout among U.S. medical students, residents, and early career physicians relative to the general U.S. population. Acad Med 89(3):443–451, 2014 24448053

Evans KH, Ozdalga E, Ahuja N: The medical education of Generation Y. Acad Psychiatry 40(2):382–385, 2016 26283527

Feeley DJ: The Triple Aim or the Quadruple Aim? Four points to help set your strategy. Line of Sight, Tuesday, November 28, 2017. Available at: http://www.ihi.org/communities/blogs/the-triple-aim-or-the-quadruple-aim-four-points-to-help-set-your-strategy. Accessed June 1, 2018.

Herzberg F, Mausner B, Snyderman BB: The Motivation to Work, 2nd Edition. New York, John Wiley, 1959

Intrator SM (ed): Living the Questions: Essays Inspired by the Work and Life of Parker J. Palmer. San Francisco, CA, Jossey-Bass, 2005

Jager AJ, Tutty MA, Kao AC: Association between physician burnout and identification with medicine as a calling. Mayo Clin Proc 92(3):415–422, 2017 28189341

Marmon LM, Heiss K: Improving surgeon wellness: the second victim syndrome and quality of care. Semin Pediatr Surg 24(6):315–318, 2015 26653167

Maslach C, Leiter MP: Understanding the burnout experience: recent research and its implications for psychiatry. World Psychiatry 15(2):103–111, 2016 27265691

Maslach C, Schaufeli WB, Leiter MP: Job burnout. Annu Rev Psychol 52:397–422, 2001 11148311

Moawad H: Are physician incomes failing? Medical Economics, October 2, 2017

National Academy of Medicine: Action Collaborative on Clinician Well-Being and Resilience. Washington, DC, National Academy of Medicine, 2018. Available at: https://nam.edu/initiatives/clinician-resilience-and-well-being. Accessed May 5, 2018.

Neff JA, McFall SL, Cleaveland TD: Psychiatry and medicine in the US: interpreting trends in medical specialty choice. Sociol Health Illn 9(1):45–61, 1987 10281530

New York Times Editorial Board: The crazy talk about bringing back asylums. The New York Times, June 2, 2018, p SR8

Relman AS: What market values are doing to medicine. Atlantic 269(3):98–102, 105–106, 1992 11651349. Available at: https://www.theatlantic.com/past/docs/politics/healthca/relman.htm. Accessed June 1, 2018.

Schaufeli WB, Enzmann D: The Burnout Companion to Study and Practice: A Critical Analysis. London, Taylor and Francis, 1998

Starr P: The Social Transformation of American Medicine: The Rise of a Sovereign Profession and the Making of a Vast Industry. New York, Basic Books, 1982

Whitten P, Love B: Patient and provider satisfaction with the use of telemedicine: overview and rationale for cautious enthusiasm. J Postgrad Med 51(4):294–300, 2005 16388172

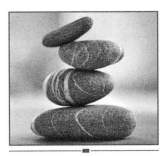

PART II

THE CONTINUUM OF STRESS, BURNOUT, AND IMPAIRMENT

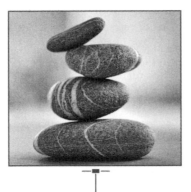

CHAPTER 3

IDENTIFYING THE CONTINUUM OF STRESS AND BURNOUT

Julie Chilton, M.D.

Andrés Martin, M.D., M.P.H.

Stress comes in many forms, durations, and intensities and can vary greatly in quality and effect. Many words are used to describe stress, including anxiety, pressure, difficulties, troubles, and worry, reflecting the challenge in creating a strict definition of this phenomenon. For instance, when the delivery of stress is parceled in just the right amounts, it can be highly motivating and even exhilarating. Occupational psychologists call this *eustress*—the adrenaline-producing ingredient that makes individuals and corporate teams ignite with innovation and creativity and zing with efficiency. Conversely, when an inflection point is reached, it can have a series of negative effects as "distress," impeding productivity and inducing a frazzled paralysis or a soul-cracking exhaustion. Yerkes and Dodson (1908) first conceptualized this spectrum of stress as a relationship between arousal and performance, as graphically depicted in their classic eponymous curve.

In this chapter, we consider stress in its many forms and its effects on human physiology, psychology, behavior, and even genetics. We review the sources of both internal and external stress, the risk factors that make individuals more vulnerable, the qualities that make cultures more toxic, and the potential moderators of stress. We specifically examine the role of stress in the practice of medicine and how it affects medical students, trainees, physicians, and, in particular, psychiatrists. Finally, we identify specific factors associated with stressed individuals who ultimately experience burnout, consider what the inflection point for full expression of the syndrome might be, and comment on the inherent challenges in drawing reliable conclusions related to the continuum of stress and burnout.

External stress is produced by an event that happens to an individual, forcing one to cope by absorbing its effect or adapting in some way. Common sources of external stress include work pressures, family problems, relationship troubles, medical issues, financial difficulties, loss of a loved one, or having too much to do. Of note, positive events such as marriage, the birth of a child, or a change in job or residence can also cause inordinate stress. Notably, research on work-life balance in medicine illuminated gender differences in the amount of stress felt by physician parents: for example, female doctors reported more stress when raising children than physician fathers (Guille et al. 2017). Psychiatrists, in particular, may have personality characteristics that predispose them to increased sensitivity to external stress in comparison with physicians in other fields (Deary et al. 1996).

Internal stress is largely created by one's interpretation of events, belief in ability to handle these pressures, and personal outlook on the future. The stress that an individual feels can be broken into underlying cognitions, physical symptoms, and subjective emotions that all contribute to behavior and actions, and thus coping ability. Although blaming an individual for a particular stress response in a dysfunctional system is wrong, there does seem to be variability in the perception of and reaction to stress between individuals. According to a Harvard Stress Management Special Report (Harvard Medical School 2018), traits and thinking styles like perfectionism, pessimism, trouble tolerating uncertainty, rigidity, an all-or-nothing attitude, and negative self-talk likely increase how stress is perceived.

Unfortunately, there is significant overlap between these characteristics known to increase the negative valence of a stressor in the general population, and the personality profile typical of medical students and physicians. Furthermore, when compared with other physicians, psychiatrists tend to rate even higher on neuroticism, openness, and agreeableness, but lower on conscientiousness, and report higher work-related emotional exhaustion (Deary et al. 1996). This combination of increased perceived job stress and neuroticism may have a negative synergy. Given that the nature of psychiatry lends itself to more intimate and thus potentially more emotionally taxing connections with patients, mental health clinicians may practice in a perfect storm of individual characteristics and occupational factors.

Biological Underpinnings of the Stress Response

The human body's neurochemical response to stress is meant to be protective; it facilitates the fight-or-flight reaction in times of danger and triggers immune responses to confront infection and promote wound healing after injury. After being exposed to an acute stressor (either physical or psychological), the sympathetic nervous system and a hormonal cascade set off by the hypothalamus trigger the release of stress hormones from the adrenal gland. More specifically, the hypothalamus releases corticotropin-releasing factor, which signals the pituitary gland to send out adrenocorticotropic hormone, causing the adrenal gland to release cortisol in tandem with epinephrine (adrenaline) and norepinephrine (noradrenaline), leading to full sympathetic activation.

It is primarily these three stress hormones (cortisol, epinephrine, and norepinephrine) that are responsible for changes in heart rate, blood pressure, muscular blood flow, pupil size, and glucose levels that are required to "fight or flee." Once cortisol reaches a certain level after a few hours, a negative feedback loop is triggered, decreasing the activity of the hypothalamus, and the system returns to its usual state with activation of the parasympathetic nervous system. Estrogen, testosterone, dopamine, and serotonin are also thought to play a role in the human stress response. Additionally, normal levels of these hypothalamus-pituitary-adrenal–axis hormones and catecholamines vary both by age and gender. Along with the corresponding stage of brain development at the time of the stress experience, these three factors are thought to create periods of vulnerability or resistance to the physiological effects of stress (Davidson and McEwen 2012; Lupien et al. 2009).

The hormones released by the adrenal glands at times of stress, glucocorticoids such as cortisol and others, can have a big impact early in life, given that optimal brain development and maturation is dependent on having just the right amount of these hormones circulating. Stress hormones can also alter transcription and gene expression; thus, abnormal levels of glucocorticoids can have long-term effects on the brain and body long after their initial effect.

Enduring Effects of Recurrent Stress: Epigenetics

The field of epigenetics focuses on stress-induced cellular modifications, such as the addition of histone tails and methyl groups, without affecting nucleotide sequence. Recent research has linked increased adverse childhood experiences of mothers to poor self-regulation in their infants (Gray et al. 2017). Given the early age at which the infant behavior was analyzed, it raises the possibility that the dysregulation was due to the effect of remote environmental stressors on maternal DNA. These cellular modifications are passed on to their offspring, perhaps explaining the dysregulation as a result of "nature" rather than "nurture." In the words of Bessel van der Kolk (2014), studies like these demonstrate how "the body keeps the score."

Thanks to the Adverse Childhood Experiences (ACE) study, we have known for nearly 30 years that distressing experiences occurring as remotely as early childhood can affect health many years later in adulthood. Examples of such stressful events include domestic violence, neglect, abuse, a caregiver with an addiction problem, or even divorce—anything that causes repeated intense activation of the stress response system. The more such experiences an individual sustains during this critical time period in childhood, the higher their "ACE score" is, and the more likely they are to exhibit high-risk behavior and develop psychiatric issues in adulthood. For instance, those study participants who had four or more adverse childhood experiences were at least four times more likely to later develop a problem with alcohol or drugs, become depressed, and make a suicide attempt (Felitti et al. 1998).

Physical consequences of prolonged, high levels of stress on the brain and human body are also well known. Cancer, cognitive impairment, autoimmune disease, cardiovascular problems, and precipitation or worsening of mental illness have been described as downstream effects of stress (Shields and Slavich 2017). Not surprisingly, ACE scores have a "graded relationship" with cancer, fractures, ischemic heart disease, and liver problems (Felitti et al. 1998). Decreased life expectancy is even an associated outcome of greater lifetime experiences of stress.

Of interest, physicians are thought to have better medical health when compared with the general population, including rates of death from stress-related cardiovascular conditions (Torre et al. 2005). However, their mental health does not fare as well (Firth-Cozens 2007), and the rate of suicide is higher in physicians than nonphysicians (Schernhammer and Colditz 2004). Some studies show that psychiatrists may be even more vulnerable to suicide than other physicians (Torre et al. 2005), but it is unclear why, and the finding is not consistently replicated. Physicians are not immune to the effects of early-life stress, and a large study of more than 700 interns identified a difficult early childhood as a risk factor for a greater increase in symptoms of depression during their first year of residency (Sen et al. 2010).

Stress and Brain Structure: Relationship to Psychopathology

Research shows that chronic stress generally has a shrinking effect on the hippocampus and frontal lobe, the amygdala increases in size as a result of prolonged adversity, and the sensitivity of specific brain regions to stress changes with age (Davidson and McEwen 2012). The hippocampus seems to be most vulnerable during childhood, the frontal cortex in adolescence, and the slow growing amygdala is affected increasingly from infancy through young adulthood. All three structures are particularly vulnerable to circulating glucocorticoids during the bookend years—the prenatal period and senescence. There is some evidence to suggest that the brain area that is most vulnerable at the time a stressor is experienced may determine which psychiatric disorder emerges. As a result, researchers speculate that given what is known about the neurological and neuroanatomical areas affected in different disorders, one might be able to predict the age at which the affected individual experienced stress (Lupien et al. 2009).

It is of interest that the brain continues to develop through the mid 20s, when critical pruning occurs. Considering that the average age of U.S. medical students at matriculation is around 25 years, the onset of significant increased stress may occur before this window of neurodevelopmental vulnerability is definitively closed in younger medical students especially (Association of American Medical Colleges 2017). However, some evidence suggests that certain interventions could "reopen" areas of plasticity in the brain, implying that it is not naïve to assume that later interventions on an individual level might "undo" effects of chronic stress (Davidson and McEwen 2012). For instance, cognitive therapy has been shown to optimize activity in the prefrontal cortex and thus inhibit amygdalar activation—the opposite of what occurs under chronic stress (DeRubeis et al. 2008). Perhaps this may partially explain why cognitive-behavioral therapy decreases suicidal thinking in interns (Guille et al. 2015).

Most depressed individuals have higher baseline glucocorticoid levels, smaller hippocampi, and decreased hippocampal function. Studies of patients with posttraumatic stress disorder (PTSD) reveal decreased hippocampal volume and function and possibly lower circulating levels of glucocorticoids, but this finding is less consistent across studies. It is also unclear whether these differences are due to the effect of the illness on the brain, were present from birth, or developed as a result of environmental stressors that then paved the way for depression or PTSD. For instance, if an individual was exposed to stress in early childhood, causing glucocorticoid hyposecretion, could that have been the actual cause of later neuroanatomical differences, with a downstream effect of a mental illness? Regardless, it makes sense to wonder whether increased exposure of the brain to stress hormones is damaging and to the prefrontal cortex and hippocampus in particular.

Stress and DSM-5: Effect on the Onset and Progression of Psychiatric Illness

It has been widely accepted for decades that an increase in stress or the experience of a new stressor can precipitate the onset of a mental illness or worsen a preexisting condition. Anxiety, obsessive-compulsive disorder, and tic disorders, in particular, are known to be exacerbated in times of stress. For example, a psychosocial stressor known as high *expressed emotion*—critical attitudes or emotional overinvolvement of key family members toward a relative with mental illness—is thought to be a major risk factor for both relapse and symptom worsening in schizophrenia, mood disorders, and eating disorders (Butzlaff and Hooley 1998). More recently, parental attitudes and interactive styles characteristic of high expressed emotion also have been linked to worse outcomes for adolescents with mental illness. When "toxic family stress" is "frequent, sustained and uncontrollable" in youth, researchers observe not only a psychological impact but also neurological and biological effects such as increased cortisol levels, cell death, and decreased neurogenesis (Peris and Miklowitz 2015).

In this context, all mental illnesses can be viewed as stress related, at least in part. Rather than having one typical mental or emotional effect, experiencing chronic stress or an acute stressor can precipitate sequelae as diverse as psychotic, manic, anxious, angry, or depressive symptomatology. However, DSM-5 (American Psychiatric Association 2013) has a specific section devoted to this topic: "Trauma-and Stressor-Related Disorders." Various permutations of the following conditions (based on severity, duration, and associated symptoms) are organized within this category: reactive attachment disorder, disinhibited social engagement disorder, PTSD, acute stress disorder, adjustment disorders, and multiple specified and unspecified trauma- and stressor-related disorders. It is beyond the scope of this chapter to describe them all in detail. However, it is worth noting what the American Psychiatric Association's diagnostic experts consider to be stress-related reactions that are pathological and worthy of a specific diagnosis of mental illness.

From Trauma-Related Psychopathology, Including Vicarious Trauma, to Burnout

Traumatic events happen unexpectedly and suddenly. They are not a normal experience of everyday life and imply a danger to life or limb (Bui et al. 2014). Childhood trauma expert Lenore Terr (1995) described two kinds of trauma: a time-limited single event such as living through a hurricane or rape is classified as Type I trauma, whereas Type II describes a repeated or more chronic traumatic experience, such as being a prisoner of war or a displaced refugee. The stressor required for a diagnosis of PTSD or acute stress disorder in DSM-5 does not have to be directly experienced by the individual with PTSD. Rather, learning of a loved one's experience of trauma can count as well, so long as the effect is still outside of the normal range of human experience. In this sense, vicarious trauma experienced by medical personnel can at times also meet the criteria for trauma.

After the experience of an acute stressor, if symptoms persist for at least 2 days but not more than 4 weeks, the duration criteria for an acute stress disorder diagnosis is met. These required symptoms include intrusive thoughts, symptoms of dissociation, avoidance of traumatic reminders, and hyperarousal. Prevalence estimates for acute stress disorder vary, but generally less than 20% of individuals who experience an acute stressor meeting the criteria develop an acute stress disorder (Bui et al. 2014). At one time, the diagnosis of acute stress disorder was thought to be a fairly reliable indicator that PTSD would follow, but more recent research has not shown that to be the case.

PTSD is diagnosed when trauma-related symptoms are intrusive, reminders are avoided, and a state of hyperarousal persists longer than a month after the trauma ends. Lifetime prevalence rates of PTSD in the general population are thought to be less than 10%. In circumstances of mass casualties, doctors often report symptoms of PTSD. In more typical day-to-day clinical circumstances, acute stressors and chronic exposure to trauma can also occur. Resident physicians report rates of PTSD higher than the public, and female trainees may be at increased risk compared with their male colleagues. Protective factors may include having a partner and social support (Klamen et al. 1995).

Experiencing death and adverse outcomes is commonly recognized as traumatic for physicians, whereas making medical errors is less often acknowledged as significantly distressing for doctors. Dr. Albert Wu coined the term *second victim* to describe the effect that medical errors have on physicians, often leading to depression, PTSD, guilt, shame, feelings of inadequacy, and a loss of confidence (Helo and Moulton 2017). Sadly, medical errors are also risk factors for later suicide completion among physicians (Gold et al. 2013).

There is relative agreement on definitive criteria for PTSD, acute stress disorder, and depression, but much less consensus exists regarding what constitutes burnout. As a result, drawing meaningful conclusions about how these syndromes or illnesses are similar or different from burnout based on physiological or neuroanatomical studies is premature.

Resiliency Training and Personality Profiles: From Blaming the Victim to Preventing Burnout

Nature and nurture, personality and environment, and individual thinking styles and job culture all interact to create outcomes related to both the quality and quantity of a stressor and an individual's reactivity to it. It is the combination of an individual's ability to cope and the degree of stress experienced that produces either successful adaptation or untenable negativity. In fact, good parenting involves *allowing* children to experience stress. With exposure to mild stressors early and often, most children learn that they need not avoid situations that make them a bit anxious, and they develop increasing confidence over time in their ability to handle stress. These observations are backed by animal studies that reveal that early exposure to mild levels of stress leads to decreased behavioral and hormonal anxiety responses later in life, possibly serving as a sort of inoculating effect (Davidson and McEwen 2012).

The concept of resilience is rooted in this idea that an individual's reaction to stress is not only dependent on the intensity of a stressor but also on the subjective interpretation of that stressor and that individual's ability to cope. However, *resilience* is a controversial topic in medicine. Opponents of the term argue that focusing on increasing resilience among doctors lays the blame of burnout at the feet of the physician. Proponents suggest that although organizational, cultural, and systemic issues make up the larger part of the problem in healthcare, maximizing personal resilience can improve coping until more sweeping changes are implemented on the macro level.

Recent occupational research shows that more resilient workers, when compared with workers with less resilience, are protected from some adverse effects of high-stress jobs—those with low control, high demand, and minimal support (Shatté et al. 2017). Additionally, skills that increase resilience are not necessarily personality traits present from birth but rather can be acquired or "taught." A recent meta-analysis of resiliency training programs shows a small effect when their intention is prevention of stress-related work issues and larger but still modest effects with secondary stress management interventions whose aim is to decrease negative outcomes after they occur (Vanhove et al. 2016).

The objective of resiliency training programs in medicine should not be to make doctors better able to cope with a permanently toxic culture and impossible system. Rather, it should be to bolster the baseline mental health of physicians, given known vulnerabilities, and impart helpful coping tools in the inevitable case that bad things happen. According to Michael Myers, an expert on the mental health of physicians, resilience is "a life force that promotes regeneration and renewal in people…the ability to confront adversity and still find hope and meaning in one's life" (Myers 2017, p. 60). Researchers studying the phenomenon generally, rather just in relation to medicine, state that "our preferred definition of resilience represents a constellation of characteristics that protect individuals from the potential negative effect of stressors" (Robertson et al. 2015, p. 534).

For years, research on the personality traits of doctors has revealed a profile that may be a setup for experiencing the more negative aspects of stress. Although not all doctors share these vulnerabilities, and there are not enough large-scale studies to make sweeping generalizations about physicians as a whole, there is some evidence of a higher frequency of these traits in medical professionals. When several of these characteristics exist in an individual under stress, the combination can create a perfect storm. Perfectionism is widely accepted to be a common trait in doctors, both with beneficial and maladaptive potential. When accompanied by the "compulsive triad" of self-doubt, feelings of guilt, and an exaggerated sense of responsibility, it can be particularly detrimental to physicians (Myers and Gabbard 2008). Additionally, high levels of neuroticism, conscientiousness, and obsessiveness are thought to be characteristic of doctors.

Pessimism (or looking at things through "negative-colored glasses") is a well-studied contributor to stress. A related concept from the anxiety treatment literature is "catastrophizing," or a tendency to overpredict the likelihood of the worst-case scenario. One can imagine how predicting negative outcomes more frequently might lead an individual to feel chronically overwhelmed, hopeless, sad, or even suicidal. Accordingly, changing this type of thought distortion is one of the basic tenets of CBT—an evidence-based treatment for both anxiety and depression. Being an excellent physician often requires guarding against the worst possible outcome through watchful prevention and treatment. As a result, a healthy amount of negative prognosticating can be difficult to cultivate.

Similar to this concept is *neuroticism,* a term that describes interpreting scenarios through a threatening lens and feeling a bigger "emotional load" over minor frustrations than most people. It is easy to understand how exaggerating the negative valence of even mildly distressing experiences might make someone experience more stress and feel overwhelmed. Not surprisingly, high neuroticism in physicians was associated with a threefold increase in the likelihood of later depression (Støen Grotmol et al. 2013).

Perfectionism is another major contributor to internal stress. In some families with exceptionally high expectations or when there is little expressed love or meaningful validation, children can feel from a young age that they have to work very hard to please their parents. This situation is a setup for developing a sense of "never being good enough" that can develop into maladaptive perfectionism down the road. Some individuals parented by supportive caregivers with manageable expectations develop this insecurity for different reasons, and yet others are just born that way. Studies show that physicians are highly perfectionistic and especially at risk for suicide after making a medical error or perceiving that others think they made an error (Gold et al. 2013). This sad statistic reflects both how important and fragile the identity of "infallible doctor" may be to physicians.

Impostor syndrome—a psychological phenomenon originating in perfectionism—is fueled by self-doubt, low self-esteem, and all-or-nothing thinking that culminates in the individual feeling like a fraud. When something goes well, these individuals feel it is due to luck or other reasons, but when things go poorly, it is entirely their fault. Physicians and trainees often relate this sentiment of self-criticism, not feeling as capable as their peers, living in constant fear of making a mistake, and rarely being satisfied with what they have achieved, when trying to articulate why doctoring is so hard. In British medical students, self-criticism was a predictor for the development of depression several years later, independent of workload (Brewin and Firth-Cozens 1997).

Learning to tolerate uncertainty is imperative in medicine. Once trainees develop this ability, they can begin to make timely decisions in spite of what is not known and accept that their actions may not always lead to positive outcomes for each patient. Experts state that this learning objective is "the key issue facing medical education" (Bleakley and Brennan 2011). Curricular design can accomplish this task by exposing students to ambiguous clinical situations, facilitating their management with appropriate supervision, and building tolerance, as evidenced by a United Kingdom study comparing cohorts from medical schools with different curricula (Bleakley and Brennan 2011).

Similarly, the way trainees view stressful situations likely creates variability in the intensity of the clinical scenarios they can handle. For instance, some medical students might feel exhilarated by a new challenge rather than being overwhelmed. Harvard Business School Professor Allison Wood Brooks (2014) terms this malleability "the anxiety reframe" or "anxious reappraisal," which describes effectively coaching the mind into feeling excited instead of anxious when faced with a difficult or potentially embarrassing task.

Interestingly, when stressed individuals tell themselves instead to feel excited, the body remains as physiologically aroused as when feeling anxious, but the mind interprets it more positively. The usual refrain "calm down, just relax" is a much harder alternative command for the body to obey because it has to decrease heart rate, slow breathing, and turn off the hormonal release induced by the stressor. As a result, this reinterpretation of stress through the excitement technique—wherein a "threat mind-set" is turned into an "opportunity mind-set"—led to improved performance compared with simply remaining anxious or attempting to become calm (Brooks 2014).

Even though the tasks assigned in the Brooks (2014) research just described were low risk and in artificial environments (singing a karaoke song in front of strangers, doing math problems, and giving a speech), there exist some commonalities with research on the ability of medical students to tolerate stress. For instance, having a mentor frame a clinical experience in a supportive and nonthreatening way that emphasizes learning (rather than dichotomous pass-fail mastery with the potential for humiliation) could increase the likelihood of a trainee feeling excited rather than terrified prior to a new rotation. Additionally, introducing this concept to medical students and trainees might also benefit their perceived need for control: there does exist an intervention that is within their power to change their experience of a situation.

Whether or not stress tolerance measures should be implemented as part of the burnout solution in medicine, medical school curricula have long employed thoughtful incremental increases in exposure to stress in their training philosophies. Level of responsibility for patient care is increased in a stepwise hierarchical fashion, as is exposure to high-acuity traumatic clinical scenarios. In a meta-analysis of studies on the effect of stress prevention on Canadian medical students, curricula with stress management programs showed decreased levels of depression and anxiety in their students as well as improved resolution of role conflicts and increased use of coping strategies (Shapiro et al. 2000).

The Challenge of Measuring Stress in the Changing Practice of Medicine

Unfortunately, the experience of stress in medicine is worsening. Given the changes that have affected medical practice in the past few decades, through the Triple Aim and other initiatives, this fact is not surprising. Many studies have illuminated well-known factors associated with increased levels of stress in medicine. One common grievance of physicians is increased use of the electronic health record and the time away from clinical duties it requires. Doctors also increasingly report not practicing at the top of their license (i.e., working to the full extent of education and training) and performing more clerical duties than in the past. Malpractice suits are a more frequent occurrence, and fear of litigation is a more prevalent concern than before. Finally, insurance reimbursement for physician services has decreased, and midlevel providers with less education are being increasingly put to work in roles previously reserved for doctors. These developments likely contribute to the sentiments of doctors that they are valued less by the healthcare industry and held in lower esteem by the general public.

The fact that stress takes many forms is precisely what makes it hard to study, measure, and compare across groups and situations—a problem inherent also in the study of burnout. Many instruments have been created and are used for stress measurement in studies. Some assessment tools are self-report questionnaires, others are semistructured interviews, and yet others are automated inventories. The Perceived Stress Scale is a commonly used, short, free self-report tool that only measures general perceived stress over the past month. Higher scores on the Perceived Stress Scale have been linked to a decreased likelihood of adequate glucose control in diabetes, lower smoking cessation, increased vulnerability to depressive symptoms, and more colds (Cohen 1994). The Life Events Checklist is another self-report questionnaire that screens for discrete stressful experiences over the lifetime, not just in the past month, and is also available on the Internet (Blake et al. 1995). The Life Events and Difficulties Schedule and the UCLA Life Stress Interview are investigator based, and thus gold standards, but they are expensive, require trained clinicians, and only assess the prior 1–2 years (Shields and Slavich 2017).

Occupational stress—or the toll work takes on an individual—is also measured by a number of instruments, making comparisons between work climates and employee groups difficult. The Professional Quality of Life Scale (Stamm 2009) assesses the effects—both positive and negative—of being a helping professional and is available free in 24 languages. Expanded from a seven-item questionnaire originally intended for doctors and medical students, the nine-item eWellBeing Index (eWBI) is short, free, and picks up on several current domains affected by workplace stress rather than just burnout or depression. Instruments specific to physicians are the Approaches to Work Questionnaire for Physicians and Workplace Climate Questionnaires for

Physicians and the American Psychiatric Association Physician Well-Being Index.

Research on antecedents of job burnout reveal potentially problematic characteristics from three realms—organization, individual, and work (Chen et al. 2012). By identifying what conditions or characteristics reliably lead to burnout, one might be able to then determine the root cause. Historically, *job burnout* is thought to be "induced by the misfit between individual personality and work or organizational characteristics" (Chen et al. 2012, p. 804). If such a high number of physicians and trainees are actually burned out, as is reported (some 50% of U.S. physicians on average), there must be factors other than personality structure also at play, despite the obvious vulnerabilities associated with the "stereotypical physician personality."

The key question is at what point does stress become burnout? Answering this question with some confidence requires several issues to be resolved. First, there is no uniformly accepted definition of exactly what burnout is and is not—how it is different from extreme stress, job-related PTSD, or even depression. Maslach et al. (1996) identified the triad of emotional exhaustion, depersonalization, and decreased sense of personal achievement to define the syndrome. However, burnout experts recently attempted a meta-analysis of 182 studies of physician burnout, which devolved into a systematic review after they recognized more than 140 heterogeneous definitions were used between studies, among other problematic inconsistencies, making scientific comparison impossible (Rotenstein et al. 2018).

In fact, there is even disagreement around whether personal achievement is a valid component of burnout or whether emotional exhaustion and depersonalization should be the lone criteria. Additionally, whether burnout exists on a spectrum or is a dichotomy muddies the diagnostic clarity. To worsen matters, there is no absolutely agreed upon burnout assessment scale. Commonly used measures include the Maslach Burnout Inventory, the Oldenberg Burnout Inventory, and the Copenhagen Burnout Inventory, although the Maslach Burnout Inventory is used in greater than 90% of global research. This instrument was not intended to be used as a diagnostic tool; the numeric cutoffs are not legitimate indicators of the difference between burned out or not nor of the degree to which one is or is not affected by burnout. Further controversy exists around its specific utility for healthcare professionals and whether it serves as an accurate tool for comparisons between different types of medical and clinical personnel and across cultures and between countries (Doulougeri et al. 2016).

Confronting the Elusive Risk of Burnout

If we cannot reliably define, diagnose, measure, or compare burnout, how can we definitively say what it is or is not as it relates to the experience of stress? There do seem to be some commonalities that describe the experience qualitatively. Descriptors such as "a crisis in values" (Doulougeri et al. 2016) and "an erosion of the soul" (Myers and Gabbard 2008) have been used to describe the gestalt of burnout, implying that the problem lies with the individual, which misses the mark according to recent research. Alternatively, there may be some inferences that could be drawn about components of burnout based on interventions that reduce burnout symptoms. For now, it seems we may need to accept that a precise definition is illusory; we do not have enough information to accurately capture the severe depletion felt by medical personnel around the globe with one simple definition, but any attempt should not imply that the individual affected is at fault.

So, what do we have? It seems there are a few consistent situational and occupational characteristics that reliably predict the toxicity of an environment. These indicators can help us predict the situations that will likely be unbearable to most individuals and perhaps give us some clue as to what causes the inflection point from stress tolerance into stress exhaustion. Unfortunately, it is what we have learned from the accounts of those who endured the most extreme stress that may offer some answers. Both survivors of concentration camps and former prisoners of war describe certain factors of their detainment that decreased physical and psychological morbidity and mortality during torture and severe deprivation.

These are the most extreme examples of stress we have in recent history, and it is imperative to not trivialize torture or overdramatize the stress of the medical culture by making such facile comparisons. However, similarities do exist between what individuals in both situations articulate helped them to cope. Additionally, there are some parallel findings between what research shows can decrease burnout in medicine and what factors improved stress tolerance during the unfathomable cruelty of both the concentration camps and wartime captivity of the twentieth century. Having a sense of control, not losing hope, having a sense of purpose, and being able to share the experience through social communication all seem key to surviving stress, whether just unpleasant or completely unfathomable.

Seeking social support is a known component of active coping closely tied to resiliency, especially when it is solution focused. When either cultural or systemic factors prevent physicians and trainees from supporting each other through shared stressful experiences, they likely end up feeling alone and not realizing that others might be similarly stressed. In addition to psychological benefits, naming stress by sharing it verbally has also been shown to shift the brain's focus from the amygdala to the prefrontal cortex. Not surprisingly, studies of peer support in medicine show positive effects on wellness, professional relationships, career, and personal relationships (Sanchez et al. 2016).

These observations correlate with findings from wartime imprisonment as well. The most effective coping mechanism reported by the 566 United States Navy prisoners of war from the Vietnam War was communication (Wood and Sexton 1997). The late Senator John McCain related how critical any form of human interaction was to him while being held in solitary confinement: "The most important thing for survival is communication with someone, even if it's only a wave or a wink, a tap on the wall, or to have a guy put his thumb up. It makes all the difference" (McCain 1973, p. 10). From a scientific perspective, this makes sense. For instance, a well-known study revealed the moderating effects of holding a partner's hand during an aversive stressor—the anterior insula and ventral anterior cingulate cortex were less affected by the negative stimulus as a result (Coan et al. 2006).

In *Why Physicians Die by Suicide*, Michael Myers defines *resilience* as "the ability to confront adversity and still find hope and meaning in one's life" (Myers 2017, p. 60). It is not surprising, then, that physicians who define medicine as a calling are less likely to experience burnout (Yoon et al. 2017). In fact, studies show that by allowing physicians to devote just 20% of their work week to whatever they are most passionate about, burnout can be averted. McCain (1973) found that it was his patriotism and love for family that kept him going. Victor Frankl (1946) also made a similar observation in *Man's Search for Meaning,* recognizing that a Nietzsche quote proved prophetic for the mortality of prisoners in concentration camps:

> "He who has a *why* to live for can bear with almost any *how*," could be the guiding motto for all psychotherapeutic and psychohygienic efforts regarding prisoners. Whenever there was an opportunity for it, one had to give them a *why*—an aim—for their lives, in order to strengthen them to bear the terrible *how* of their existence. Woe to him who saw no more sense in his life, no aim, no purpose, and therefore no point in carrying on. He was soon lost. (p. ix)

Even though mindfulness interventions often elicit skepticism from physicians and trainees, empirical evidence shows that these interventions decrease negative ruminations and allow the mind to become calm. One study of mindfulness-based stress reduction (MBSR) showed that after only 8 weeks of meditation training, right-amygdalar gray matter volume decreased significantly and in correlation with reductions in perceived stress. The authors hypothesized "that an active re-learning of emotional responses to stress (such as taught in MBSR) can lead to beneficial changes in neural structure and well-being even when there is presumably no change in the person's external environment" (Hölzel et al. 2010, p. 15). Furthermore, a meta-analysis revealed that MBSR interventions may be more effective in healthcare practitioners than in other populations under stress (Khoury et al. 2015).

Having the ability to turn down the cognitive chaos of negative thoughts likely also creates a sense of internal control. Neurofunctional studies show that having a sense of control engages the prefrontal cortex, and having no sense of control enhances amygdalar function (Arnsten 2015). These techniques may have additional psychological utility by allowing physicians to have an internal mental boundary that prevents unwanted entry of work stress during time off.

In John McCain's firsthand account of wartime imprisonment, he recounted how important it was for him to keep his mind busy during solitary confinement—memorizing 300-plus names of prisoners of war, writing plays and poems in his head, and thinking through the historical events of the twentieth century he had studied in college. Perhaps these memory games were meditative and also provided a world where he was still in charge. A world that he filled with reflections on his passions—country and kin—and one in which abuse and torture gained no admission, and so he was able to maintain some sense of internal control.

Conclusion

Prolonged, intense, and negative stress is never good, but there seem to be several additional characteristics of the experience that may determine when and if stress evolves into burnout. When physicians and trainees are exposed to the chronic stress of the medical culture, there are certain individual factors that increase the risk of adverse outcomes. Changing negative, self-critical, and perfectionistic thinking styles could likely protect physicians from stress to a degree. Anticipating challenges with excitement rather than fear, mindfulness training, and learning to tolerate uncertainty may increase coping. Environmental characteristics can either mitigate some of these vulnerabilities or push medical students and doctors from the stressed zone into burnout. Stressful work environments that allow physicians little control and limited social support likely diminish resilience. Conversely, having a sense of purpose or meaning and pursuing one's passion at least 1 day a week is protective. The future lies not just in learning more about what humans need to survive adverse conditions and prevent negative stress-related outcomes but in proactively creating workplace environments where thriving is the most likely outcome for our physicians and trainees.

KEY POINTS

- Stress and arousal can be helpful, but only up to a point, after which they can quickly become a burden and liability.

- The stress response is mediated in the short term by the hypothalamus-pituitary-adrenal axis. Recurrent stress can lead to psychopathology and even to enduring epigenetic changes.

- Physicians face common stressors in their daily practice: chronic fatigue, overwork, decreased sleep, vicarious trauma, and medical errors. Acknowledging these occupational stressors and addressing them with systemic change is the intervention of most importance.

- Perfectionism, pessimism, and neuroticism are common personality traits among physicians, which can increase their vulnerability for adverse stress responses.

- Retaining a sense of control and purpose and being able to share experiences through social engagement may be protective and can buffer the effects of toxic work environments until widespread system change is accomplished.

References

American Psychiatric Association: Diagnostic and Statistical Manual of Mental Disorders, 5th Edition. Arlington, VA, American Psychiatric Association, 2013

Arnsten AF: Stress weakens prefrontal networks: molecular insults to higher cognition. Nat Neurosci 18(10):1376–1385, 2015 26404712

Association of American Medical Colleges: Age of applicants to U.S. medical schools at anticipated matriculation by sex and race/ethnicity, 2014–2015 through 2017–2018. Washington, DC, American Association of Medical Colleges, 2017. Available at: https://www.aamc.org/download/321468/data/factstablea6.pdf. Accessed October 21, 2018.

Blake DD, Weathers FW, Nagy LM, et al: The development of a clinician-administered PTSD scale. J Trauma Stress 8:75–90, 1995

Bleakley A, Brennan N: Does undergraduate curriculum design make a difference to readiness to practice as a junior doctor? Med Teach 33(6):459–467, 2011 21609175

Brewin CR, Firth-Cozens J: Dependency and self-criticism as predictors of depression in young doctors. J Occup Health Psychol 2(3):242–246, 1997 9552294

Brooks AW: Get excited: reappraising pre-performance anxiety as excitement. J Exp Psychol Gen 143(3):1144–1158, 2014 24364682

Bui E, Ohye B, Palitz S, et al: Acute and chronic reactions to trauma in children and adolescents, in IACAPAP Textbook of Child and Adolescent Mental Health. Edited by Rey JM and Martin A. Geneva, Switzerland, International Association for Child and Adolescent Psychiatry and Allied Professions, 2014. Available at: http://iacapap.org/wp-content/uploads/F4-PTSD-2014.pdf. Accessed October 7, 2018.

Butzlaff RL, Hooley JM: Expressed emotion and psychiatric relapse: a meta-analysis. Arch Gen Psychiatry 55(6):547–552, 1998 9633674

Chen H, Wu P, Wei W: New perspective on job burnout: exploring the root cause beyond general antecedents analysis. Psychol Rep 110(3):801–819, 2012 22897086

Coan JA, Schaefer HS, Davidson RJ: Lending a hand: social regulation of the neural response to threat. Psychol Sci 17(12):1032–1039, 2006 17201784

Cohen S: Perceived Stress Scale. Menlo Park, CA, Mind Garden, 1994. Available at: http://www.mindgarden.com/documents/PerceivedStressScale.pdf. Accessed September 23, 2018

Davidson RJ, McEwen BS: Social influences on neuroplasticity: stress and interventions to promote well-being. Nat Neurosci 15(5):689–695, 2012 22534579

Deary IJ, Agius RM, Sadler A: Personality and stress in consultant psychiatrists. Int J Soc Psychiatry 42(2):112–123, 1996 8811395

Delva MD, Kirby JR, Knapper CK, et al: Postal survey of approaches to learning among Ontario physicians: implications for continuing medical education. BMJ 325(7374):1218, 2002 12446540

DeRubeis RJ, Siegle GJ, Hollon SD: Cognitive therapy versus medication for depression: treatment outcomes and neural mechanisms. Nat Rev Neurosci 9(10):788–796, 2008 18784657

Doulougeri L, Georganta K, Montgomery A, et al: "Diagnosing" burnout among healthcare professionals: can we find consensus? Cogent Med 3(1), 2016 Epub

Felitti VJ, Anda RF, Nordenberg D, et al: Relationship of childhood abuse and household dysfunction to many of the leading causes of death in adults. The Adverse Childhood Experiences (ACE) Study. Am J Prev Med 14(4):245–258, 1998 9635069

Firth-Cozens J: Improving the health of psychiatrists. Adv Psychiatr Treat 13(3):161–168, 2007

Frankl V: Man's Search for Meaning: An Introduction to Logotherapy. Austria, Verlag für Jugend und Volk, 1946

Gold KJ, Sen A, Schwenk TL: Details on suicide among US physicians: data from the National Violent Death Reporting System. Gen Hosp Psychiatry 35(1):45–49, 2013 23123101

Gray SAO, Jones CW, Theall KP, et al: Thinking across generations: unique contributions of maternal early life and prenatal stress to infant physiology. J Am Acad Child Adolesc Psychiatry 56(11):922–929 2017 29096774

Guille C, Zhao Z, Krystal J, et al: Web-based cognitive behavioral therapy intervention for the prevention of suicidal ideation in medical interns: A randomized clinical trial. JAMA Psychiatry 72(12):1192–1198, 2015 26535958

Guille C, Frank E, Zhao Z, et al: Work-family conflict and the sex difference in depression among training physicians. JAMA Intern Med 177(12):1766–1772, 2017 29084311

Harvard Medical School: Stress Management: Enhance Your Well-Being by Reducing Stress and Building Resilience. A Harvard Medical School Special Report. Boston, MA, Harvard Health Publishing, 2018. Available at: https://www.health.harvard.edu/mind-and-mood/stress-management-enhance-your-well-being-by-reducing-stress-and-building-resilience. Accessed September 13, 2018.

Helo S, Moulton CE: Complications: acknowledging, managing, and coping with human error. Transl Androl Urol 6(4):773–782, 2017 28904910

Hölzel BK, Carmody J, Evans KC, et al: Stress reduction correlates with structural changes in the amygdala. Soc Cogn Affect Neurosci 5(1):11–17, 2010 19776221

Khoury B, Sharma M, Rush SE, et al: Mindfulness-based stress reduction for healthy individuals: a meta-analysis. J Psychosom Res 78(6):519–528, 2015 25818837

Klamen DL, Grossman LS, Kopacz D: Posttraumatic stress disorder symptoms in resident physicians related to their internship. Acad Psychiatry 19(3):142–149, 1995 24442586

Lupien SJ, McEwen BS, Gunnar MR, et al: Effects of stress throughout the lifespan on the brain, behaviour and cognition. Nat Rev Neurosci 10(6):434–445, 2009 19401723

Maslach C: Burned-out. Hum Behav 9:16–22, 1976

Maslach C, Jackson S, Leiter MP: Maslach Burnout Inventory Manual, 3rd Edition. Palo Alto, CA, Consulting Psychologists Press, 1996

McCain JS: John McCain, prisoner of war: a first-person account. U.S. News and World Report, May 1973. Available at: https://www.usnews.com/news/articles/2008/01/28/john-mccain-prisoner-of-war-a-first-person-account. Accessed September 8, 2018.

Myers MF: Why Physicians Die by Suicide: Lessons Learned From Their Families and Others Who Cared. New York, Michael F. Myers, 2017

Myers MF, Gabbard GO: The Physician as Patient: A Clinical Handbook for Mental Health Professionals. Washington, DC, American Psychiatric Publishing, 2008

Peris TS, Miklowitz DJ: Parental expressed emotion and youth psychopathology: new directions for an old construct. Child Psychiatry Hum Dev 46(6):863–873, 2015 25552241

Robertson IT, Cooper CL, Sarkar M, et al: Resilience training in the workplace from 2003 to 2014: a systematic review. Journal of Occupational and Organizational Psychology 88(3):533–562, 2015

Rotenstein LS, Torre M, Ramos MA, et al: Prevalence of burnout among physicians: a systematic review. JAMA 320(11):1131–1150, 2018 30326495

Sanchez LT, Candilis PJ, Arnstein F, et al: Effectiveness of a unique support group for physicians in a physician health program. J Psychiatr Pract 22(1):56–63, 2016 26813489

Schernhammer ES, Colditz GA: Suicide rates among physicians: a quantitative and gender assessment (meta-analysis). Am J Psychiatry 161(12):2295–2302, 2004 15569903

Sen S, Kranzler HR, Krystal JH, et al: A prospective cohort study investigating factors associated with depression during medical internship. Arch Gen Psychiatry 67(6):557–565, 2010 20368500

Shapiro SL, Shapiro DE, Schwartz GER: Stress management in medical education: a review of the literature. Acad Med 75(7):748–759, 2000 10926029

Shatté A, Perlman A, Smith B, et al: The positive effect of resilience on stress and business outcomes in difficult work environments. J Occup Environ Med 59(2):135–140, 2017 28002352

Shields GS, Slavich GM: Lifetime stress exposure and health: a review of contemporary assessment methods and biological mechanisms. Soc Personal Psychol Compass 11(8):e12335, 2017 28804509

Stamm BH: Professional Quality of Life: Compassion Satisfaction and Fatigue Version 5 (ProQOL). Copyright B. Hudman Stamm, 2009. Available at: https://proqol.org/uploads/ProQOL_5_English.pdf. Accessed November 18, 2018.

Støen Grotmol K, Gude T, Moum T, et al: Risk factors at medical school for later severe depression: a 15-year longitudinal, nationwide study (NORDOC). J Affect Disord 146(1):106–111, 2013 23017539

Terr LC: Childhood traumas, in Psychotraumatology: Key Papers and Core Concepts in Post-Traumatic Stress. The Springer Series on Stress and Coping. Edited by Everly Jr GS, Lating JM. Boston, MA, Springer, 1995 pp 301–320

Torre DM, Wang NY, Meoni LA, et al: Suicide compared to other causes of mortality in physicians. Suicide Life Threat Behav 35(2):146–153, 2005 15843332

van der Kolk B: The Body Keeps the Score: Brain, Mind, and Body in the Healing of Trauma. New York, Penguin Books, 2014

Vanhove AJ, Herian MN, Perez AL, et al: Can resilience be developed at work? A meta-analytic review of resilience-building programme effectiveness. J Occup Organ Psychol 89(2):278–307, 2016

Wood DP, Sexton JL: Self-hypnosis training and captivity survival. Am J Clin Hypn 39(3):201–211, 1997 9037797

Yerkes RM, Dodson JD: The relation of strength of stimulus to rapidity of habit-formation. Journal of Comparative Neurology 18(5):459–482, 1908

Yoon JD, Daley BM, Curlin FA: The association between a sense of calling and physician well-being: a national study of primary care physicians and psychiatrists. Acad Psychiatry 41(2):167–173, 2017 26809782

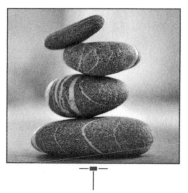

CHAPTER 4

UNDERSTANDING BURNOUT AND ITS POTENTIAL EFFECTS ON CLINICAL CARE

Sheila LoboPrabhu, M.D.

Hillary Rouse, M.A.

Victor Molinari, Ph.D.

Professional burnout is a phenomenon that occurs after an extended period of overwhelming work-related stress that results in the depletion of physical and emotional resources (Hammond et al. 2018). Burnout is not considered a state that a professional has reached but is a syndrome that evolves over time. There is considerable evidence that professional burnout is a medical condition, potentially overlapping with major depressive disorder, but there are currently no diagnostic criteria in DSM-5 (American Psychiatric Association 2013). The ICD-10 has recently recognized burnout as a life management problem and as a factor influencing health status. In the ICD, burnout is defined as a vital state of exhaustion (World Health Organization 2016). Although this definition helps to create a standard for what burnout encompasses, the term *burnout* is used and defined inconsistently by researchers who attempt to assess it, thus influencing the validity of study findings.

Burnout can occur in any type of job but is more common among healthcare workers. Negative reactions to work demands, in addition to interpersonal stressors, is one of the key reasons for the development of professional burnout (Rodriguez and Carlotto 2017; Rupert and Kent 2007). Burnout is also thought to be the result of internal conflict regarding the discrepancy between what professionals believe their job entails and what it truly does (Di Benedetto and Swadling 2014; Gilbert and Daloz 2008). Three separate but related dimensions define professional burnout. These dimensions include emotional exhaustion, depersonalization, and reduced sense of personal accomplishment (Domaney et al. 2018; Gül et al. 2017; Kumar 2011). Physicians who are burned out experience decreased mental energy with emotional exhaustion (Rupert and Morgan 2005). They can no longer give of themselves, resulting in detachment from patients and a sense of cynicism. Depersonalization causes physicians to feel devalued, replaceable, and meaningless, creating a low sense of personal accomplishment. All dimensions are critical in understanding the multidimensional nature of this syndrome.

Emotional exhaustion is the first dimension of burnout, and it is viewed as the most influential on the future development of burnout. Emotional exhaustion encompasses both physical and mental exhaustion; professionals feel that they are emotionally worn out and overextended because of work demands (Garcia et al. 2016). Emotional exhaustion is thought to be the stress dimension of burnout because it has been found to be highly correlated with stress levels in professionals. This dimension may be central to burnout because it mediates the effects of stress on the development of the other dimensions of burnout (Ben-Zur and Michael 2007; Rupert and Kent 2007). It has been argued that it does so by acting as a brake in some cases to help the burned-out physician slow down when he or she may not know how or when to appropriately rest in order to engage in self-care (Kumar 2011). Emotional exhaustion is also associated with the development of depersonalization because the exhaustion experienced can lead to distancing oneself from patients and work (Ben-Zur and Michael 2007).

The second dimension of burnout is depersonalization, and the development of this symptom can be an ethical challenge for professionals who have an obligation to treat their patients to the best of their abilities. Depersonalization, or cynicism (Domaney et al. 2018), is the interpersonal dimension of burnout (Ben-Zur and Michael 2007) in which healthcare workers stop considering their colleagues, students, and patients as people and instead treat them as objects. This dimension includes the adoption of callous, indifferent, and negative attitudes as well as detached and impersonal relationship styles. These feelings may also reflect a sense that patients are to blame for their difficulties, further driving negative attitudes. It is believed that depersonalization develops because professionals create a protective distance from work demands to shield themselves against further "emotional drowning" (Garcia et al. 2016).

Personal accomplishment is the final dimension of burnout; this relates to the self-evaluation concept of burnout (Ben-Zur and Michael 2007). A reduced sense of personal accomplishment encompasses negative attitudes or judgments about one's work, specifically about one's efforts, skills, and professional achievements. This includes dissatisfaction with how one is performing at work and feeling ineffective at fulfilling one's job responsibilities. This reduced sense of accomplishment also leads the professional to feel incompetent, inadequate, and unproductive (Garcia et al. 2016; Kumar 2011).

Research suggests that exhaustion and cynicism are more closely related to each other than to reduced professional efficacy (Kim and Ji 2009) and are therefore more frequently seen as the essential features of professional burnout.

Physicians today work long hours, often in an atmosphere of bureaucratic regulation and overwork, with these being two of the major causes of burnout. Compared with other physicians, psychiatrists as a group experience more stress due to these organizational constraints, as well as more clinical demands on their time. The stress typically occurs as a function of administrative pressure placed on psychiatrists via the context of their job. This includes school, Veterans Affairs/military, and hospital administrations. The stress experienced by psychiatrists also occurs more frequently because of the lack of positive feedback, poor working environments, and negative characteristics of patients and their relatives. Stress is particularly prevalent after a patient suicide (Fothergill et al. 2004). Yet even with the high levels of stress reported, psychiatrists are found to have higher levels of job satisfaction and moderately lower levels of burnout compared with other medical and surgical specialties (Kumar 2008; Medscape 2018).

Professional burnout is a very serious problem within our healthcare system today, with more than 50% of the physicians in the United States currently experiencing at least one of the dimensions of burnout. Because of the emotional nature of physicians' jobs, they are at an increased risk for chronic stress and therefore the development of burnout. Burnout occurs not only in different times of a physician's career but also during medical school and postgraduate resident years. The work-related effects of burnout are enormous, with increased risk of medical errors, poor performance, and decreased professional empathy. In addition, psychiatrists are more likely to either find a new career or retire early because of burnout (Domaney et al. 2018; Kumar 2011).

Prevalence Rates

According to the Medscape *National Physician Burnout and Depression Report* (Medscape 2018), 15,543 U.S. physicians from 29 different specialties reported that 42% of them were burned out, 12% reported "feeling down," and 3% reported being clinically depressed. Forty-eight percent of female physicians reported burnout versus 38% of male physicians. This is likely due to the higher likelihood of female physicians needing to balance both work and home responsibilities, compared with male physicians. The burnout rate was 35% for the youngest group of physicians ages 28–34; it increased to 43% for those between ages 35 and 44 and to 50% for those between ages 45 and 54 and then decreased to 41% for the 55–69 age group. The highest burnout rates were reported by intensivists and neurologists (48%), whereas the lowest burnout rates were reported by plastic surgeons (23%). In this report, psychiatrists reported a 36% rate of burnout, but in other research this number is reported as high as 40%–70% (Domaney et al. 2018). The American Psychiatric Association survey of 1,500 psychiatrists found that 74% had an Oldenburg burnout score indicating that they were burned out (Everett 2018). Some studies suggest that psychiatrists represent a group of physicians who may be at particularly high risk for developing burnout compared with other physicians, either because of the nature of their work or because of their personality structure. When investigating the outcomes of burnout among psychiatrists compared with other physicians, it is found that they are at an increased risk for extreme levels of stress, future diagnoses of mental illness, and suicide (Fothergill et al. 2004; Gül et al. 2017; Kumar 2011). The "serious stress syndrome" of burnout is a state of ill-being that is defined by the work-related symptoms of exhaustion, cynicism, and decreased professional efficacy (Maslach et al. 1996). This syndrome has been extensively researched since it was originally described in the literature in the 1970s (Leiter et al. 2014). However, other studies report that psychiatrists are less burned out than other specialties and that they report a better professional/personal life balance (Medscape 2018), perhaps because their training emphasizes the understanding of stress and its effects and how to implement stress-reducing strategies.

Factors Related to Burnout

SYMPTOMS OF BURNOUT IN PSYCHIATRISTS

Because of the various aspects that can influence the development of burnout, a burned-out psychiatrist can present with a variety of symptoms. As with most defense mechanisms, these symptoms may serve both adaptive and maladaptive functions. The defense may be adaptive by helping to protect the psyche against damage when there is "no way out" (Angyal 1965). However, this may come at the price of poor psychological well-being, fatigue, apathy, dysphoric mood, a sense of helplessness, and negative changes in attitude toward one's life and job. These negative changes in attitude include a loss of idealism, reduced work goals, greater self-interest, and increasing sense of emotional detachment from patients and families (Kumar et al. 2005). When examining the symptoms associated with burnout, there is consistency between those found in physicians in other fields and in psychiatrists. These symptoms include physical symptoms such as chronic fatigue, headache, frequent sickness, insomnia, rapid pulse, and gastrointestinal symptoms such as nausea, ulcers, heartburn, and weight gain or loss. These symptoms also include psychological symptoms such as irritability, anxiety, depression, decreased libido, poor concentration, excessive criticism, suicidal ideation, and cognitive distortions of perfectionism and the need to control everything (Hammond et al. 2018).

Physician burnout is typically reflected in psychological and physical manifestations, but it also can affect the physician's spirituality. Burnout can be associated with doubts in spiritual beliefs or personal values, anger and bitterness at God, and possible withdrawal from religion (Franke 1999). In care delivery systems where attention to the patient's spiritual needs is especially important, such as in critical care units, intensive care, or hospice, a burned-out physician may not be able to pay attention to the patient's spiritual needs when the physician has spiritual doubts or issues of his or her own.

ETIOLOGY OF BURNOUT

Stress is a consequence of the determination that the demands of one's current environment exceed available coping abilities. *Coping* is defined as cognitive and behavioral regulatory attempts to address both internal and external demands that have been judged as straining one's current available resources (Montero-Marín et al. 2009). As noted in the previous subsection, symptoms of burnout can be both adaptive and maladaptive. Not all attempts by professionals to adapt to the environment are successful. Burnout develops as a consequence of professionals failing to use adequate coping mechanisms when attempting to adapt or protect themselves from workplace-related stress. Rupert et al. (2015), in their study of psychologists' coping strategies, noted that escape-avoidance or emotion-focused coping is related to higher levels of burnout. Emotion-focused strategies are associated with higher levels of depersonalization and lower personal accomplishment. However, the use of problem-focused coping strategies is more effective because it leads to greater feelings of personal accomplishment and lower levels of depersonalization. In a cross-sectional survey of university employees, Montero-Marín et al. (2014) evaluated the different coping strategies for the three subtypes of burnout:

1. The *frenetic* subtype of burnout is associated with an employee who works increasingly hard toward success to the point of exhaustion. It is associated with involvement, ambition, and overload. The coping strategy correlated with this burnout subtype is more strongly related to affective *venting*. Individuals with the frenetic subtype of burnout cope with stress by complaining about workplace organizational management, which they feel limits their goals and ambitions. This results in stress overload and a desire to quit the job.
2. In the *underchallenged* subtype, the individual experiences burnout stemming from boredom and lack of personal development due to monotonous and understimulating conditions that fail to provide satisfaction. Individuals with the underchallenged subtype of burnout often employ an avoidance coping strategy. These individuals manage stress at work by distancing themselves, depersonalization, and cynicism, which also results in a wish to leave the job.
3. The *worn-out* subtype of burnout involves giving up when faced with stress in the absence of gratification. Although individuals with this subtype of burnout have goals they want to achieve, they lack the motivation to overcome barriers to success. They feel a lack of control, unacknowledged, and neglected.

The standard definition of burnout mentioned earlier in this chapter—characterized by emotional exhaustion, depersonalization, and a reduced sense of personal accomplishment—is strongly related to the way that burnout is formulated here through the dimensions of overload, lack of development, and neglect within the frenetic, underchallenged, and worn-out subtypes. Overload, in particular, involves individuals feeling as if they are risking their health and personal life in chasing optimal outcomes and is strongly related to emotional exhaustion. Lack of development involves limited personal development for professionals, along with an unsatisfied desire to explore alternative opportunities through which they can strengthen their skills, and is significantly associated with cynicism. Finally, neglect involves an individual's lack of concern and professional effort when difficulties arise and is significantly related to inefficacy (Montero-Marín et al. 2014).

RISK FACTORS FOR BURNOUT IN PSYCHIATRISTS

Psychiatry is one of the medical fields that has seen the most significant and rapid transformations in recent decades. It has changed from being asylum based, for people experiencing very significant mental illnesses, to having a community focus that also incorporates people with minor mental stresses. This has led to a greater number of patients being treated, and therefore additional administrative tasks, as well as greater expectations from others about the ability to cure those with mental illness. These expectations and rapid changes have stigmatized psychiatry and stunted its growth, contributing to psychiatrist burnout (O'Connor et al. 2018). According to the *National Physician Burnout and Depression Report* (Medscape 2018), the top reasons for burnout were too many bureaucratic tasks (56%); long work hours (39%); lack of respect from employers, colleagues, and staff (26%); and electronic health records (EHRs; 24%). In addition to these organizational factors, there are multiple risks for the development of burnout that are related to the providers (family stress, personality traits) as well as to the patients they see.

Studies have consistently found that overwork, or an excessive workload, is significant in the development of burnout (Ben-Zur and Michael 2007; Di Benedetto and Swadling 2014). More specifically, about 20% of health professionals suggest that their burnout is a direct result of overwork (Gül et al. 2017). Overworking includes the number of hours worked as well as having complex and heavy caseloads and maintaining clinical competence. Also, subjective feelings of work pressure surrounding an increased demand to see more patients for higher productivity rates is seen as an additional factor that can determine whether someone feels overworked (Garcia et al. 2016; Hammond et al. 2018; Rupert and Morgan 2005). Another factor related to feeling overworked is the administrative tasks and paperwork that need completing. The amount of time spent in these activities has been found to be directly related to greater levels of emotional exhaustion and a reduced amount of personal accomplishment (Garcia et al. 2016). In addition to this, problems within the administration and staff are a common theme. A lack of administrative support, clinical management conflicts, negative relationships with other staff (Fothergill et al. 2004), and weak work group cohesion have all been established as risk factors. Inadequate resources, or resource issues in general, have been additionally found to increase the risk of burnout. The lack of resources could contribute directly to burnout or indirectly through low staffing levels, low pay, and low rewards (Fothergill et al. 2004; Kumar 2011; Kumar et al. 2005). Finally, one of the greatest risk factors related to the organizational level is role ambiguity, or role conflict, at the work place. This could lead to psychiatrists having self-esteem issues, perceiving that future goals are unachievable, and potentially having to take on patients whom they may not be comfortable with treating (Fothergill et al. 2004; Franke 1999).

Most healthcare systems have implemented EHRs for their practice, with the percentage of practices using EHRs jumping from 4% to 13% in 2008 and to 72% in 2012 (Hsaio and Hing 2012). The EHR is a way of recording patient data as well as garnering insurance coverage for treatment. EHR glitches have been found to be significant triggers for development of burnout. These malfunctions can lead to problems with insurance involvement as well as problems with documents being completed in the way needed for payment. The U.S. government created financial incentives for investment in EHRs and their "meaningful use." However, the Minimizing Error Maximizing Outcome (MEMO) study by Babbott et al. (2014) has shown that although job stress is modestly reduced for those physicians with advanced EHR systems, greater levels of stress with reduced feelings of job satisfaction can be found with moderate use of a variety of EHR functions. Time pressure was associated with poor physician outcomes, mainly in those physicians using a high number of EHR functions. These negative outcomes are mediated by increasing cognitive demands on the physician, information overload, and "information chaos." Physicians struggle to balance an increase in tasks needing to be completed during the patient visit, with no increase in time allotted to fill out the EHRs. A recent study by Domaney et al. (2018) reported that resident physicians' time with EHRs has been increasing dramatically, as residents are spending 43% of their time at their workstations. Furthermore, the study found that there was a significant relationship between the total hours of EHR use and burnout. This suggests that the EHR may not be as beneficial for physicians as was originally envisioned.

Personal factors leading to burnout can be financial pressures, family pressures, lack of time, fear of malpractice litigation, and work-home conflict. Specifically related to family, research has established that marital status is generally not associated with work stress but having children is. By law, health service professionals are also not allowed to discuss anything about their patients with nonprofessionals such as family or friends. This leaves little or no opportunity to share emotional reactions to their work experiences, and this has been found to be a major determinant for future burnout (Emery et al. 2009). The culture of medicine also causes physicians to view emotion as a weakness, dictates that patients' needs should always come first, encourages physicians to sacrifice their own needs, and often causes physicians to be unable to recognize their own needs or to ask for help. Psychiatrists especially feel responsible for the day-to-day lives of others, trying to maintain constructive relationships with patients—including challenging or difficult ones—and dealing with problems and emotional concerns. Burnout causes physicians to engage in unethical behavior and boundary violations. One boundary violation commonly seen is an overinvolvement of the psychiatrist with patients. This has been found to be related to higher levels of emotional exhaustion and depersonalization but also to an enhanced sense of personal accomplishment (Rupert and Morgan 2005). During times of severe stress such as relationship problems, grief from a major loss, financial difficulties, or malpractice litigation, physicians are at risk for burnout and engaging in ethical violations.

Personality traits of psychiatrists as a group in general predispose them to a greater risk of burnout. Psychiatrists tend to be more neurotic, open, and agreeable, but they often score low on conscientiousness and their views of themselves (Ben-Zur and Michael 2007). Other personality traits predisposing them to develop burnout are perfectionism, the need to control, and overachievement. Perfectionism, in particular, is a vulnerability factor for depression, anxiety, burnout, and suicide (Beevers and Miller 2004). Perfectionism often predicts burnout because it is associated with an exaggerated sense of responsibility, leading to self-doubt and guilt (Oreskovich and Anderson 2013). It also has been found that the association between perfectionism and eventual burnout is mediated by stress. Therefore, holding these higher expectations of oneself leads to rigidity and an inability to delegate, promoting overwork and thereby exacerbating the risk for future burnout. These behaviors may result in excessive devotion to and overidentification with work, to the detriment of relationships and self-care. Those with perfectionistic ideas are less likely to recover from burnout when compared with others who are more realistic about their strengths, weaknesses, and work preferences (Emery et al. 2009). Finally, perfectionism can also predispose to suicide because fear of failure may lead to the need to completely control everything in a physician's professional and personal life. This can result in depersonalization and cynicism. The physician can become irritable and hypervigilant, experiencing insomnia, nightmares, social withdrawal, and depression.

The final risks for provider burnout come from the patients for whom psychiatrists care. Studies have identified feelings of entitlement by patients as a risk factor for occupational stress and future burnout of physicians (Franke 1999). Problems that psychiatrists often experience that lead to burnout are increased feelings of responsibility for their patients, nonreciprocated attentiveness, and having to constantly give of oneself to the patient. About three-fourths of professionals find that if their patients do not have successful outcomes, they feel more stress about their ability to perform at work (Gül et al. 2017). This could be why patient suicide is significantly implicated in mental health professional burnout (Emery et al. 2009; Fothergill et al. 2004; Kumar et al. 2005). As many as 51%–82% of psychiatrists have experienced a patient suicide, and 47% of these experienced their first patient suicide within the first 5 years of entering the field of psychiatry. This could lead to results that affect psychiatrists variably because those who are younger and less experienced are more likely to feel the greatest emotional consequences from this. The consequences of patient suicide are significantly greater for American psychiatrists compared with European psychiatrists. After a patient commits suicide, psychiatrists tend to experience feelings of anger and guilt; have low mood and irritability; experience loss of self-esteem and impaired sleep; have thoughts or a desire to commit suicide; take or consider early retirement; and exhibit reduced performance at work, with some psychiatrists completely altering the way they practice. Professional liability and threats of lawsuits may further exacerbate the psychological turmoil. In addition, violent patients who present with aggressive or threatening behaviors, including harassment and bullying, increase the risk for psychiatrist burnout (Fothergill et al. 2004; Kumar 2011). Finally, there are specific cases and diagnoses that are implicated more in psychiatrist burnout. Treating children, trauma victims, those who have psychosis, and those with a personality disorder lead to greater rates of burnout (Kumar et al. 2005). The rate of burnout is potentially higher when working with these populations because they tend to require more time and emotional energy.

PROTECTIVE FACTORS AGAINST BURNOUT

Certain factors are protective against burnout. Researchers have investigated the influence of internal beliefs on burnout outcomes. They found that mental health staff who perceive their work as a calling are more motivated in their careers and show lower rates of burnout. The sense of calling is believed to help staff maintain their clinical commitment by continually restoring meaning and intrinsic reward within their job, even when facing negative events (Yoon et al. 2017). Relative to this, personal beliefs about the effectiveness of psychotherapy and pharmacotherapy can influence staff attitudes toward the job, as well as foster therapeutic success, which can indirectly influence job satisfaction (Ballenger-Browning et al. 2011). In addition to beliefs related to their job, cognitive strategies can influence the development of burnout, specifically the dimension of depersonalization. In a study of psychologists, it was found that mental health staff who preserve a sense of control, reflect on positive work experiences, maintain a balance between work and personal lives, and retain self-awareness are less likely to be cynical toward patients (Rupert et al. 2015). Furthermore, autonomy in their work leads physicians to be able to resist stress better, to avoid counterproductive behaviors, to maintain a sense of importance in their job, and to be satisfied with their employment (Madathil et al. 2014). Reflection on experiences includes both internally within oneself as well as with superiors. Supervisor support of processing experiences with patients is positively related to personal accomplishment and negatively related to emotional exhaustion and depersonalization. Time spent conducting therapy could be indirectly related to the psychiatrist's ability to reflect on satisfying experiences because the psychiatrist would have more interactions to review. Research suggests that more time in therapy with patients is positively correlated with personal accomplishment and that maintaining empathy in the therapeutic relationship can significantly help to prevent burnout (Kumar et al. 2005; Rupert and Morgan 2005). The ability to sustain a balance between one's career and home life is influential because there is a bidirectional effect on the development of burnout and the development of family conflict. Also, social and family supports are protective against burnout. Finally, being mindful of oneself can assist in identifying and challenging unhelpful beliefs and negative behaviors that may be early signs of burnout. Cultivating alternative beliefs and more positive behaviors can result in better physician mental health, which will ultimately decrease the risk of burnout (Emery et al. 2009).

There are specific factors that a psychiatrist can control to help protect against burnout. Certain types of coping strategies can help to reduce the risk of burnout. Psychiatrists who use problem-focused coping strategies, compared with escape-avoidance and emotion-focused coping, experience significantly reduced levels of depersonalization and greater levels of personal accomplishment (Ben-Zur and Michael 2007). Lifestyle factors that include paying attention to, and being satisfied with, one's life outside of work and engaging in self-care activities are also known to be protective against burnout. Lifestyle factors that involve teaching classes or mentoring students have consistently been found to prevent burnout, perhaps by increasing one's sense of personal accomplishment and generativity. Self-care behaviors include self-awareness, self-acceptance, cognitive coping skills, and career-sustaining behaviors. Career-sustaining behaviors that have been identified as preventive mechanisms against burnout include exercise, social activities, mindfulness, and taking breaks between therapy sessions to collect one's thoughts. These protective factors tend to correlate significantly with reduced levels of emotional exhaustion and greater levels of personal accomplishment (Di Benedetto and Swadling 2014; Kumar et al. 2005).

Workplace social support, feedback from supervisors, and job autonomy all serve as buffers against burnout. In addition to these protective factors, research has established that certain working environments are better than others at protecting against burnout. For psychiatrists, those working in a private work setting have lower levels of burnout. This could be associated with the setting or to the fact that psychiatrists in these settings tend to have less work stress, higher income, and more direct therapy hours and to be of older age (Emery et al. 2009). Psychiatrists feel more control over their work if they are either in a solo or in an independent group practice. In addition, these practitioners are more likely to have private-pay patients. Independent group practitioners are less likely to deal with dangerous or threatening patients as well, resulting in a decreased risk of burnout (Rupert and Morgan 2005).

Consequences of Burnout

Even with extensive research on outcomes of burnout in psychiatrists, the consequences remain unclear. Consequences for the psychiatrist can be profound when burnout is not properly managed, and burnout can lead to impaired mental and physical health as well as the development of negative behaviors. With increasing burnout, psychiatrists are at an elevated risk for depression, anxiety, interpersonal conflict, and a loss of sense of self. The most significant consequence related to mental health for these professionals is a heightened risk of suicidal ideation and attempted suicide. Also related to one's mental status, physicians with burnout, including psychiatrists, complain about impaired cognitive functioning and abilities (Domaney et al. 2018; Gül et al. 2017; Kumar 2011). Because burnout can lead to many physiological changes that are associated with these somatic symptoms, if these symptoms continue over time, then the individual may be at risk for significant physical illness. These include hypertension, coronary heart disease, obesity, irritable bowel syndrome, and even the risk of dementia (Hammond et al. 2018). In addition to such negative physical and mental health outcomes, psychiatrists as a group are more at risk for dysfunctional or risky behaviors, including use of alcohol and drugs as well as boundary violations

(Gül et al. 2017; Kumar 2011). These behaviors tend to result in strain and conflict with current relationships, including those with their family, friends, and coworkers. Also, because of the nature of their work, psychiatrists are more likely to develop sexual relationships with their patients, compared with other disciplines (Gül et al. 2017; Kumar 2011). Overall, the consequences associated with burnout can lead to a significant reduction in the quality of life for psychiatrists (Gilbert and Daloz 2008).

Effects of Burnout on Clinical Care

Psychiatrist burnout can have a profound impact on the physician's occupational functioning, leading to costs for the organization they work for and possible harm to their patients (Rupert and Morgan 2005). It has been consistently found that burnout is more than likely to lead to a reduction in the quality of medical care by physicians and a reduction in the commitment to their job (Garcia et al. 2016; Kumar 2011). The decreased quality of care directly influences the patient in a negative way, resulting in decreased patient satisfaction (Domaney et al. 2018; Kumar 2011; West et al. 2016). The quality of care is thought to be dramatically reflected in an increased risk of medical errors as well as deviation from best practice guidelines. Indeed, a recent systematic review and meta-analysis of 47 studies conducted across varied countries indicated that physician burnout is associated with lowered professionalism, increased incidents regarding patient safety, and reduced patient satisfaction (Panagioti et al. 2018). These medical errors are associated with poor documentation and record keeping, procrastination and missing of deadlines, lack of empathy, and a preoccupation with one's current state (Domaney et al. 2018; Gül et al. 2017). Deviations from best practice guidelines occur when the physician intentionally reduces the time spent in patient care or tries to avoid patients, when the physician has emotional outbursts, or when the physician engages in self-disclosure to their patients for the physician's own well-being (Yoon et al. 2017). Recent research has found that if those physicians who are experiencing some burnout have even the smallest additional increase in their level of burnout, they are significantly more likely to report greater self-perceived major medical errors and self-perceived poorer quality of work (West et al. 2016).

Physician burnout can dramatically affect the organization. Related to quality of work, there is a striking decrease in the productivity of burned-out physicians that is related to a loss of motivation and commitment to their field. There is a significant increase in physicians' desire to leave their position, and sometimes the medical community. It is therefore not surprising that physician turnover is found to be a direct result of burnout. With a high turnover rate, organizations lose staff who may be extremely skilled because of their experience and conscientiousness and may therefore retain employment of only the remaining staff who may be of lower quality. If physicians remain at their practice, those with burnout are more likely to be consistently tardy or absent and more likely to limit the number of hours they work per week (Kumar 2011; Yoon et al. 2017). Physicians who are feeling unwell can either report to work in a medically ill state (often referred to as "presenteeism") or take time off. This can cause slowed or altered delivery of patient care. Recurrent tardiness or absenteeism results in decreased patient access to care, increased need for cross coverage by physicians who may have never cared for the patient before, and elevated risk of medical errors. Overall, physicians who have invested a great number of years training for their position often will lose sight of the goals that they have worked so hard to achieve directly because of burnout (Di Benedetto and Swadling 2014).

According to the American Medical Association (Shanafelt et al. 2017), physician burnout can lead to significant costs for an organization, with the average costs ranging from $500,000 to more than $1 million per physician. The current annual projected cost of U.S. physician turnover due to burnout is $6,136,364. These financial repercussions are directly related to the organization having to recruit and replace the physician once they have left the practice as well as the cost of incentives offered to the new physician joining the practice. This includes sign-on bonuses, lost billings, and ramp-up costs. If a burned-out physician decides to stay, the financial burden is due to reducing the physician's clinical hours to only part-time. There are also indirect financial consequences that occur because of physician burnout. These include the indirect costs of medical errors resulting in more medical treatment for patients and potentially higher malpractice lawsuit risks. In addition to this, physician burnout can lead to reduced patient satisfaction, which can result in damage to the organization's name, with fewer patients returning to the organization (Sinsky et al. 2017).

Because psychiatrists use themselves as healing "tools" in their clinical work (Kumar 2007), any major disruptor to the psychiatrist's emotional state can have immediate and lasting effects on clinical care by directly affecting the patient. A burned-out psychiatrist who is emotionally labile is not a good role model and may violate ethical standards by engaging in angry, belittling, or hostile behavior. A psychiatrist behaving in an emotionally exhausted, avoidant, or distancing manner can elicit feelings of rejection and neglect in patients who are already vulnerable to stigma by the very nature of their illness. Depersonalization in psychiatrists can cause lack of empathy and viewing the patient as an object, as well as emotional distancing or disengagement from patients. This is a particularly risky frame of mind and behavior for a healer who has a fiduciary responsibility toward vulnerable patients in distress. Emotional exhaustion predisposes burned-out psychiatrists to stop listening because of their depleted emotional resources. This can lead to impaired professional abilities because the psychiatrist is more likely to miss important clues to the patient's emotional state. Finally, a low sense of personal accomplishment can place psychiatrists at risk for anxiety and depression, conditions for which they are already vulnerable.

Illness Versus Impairment

Illness is simply the existence of disease. However, impairment is a functional classification and implies the inability of the person affected by the disease to perform specific activities. An illness such as anxiety, depression, or substance abuse can lead to impairment. However, an ill person may not necessarily be impaired. This is a crucially important distinction. The Federation of State Medical Boards (2011, p. 5) *Policy on Physician Impairment* defines *impairment* as the inability of a licensed physician to practice medicine with reasonable skill and safety as the result of 1) mental disorder; or 2) physical illness or condition, including but not limited to those illnesses or conditions that would adversely affect cognitive, motor, or perceptive skills; or 3) substance-related disorders including abuse and dependency of drugs and alcohol.

Burnout can be accompanied by anxiety, depression, and possibly alcohol or substance use disorders. It is a slippery slope from burnout to illness and then impairment. Physicians who reach out for help or who are referred for treatment by concerned family, friends, colleagues, or hospitals may be able to secure help before engaging in unethical behavior or patient harm.

Depression Versus Burnout

Depression is a mood disorder characterized by persistent sad, anxious, hopeless, or pessimistic feelings and results in a loss of interest or pleasure in activities, as well as several other symptoms (American Psychiatric Association 2013). Besides genetic risk, chronic stress is considered to be one of the most influential factors related to whether someone develops a depressive disorder. Burnout is not classified as a mood disorder but can present in a way in which the person is persistently sad, anxious, hopeless, or pessimistic because of a current occupational situation. Burnout typically presents as a loss of desire or interest in persisting at tasks at the workplace. Therefore, burnout may be highly associated with depression because of the overlap in symptomatology, but the relationship is multifaceted and poorly understood (Kumar et al. 2005; Orosz et al. 2017). Lower levels of burnout may not overlap as much with depressive symptoms, but with increasing severity of burnout, the risk for a diagnosis of depression is great. In addition to the presentation of related symptoms, recent studies have found it to be extremely difficult to discriminate between the two at the physiological and neurological levels (Orosz et al. 2017). Given the similarity in symptoms and the evidence for stress as a key determinant for the development of symptoms associated with both conditions, one can conclude that burnout and depression may be much more similar than originally perceived.

Although the overlap between depression and burnout seems to be great, there are also some aspects of each that are significantly different. Depression affects all aspects of life, whereas burnout is conceived to affect only one's occupation. Indeed, those with depression may have anhedonia, whereas those with burnout are still capable of enjoying activities outside of work. The three dimensions of burnout closely correlate with each other, but only the dimension of emotional exhaustion seems to be strongly correlated with the negative affect associated with depression. One of the defining differences between depression and burnout concerns feelings of superiority and status. Individuals who are depressed have a significant reduction in their sense of superiority and feel that they have lost their status. In those experiencing burnout, research has found that they may retain these feelings because they are still attempting to obtain status and gain superiority in their workplace. This shows a key difference between these individuals with regard to their motivation (Brenninkmeyer et al. 2001; Kumar et al. 2005) and suggests that burnout is an active process that, depending on its persistence, can be prodromal to depression.

Compassion Fatigue and Vicarious Traumatization Versus Burnout

In physicians, specifically those in the mental health field, burnout is sometimes mistaken for compassion fatigue or vicarious traumatization. *Compassion fatigue* is a phenomenon that occurs as a direct result of the emotional strain from working intensively with exacting patients. Compassion fatigue can be conceptualized as a type of burnout that is typically associated with the "cost of caring" for others. *Vicarious traumatization,* or secondary traumatic stress, is a very severe form of compassion fatigue that develops by indirect exposure to a traumatic event through the firsthand recollection of events by the traumatized patient. The most significant difference is in how each develops; burnout is typically progressive, whereas compassion fatigue and vicarious traumatization often emerge suddenly (Di Benedetto and Swadling 2014; Linneroot et al. 2011).

Compassion fatigue is different from burnout in that it is caused by empathy and encompasses more advanced psychological disruption (Kumar 2011; Linneroot et al. 2011). Compassion fatigue, especially vicarious traumatization, is much more common in physicians who work with patients who have experienced trauma. This includes combat-related trauma seen in military personnel and trauma from abuse in children and adults, along with other trauma-related events. Risk factors for physicians to develop compassion fatigue include younger age, higher motivation, personal life stressors, lack of social support, higher idealism, cumulative grief from multiple losses either within or outside of work, and prolonged exposure to stressful environments. The symptoms of compassion fatigue are found across seven domains: cognitive, emotional, behavioral, personal relations, work performance, somatic, and spiritual (Linneroot et al. 2011). Regarding cognitive symptoms, professionals with compassion fatigue typically experience disorientation, apathy, lowered concentration, and preoccupation with the trauma. Emotional symptoms typically reflect powerlessness, anxiety, guilt, shock, helplessness, sadness, and anger. Irritability, poor sleep, nightmares, isolation, hypervigilance, and appetite changes are behavioral symptoms. The quality of personal relationships and performance at work decreases. The somatic symptoms associated with compassion fatigue are headaches, dizziness, sweating, rapid heartbeat, impaired immune system functioning, and difficulty breathing. Finally, spiritual symptoms include loss of faith, loss of purpose, questioning life's meaning, and questioning one's own religious beliefs (Meier et al. 2001).

Vicarious traumatization occurs with increasing contact with the individual who experienced the trauma as well as the intensifying detail surrounding the experience. The physician may develop vicarious traumatization because of repeated exposure to the graphic and violent imagery that the patient presents with or because of countertransference issues. Vicarious traumatization is its own form of compassion fatigue because of the overlapping nature of these symptoms with those that are commonly seen in posttraumatic stress disorder. The overlapping symptoms are avoidance and intrusion, as well as the possibility of the development of arousal after exposure to an incident that is related to what has been discussed. Other symptoms associated with vicarious traumatization include avoidance of social contact, irritability, becoming judgmental or argumentative, depression, anxiety, impatience, disconnection, low motivation, and low self-image (Linneroot et al. 2011; Kumar 2011).

Conclusion

Research on professional burnout has mostly investigated the development, progression, and outcomes of burnout. Very few studies have looked at preventive or secondary interventions. Burnout has serious and important personal, professional, and ethical implications. Because of the multidimensional nature of burnout, interventions should be aimed at both individual and systemic environmental contexts (Rodriguez and Carlotto 2017). The most effective intervention thus far appears to be initiatives sponsored by medical societies for physicians to become aware of symptoms that are associated with the dimensions of burnout, as well as to empower them to be involved with their professional organizations to reduce triggers associated with burnout. Interventions are thought to be most successful when they foster resilience and mindfulness, for example, stress management courses, duty hour limitation, and small group discussions. However, although findings are nondefinitive, the substance of the research suggests that individual-directed and work-directed group interventions combined may be the most influential in helping to reduce physician burnout (Deb 2017; Kumar 2011; West et al. 2016). The ultimate goals of these interventions should be to advance excellence in the physician and organization, enrich the quality of physician-patient relationships, and modify the outlook of physicians themselves (Deb 2017).

KEY POINTS

————————■————————

- Burnout is a condition that occurs in many physicians.
- The three main dimensions of burnout include emotional exhaustion, depersonalization, and reduced sense of personal accomplishment.
- Burnout occurs when professionals use ineffective coping strategies to protect themselves from workplace-related stress.
- Risk factors for psychiatrist burnout include organizational variables (too many bureaucratic tasks, long work hours), personal stressors (financial, work-home conflict), personality traits (perfectionism, low self-esteem), and patients for whom they care (increased sense of responsibility for their patient, having to constantly give of oneself to the patient).
- Internal beliefs regarding the effectiveness of their professional services, autonomy, a balanced home/family life, family support, and active problem-focused coping are protective factors against physician burnout.

————————■————————

References

American Psychiatric Association: Diagnostic and Statistical Manual of Mental Disorders, 5th Edition. Arlington, VA, American Psychiatric Association, 2013

Angyal A: Neurosis and Treatment: A Holistic Theory. Hoboken, NJ, John Wiley and Sons, 1965

Babbott S, Manwell LB, Brown R, et al: Electronic medical records and physician stress in primary care: results from the MEMO Study. J Am Med Inform Assoc 21(e1):e100–e106, 2014 24005796

Ballenger-Browning KK, Schmitz KJ, Rothacker JA, et al: Predictors of burnout among military mental health providers. Mil Med 176(3):253–260, 2011 21456349

Beevers CG, Miller IW: Perfectionism, cognitive bias, and hopelessness as prospective predictors of suicidal ideation. Suicide Life Threat Behav 34(2):126–137, 2004 15191269

Ben-Zur H, Michael K: Burnout, social support, and coping at working among social workers, psychologists, and nurses: the role of challenge/control appraisals. Soc Work Health Care 45(4):63–82, 2007 17954449

Brenninkmeyer V, Van Yperen N, Buunk B: Burnout and depression are not identical twins: is decline of superiority a distinguishing feature? Pers Individ Dif 30(5):873–880, 2001

Deb A: Practical considerations in addressing physician burnout. Continuum (Minneap Minn) 23(2, Selected Topics in Outpatient Neurology):557–562, 2017 28375919

Di Benedetto M, Swadling M: Burnout in Australian psychologists: correlations with work-setting, mindfulness and self-care behaviours. Psychol Health Med 19(6):705–715, 2014 24279368

Domaney N, Torous J, Greenberg W: Exploring the association between electronic health record use and burnout among psychiatry residents and faculty: a pilot survey. Acad Psychiatry 42(5):648–652, 2018 29785625

Emery S, Wade T, McLean S: Associations among therapists' beliefs, personal resources, and burnout in clinical psychologists. Behav Change 26(2):83–96, 2009

Everett A: Combating compassion fatigue and burnout: interview with Anita Everett M.D., part 1. Medical Bag, May 25, 2018. Available at: https://www.medicalbag.com/lifestyle/compassion-fatigue-burnout-apa-president-interview/article/768679/. Accessed November 25, 2018.

Federation of State Medical Boards: Policy on Physician Impairment. Washington, DC, Federation of State Medical Boards, 2011

Franke J: Stress burnout and addiction. Tex Med 95(3):42–52, 1999 10932634

Fothergill A, Edwards D, Burnard P: Stress, burnout, coping and stress management in psychiatrists: findings from a systematic review. Int J Soc Psychiatry 50(1):54–65, 2004 15143847

Garcia HA, McGeary CA, Finley EP, et al: The influence of trauma and patient characteristics on provider burnout in VA post-traumatic stress disorder specialty programmes. Psychol Psychother 89(1):66–81, 2016 25643839

Gilbert D, Daloz L: Disorders associated with burnout and causal attributions of stress among health care professional in psychiatry. Eur Rev Appl Psychol 58(4):263–274, 2008

Gül A, Gül H, Özkal UC, et al: The relationship between sluggish cognitive tempo and burnout symptoms in psychiatrists with different therapeutic approaches. Psychiatry Res 252:284–288, 2017 28288439

Hammond TE, Crowther A, Drummond S: A thematic inquiry into the burnout experience of Australian solo-practicing clinical psychologists. Front Psychol 8:1996, 2018 29403402

Hsaio CJ, Hing E: Use and Characteristics of Electronic Health Record Systems Among Office-Based Practices: United States, 2011–2012 (NCHS Data Brief, No 111). Hyattsville, MD, U.S. Department of Health and Human Services, Centers for Disease Control and Prevention, National Center for Health Statistics, 2012

Kim H, Ji J: Factor structure and longitudinal variance of the Maslach Burnout Inventory. Res Soc Work Pract 19(3):325–340, 2009

Kumar S: Burnout in psychiatrists. World Psychiatry 6(3):186–189, 2007 18188444

Kumar S: Job satisfaction among psychiatrists: an urgent area for research. Mental Health Review Journal 13(3):16–23, 2008

Kumar S: Burnout and psychiatrists: what do we know and where to from here? Epidemiol Psychiatr Sci 20(4):295–301, 2011 22201205

Kumar S, Hatcher S, Huggard P: Burnout in psychiatrists: an etiological model. Int J Psychiatry Med 35(4):405–416, 2005 16673840

Leiter MP, Bakker AB, Maslach C: The contemporary context of job burnout, in Burnout at Work: A Psychological Perspective. Edited by Leiter MP, Bakker AB, Maslach C. Hove, Sussex, Psychology Press, 2014, pp 1–9

Linneroot PJ, Mrjenovich AJ, Moore BA: Professional burnout in clinical military psychologists: recommendations before, during, and after deployment. Prof Psychol Res Pr 42(1):87–93, 2011

Madathil R, Heck NC, Schuldberg D: Burnout in psychiatric nursing: examining the interplay of autonomy, leadership style, and depressive symptoms. Arch Psychiatr Nurs 28(3):160–166, 2014 24856267

Maslach C, Jackson S, Leiter M: Maslach Burnout Inventory Manual, 3rd Edition. Palo Alto, CA, Consulting Psychologists Press, 1996

Medscape: National Physician Burnout and Depression Report 2018. New York, Medscape, 2018. Available at: https://www.medscape.com/slideshow/2018 -lifestyle-burnout-depression-6009235. Accessed May 6, 2018.

Meier DE, Back AL, Morrison RS: The inner life of physicians and care of the seriously ill. JAMA 286(23):3007–3014, 2001 11743845

Montero-Marín J, García-Campayo J, Mosquera Mera D, et al: A new definition of burnout syndrome based on Farber's proposal. J Occup Med Toxicol 4:31, 2009 19948055

Montero-Marín J, Prado-Abril J, Piva Demarzo MM, et al: Coping with stress and types of burnout: explanatory power of different coping strategies. PLoS One 9(2):e89090, 2014 24551223

O'Connor K, Muller Neff D, Pitman S: Burnout in mental health professionals: a systematic review and meta-analysis of prevalence and determinants. Eur Psychiatry 53:74–99, 2018 29957371

Oreskovich M, Anderson J: Physician personalities and burnout. Bull Am Coll Surg 98(6):40–42, 2013 23789198

Orosz A, Federspiel A, Haisch S, et al: A biological perspective on differences and similarities between burnout and depression. Neurosci Biobehav Rev 73:112–122, 2017 27993607

Panagioti M, Geraghty K, Johnson J, et al: Association between physician burnout and patient safety, professionalism, and patient satisfaction: a systematic review and meta-analysis. JAMA Intern Med 178(10):1317–1330, 2018 30193239

Rodriguez S, Carlotto M: Predictors of burnout syndrome in psychologists. Estudos de Psicologia 34(1):141–150, 2017

Rupert PA, Kent JS: Gender and work setting differences in career-sustaining behaviors and burnout among professional psychologists. Professional Psychology: Research and Practice 38(1):88–96, 2007

Rupert PA, Morgan DJ: Work setting and burnout among professional psychologists. Professional Psychology: Research and Practice 36(5):544–550, 2005

Rupert PA, Miller AO, Dorociak KE: Preventing burnout: what does the research tell us? Professional Psychology: Research and Practice 46(3):168–174, 2015

Shanafelt TD, Dyrbye LN, West CP: Addressing physician burnout: the way forward. JAMA 317(9):901–902, 2017 28196201

Sinsky C, Shanafelt T, Murphy M, et al: Creating the Organizational Foundation for Joy in Medicine: Organizational Changes Lead to Physician Satisfaction. Chicago, IL, American Medical Association, 2017

West CP, Dyrbye LN, Erwin PG, et al: Interventions to prevent and reduce physician burnout: a systematic review and meta-analysis. Lancet 388(10057):2272–2281, 2016 27692469

World Health Organization: Z73.0: Burn-out, in International Statistical Classification of Diseases and Related Health Problems, 10th Revision: Version for 2016. Geneva, Switzerland, World Health Organization, 2016. Available at: http:// apps.who.int/classifications/icd10/browse/2016/en#/Z73.0. Accessed July 26, 2018.

Yoon JD, Daley BM, Curlin FA: The association between a sense of calling and physician well-being: a national study of primary care physicians and psychiatrists. Acad Psychiatry 41(2):167–173, 2017 26809782

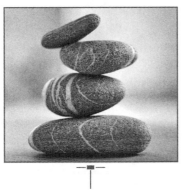

CHAPTER 5

FROM BURNOUT TO IMPAIRMENT

The Slippery Slope

Laurel E.S. Mayer, M.D.

At every step in the pathway to becoming a successful physician, from premed student to medical student to resident to fellow to independent practitioner, hard work, persistence, and sterling credentials are required. Critical in this process is a strong desire to make a significant contribution to other people experiencing distress, along with the ability to tolerate the emotional demands of providing services to them (Leiter and Durup 1994). It is this very desire, at least in part, that serves as a vulnerability to burnout. *Burnout,* described in detail in Chapter 1, "The History of Burnout in Society, Medicine, and Psychiatry," is a work-related syndrome specific to human service professionals, defined by a constellation of three primary components: emotional exhaustion, depersonalization, and decreased perceived personal accomplishment. It has been described as a prolonged response to chronic interpersonal stressors on the job (Maslach and Leiter 2017). Burnout differs from depression (see Chapter 6, "Physician Depression and Suicide") in that it is not a problem rooted within a person but of the social/professional environment in which they work. Viewed from another perspective, however, burnout is also an individual response to systemic problems (C. Bernstein, personal communication, September 23, 2018).

Burnout Has Consequences for Patient Care

As described in detail in chapter 4, "Understanding Burnout and Its Potential Effects on Clinical Care," it is becoming increasingly well documented that burnout has consequences, both professional and personal. Burnout impacts patient care practices and attitudes (Shanafelt et al. 2002). Physicians with burnout are more likely to report discharging patients to "make the service manageable" and less likely to fully discuss treatment options or answer patients' questions. Physicians with burnout compared with physicians who do not have burnout are more likely to self-report medical errors. Whether burnout contributes to an increased rate of actual errors is less clear. In a study by Fahrenkopf et al. (2008), depression, but not burnout, was associated with increased rates of medical errors. Physicians with burnout may be more concerned about making mistakes, may magnify the significance of minor incidents, or experience more "near misses," but additional study is needed to fully evaluate the relationship between burnout and medical errors.

Physicians with burnout compared with those without burnout receive lower patient satisfaction scores, have decreased productivity, and are more likely to leave their jobs, thus contributing to higher physician turnover (Shanafelt and Noseworthy 2017; Williams et al. 2001). On the personal side, burnout is associated with increased substance use, impaired relationships, depression, and suicide (Shanafelt and Noseworthy 2017). One might argue that physicians, because of their extensive training and dedication, are able to continue to provide excellent medical care to their patients despite the personal consequences of burnout. However, on the professional side, the impact of burnout on patient care and patient care attitudes is measurable and significant. This begs the question: At what point does the physician with burnout become impaired?

VIGNETTE I: THE BURNED-OUT PSYCHIATRIST

The consult-liaison service has been unusually busy for the past 6 months with many complicated, medically ill patients. Because of the complexity and volume of the consults, you've been staying late more nights than not, writing detailed notes and trying to take the best care of the patients you can. The medicine team is similarly overworked and stressed, and they've just called a new consult for "rule out depression" in a 65-year-old man with a history of alcohol use disorder and end-stage cirrhosis who is awaiting a liver transplant. You think about how tired you are, how tired you are of hearing about chronic problems, and you wonder why people don't take better care of themselves. You enter the room to introduce yourself and begin your evaluation, and the patient yells at you that he doesn't need a psychiatrist, he's "not crazy" and refuses to talk to you. After a visible sigh and deep breath, you respond that his doctor "is worried about him and thought [you] might be able to help." You continue, "but your doctor must have been mistaken" and you turn to leave the room. The patient asks you to wait, but you will not reinforce his bad behavior by granting his request. You tell him how busy you are with other patients, and you'll come back later. You are curt with the medicine intern who asked about the outcome of the evaluation and spend 10 minutes trying to document in the electronic health record (EHR), that the patient refused your visit. You suggest to your division chief that she should consider arranging another in-service training to the medicine department about proper procedure for calling consults.

What Is Impairment?

The Federation of State Medical Boards makes an important distinction between "illness" and "impairment." *Illness* is a disease. Impairment is a functional classification. It exists on a continuum, and its severity can change over time. *Impairment* is defined as the "inability of [a physician] to practice medicine with reasonable skill and safety" (Federation of State Medical Boards 2011, p. 7). It is important to recognize that illness can exist without impairment, although untreated illness is likely to progress to impairment.

What Is a Mental Disorder?

According to DSM-5 (American Psychiatric Association 2013),

> A mental disorder is a syndrome characterized by *clinically significant* disturbance in an individual's cognition, emotion regulation, or behavior that reflects a dysfunction in the psychological, biological, or developmental processes underlying mental functioning. Mental disorders are usually associated with significant distress or disability in social, occupational, or other important activities. *An expectable or culturally approved response to a common stressor or loss, such as the death of a loved one, is not a mental disorder.* (p. 20; emphasis added)

Burnout is not currently a diagnosis included in DSM-5, but by examining the critical elements of a mental disorder, we may more effectively understand the construct of burnout and its significance.

1. To be considered a mental disorder, symptoms must be of "clinical significance." What is clinical significance? Two components are described: distress and functional impairment. *Functional impairment* is defined as dysfunction in social and occupational spheres of life. Although not stated directly, the clinical significance specifier implies that a mental disorder must be associated with impairment. If burnout is associated with distress and impairment in occupational functioning and meets the "clinical significance" specifier of a mental disorder, does it merit consideration as a diagnosis?

   Burnout is certainly associated with internal distress. Emotional exhaustion feels bad. Low perceived personal accomplishment, especially in generally successful, high-achieving physicians, feels bad. Depersonalization is a psychological attempt to minimize (physically) feeling bad. There is a helplessness aspect to the distress: "Stress is just part of the job." This helplessness is compounded by those drivers of burnout that are external to the physician: the culture of medicine to put patient care above self-care, work compression, the EHR, hospital inefficiencies and bureaucracies, and hospital executives who seem to value reputation and revenues over compassionate patient care. These tensions lead to stress, anxiety, and dissatisfaction. It is less clear how this distress relates to impairment. The growing literature describing the effects of burnout on patient attitudes and patient safety would suggest that the physician with burnout is impaired. In Vignette 1, a clinician without burnout may have been better able to tolerate and address the patient's resistance to the consult, resulting in a more positive experience for both the patient and clinician. Although the patient was not overtly harmed, and the clinician does not need to be relieved of duty or reported to the medical board, burnout was a significant contributor to this suboptimal, unprofessional doctor-patient interaction. Burnout is not a dichotomous construct, but how the severity of burnout (mild, moderate, severe) correlates with level of impairment is an area for further investigation.

2. Burnout was once called "professional depression" (Firth et al. 1986). In contrast, Leiter and Durup (1994, p. 357) argued that burnout and depression are categorically different, and burnout was described because "established perspectives of clinical psychology used to explain personal distress…are not suited to explain largely interpersonal and organizational constructs." The relationship between burnout and depression is currently an unresolved, active debate (Bianchi and Schonfeld 2017; Bianchi et al. 2017; Leiter and Durup 1994; Maslach and Leiter 2016; Melnick et al. 2017) with compelling arguments on both sides (see Chapter 6, "Physician Depression and Suicide"). Those who support burnout as distinct from depression assert that burnout is not a disease, is situation specific, and is driven by a demanding work environment coupled with insufficient resources (Melnick et al. 2017). Depression, in contrast, has well-defined diagnostic criteria and most importantly occurs "context-free."

3. Consistent with this context-dependent definition, the reportedly high prevalence of burnout, and in light of the DSM-5 definition, could burnout be considered an "expectable response" to the "common stressor" of medical training and medical practice? The literature consistently describes burnout as a work-related syndrome, not as an illness.

Burnout is not a (psychiatric) diagnosis, yet there is ample evidence that burnout can have a *clinically significant* impact on patient care, attitudes toward patients, and job satisfaction. It remains unclear, however, when this impact becomes impairment. In the next sections, I consider both individual and organizational risk factors that may contribute to the progression toward impairment and elucidate opportunities to push back on the slippery slope of burnout and gain traction in achieving engagement and flourishing.

The Impaired Physician and His or Her Individual Risk Factors for Burnout

To further explore the slippery slope of burnout to impairment, perhaps it is important to examine the profile of the "impaired physician." In their book *The Physician as Patient,* Myers and Gabbard (2008) proposed that the term *impaired physician* may be misleading because it suggests a dichotomous construct in which a physician either "is" or "is not" impaired. Consistent with the Federation of State Medical Boards (2011) approach, Myers and Gabbard emphasize that impairment occurs on a continuum. A career in medicine may attract individuals with certain common psychological traits, and when these individuals are exposed to stressors inherent in the culture of medicine, the traits become "occupational hazards for virtually all physicians" (Myers and Gabbard 2008, p. 4). When considering how to reduce the prevalence and impact of burnout during medical training and practice, appreciating potential individual vulnerabilities and the stressors inherent in the practice of medicine may be a useful part of the initial approach. This process may also shed light on barriers to seeking treatment and why physicians may be more prone to wait until they are impaired, sometimes significantly impaired, rather than proactively reaching out at the first signs and symptoms of difficulty.

Profile of the "Typical Physician"

Before presenting the profile of a "typical physician," it is important to state at the outset, as Myers and Gabbard (2008) did, that those who enter and successfully pursue a career in medicine manifest a wide range of personality traits and types. The following profile is in no way intended to be an inclusive inventory of the traits of all physicians. It is intended, however, as a useful, meaningful description of common traits. As I discuss, some of these traits are adaptive in the service of caring for patients, whereas others are maladaptive, possibly leading to distress.

HIGH ACHIEVEMENT

The "physician personality" (Gabbard 1985) includes being high achieving, perfectionistic, and compulsive. Medical training is a rigorous, selective process that starts in college, if not earlier. The series of challenging educational and extracurricular requirements selects for extremely motivated, focused, high-achieving individuals. Related to high achievement is perfectionism, which itself is often confused with being driven to succeed and being perfect. Perfectionism, although often a trait desired by patients who may feel comforted by being taken care of by an infallible doctor, may come at great personal cost to the individual physician.

PERFECTIONISM

Perfectionism is not actually attainable or adaptive (Myers and Gabbard 2008, p. 5), thus the pursuit of perfection is more likely to contribute to anxiety and stress and serve as a risk factor for burnout. To the perfectionist, the absence of perfection is failure. Perfectionist physicians often have the distorted belief that others will value them only if they are perfect. This contributes to a scenario in which physicians are less likely to reveal their "mistakes" or "failures." Another side effect of the pursuit of perfection is the reduced satisfaction of real accomplishment. Praise for correctly identifying an elusive diagnosis is perceived by the physician himself or herself as "undeserved," "not a big deal," or "anyone could have done it" (although many, in fact, did not figure out the correct diagnosis). Despite feeling undeserving, these perfectionist physicians are often viewed "as physicians who can be counted on to 'get the job done, no matter what it takes'" (Myers and Gabbard 2008, p. 6). This lack of satisfaction in actual, albeit modest accomplishments could contribute to the low personal accomplishment factor of burnout.

TRIAD OF COMPULSIVENESS

Self-described and objectively measured compulsive traits are common among physicians (Gabbard 1985; Krakowski 1982) and may even facilitate success during medical training (Gazelle et al. 2015). Gabbard (1985; Myers and Gabbard 2008) described a "triad of compulsiveness"—*doubt, guilt,* and *an exaggerated sense of responsibility.* Other relevant compulsive traits include rigidity, stubbornness, excessive devotion to work, inability to delegate, and difficulty taking time off or engaging in leisure time activities. These traits are associated with the need to put patients first. This prioritization contributes to poor self-care and more ominously to a delay in recognizing one's own need for help and a delay in accessing treatment.

The first trait in the "triad of compulsiveness" is *doubt.* Self-doubt can be adaptive: it drives physicians to be thorough in diagnostic efforts, to stay current with the literature, and to be alert to novel treatment approaches. These behaviors are reinforced by patients who benefit and appreciate that their doctor is doing everything to take the very best care of them. However, for the physician, persistent self-doubt can lead to guilt, dissatisfaction, and anxiety. *Guilt* (the second trait) about overlooking an important sign or not anticipating a side effect (Myers and Gabbard 2008) can lead to anxiety and distress. The tendency to minimize successes and magnify mistakes and oversights could lead physicians to feel a sense of low perceived personal accomplishment. A strong *sense of responsibility* (the third trait) can be adaptive. An exaggerated sense of responsibility can be a vulnerability. Physicians are acutely aware of the trust bestowed on them by their patients. However, this can also lead to feeling personally responsible for every aspect and outcome related to the patient's care. The physician may have difficulty setting limits or delegating tasks to others. They may have difficulty with work-life integration, preferring to work long hours and allocating little time for their own family. They may confuse selfishness with healthy self-interest. These attitudes deny the reality that the practice of medicine actually involves teams and collaborations. Collaborations with colleagues, nurses, technicians, students, and others are essential. Even the care of the patient requires a partnership: the physician recommends treatment to the patient, and the patient must choose whether to follow the recommendations. Yet as we are well aware, patients do not always comply. Treatments may not go as planned; expected (side effects) and unexpected outcomes occur that are beyond the physician's control. Nevertheless, the physician feels guilty about possible errors or not having "done enough." With time, the physician may feel spent, underappreciated, and emotionally exhausted or cynical and jaded from seemingly one-way efforts.

Why Might Physicians Not Recognize That They Are Impaired?

Despite countless successes, when confronted with realities and challenges of practicing medicine, physicians, especially trainees, may start feeling as though they do not really belong. In the current system, students and house staff are not used to making mistakes or failing. There is reluctance to report "failures" such as being unable to complete their work without duty hour violations. This often leads to severe distress. As described, physicians and physician trainees have enormous personal strength and therefore can often "compensate" for feeling as though they do not really know enough or for worrying about being "exposed." However, this capacity can make it difficult for others to identify when these physicians are struggling and obscure their need for assistance (M. Oquendo, personal communication, May 8, 2018). This compounds their feeling isolated and alone because no one knows how they really feel. Loneliness seems to be an increasingly recognized contributor to burnout (Karaoglu et al. 2015; Rogers et al. 2016). Gender differences may contribute to help-seeking behaviors. Women physicians may be more likely than male physicians to present voluntarily for mental health care, and male physicians may need to be compelled to access help (Gunderson 2006). Others (Pitt et al. 2004), however, suggest equal rates of help seeking in male and female physicians. In addition to these internal, constitutional traits that serve as vulnerabilities and may interfere with the ability to recognize burnout in oneself, there are external influences that must also be considered.

Organizational Risk Factors for Burnout

It cannot be overstated that burnout is an individual response to *systemic* issues. As such, it is critical to consider potential organizational contributors to burnout. Shanafelt and Noseworthy (2017) have eloquently written about this. They proposed seven factors that when misaligned drive burnout and when maximized facilitate physician engagement. The proposed drivers are "workload, efficiency, flexibility/control over work, work-life integration, alignment of individual and organizational values, social support/community at work, and the degree of meaning derived from work" (p. 131).

WORKLOAD AND EFFICIENCY

The average physician demonstrates tremendous capacity for work; this capacity, however, is not without limits. Mandates to decrease inpatient length of stay and maximize revenue targets in the context of ever-changing third-party reimbursement models contribute to increases in workload. Physicians are expected to work longer hours, including more night and weekend calls. Total hours worked per week has been associated with increased risk of burnout (Shanafelt et al. 2009). Physicians with burnout reported working an average of almost 5 more hours per week than physicians who were not burned out (mean hours worked 72.1 vs. 67.5, $P=0.006$), with an increased likelihood of burnout described for each additional hour worked per week (odds ratio 1.02 [1.004–1.031], $P<0.01$) (Shanafelt et al. 2009). Residents and fellows must comply with Accreditation Council for Graduate Medical Education (ACGME)–mandated duty hour restrictions and therefore struggle with work compression.

System inefficiencies contribute and compound the stress of work overload. Although some bureaucracy is inherent in any organization, excessive inefficiency strains the system and contributes to burnout. Documentation requirements in the EHR are experienced by many as onerous, and use of an EHR or computerized physician order entry system has been associated with increased risk for burnout (Shanafelt et al. 2016).

FLEXIBILITY/AUTONOMY OVER SCHEDULE AND WORK-LIFE INTEGRATION

It has been repeatedly demonstrated that burnout is associated with decreased satisfaction in work-life balance (Shanafelt et al. 2012, 2015b,

2019b). Efforts that increase autonomy, such as controlling clinic hours (start/end times), call schedules, and flexibility in vacation time may minimize burnout (Shanafelt and Noseworthy 2017). An inflexible and rigorous work schedule may contribute to significant stress and dissatisfaction for those with family or other responsibilities outside of work. Policies that allow physicians to adjust work hours or work part-time may facilitate physician productivity, retention, and well-being.

ALIGNMENT OF INDIVIDUAL AND ORGANIZATION VALUES

Organizational climate influences burnout. Negative leadership attitudes and behaviors, lack of solicitation of input from physician staff, and poor communication reduce work satisfaction (Shanafelt et al. 2015a). The perception of profits over quality patient care also leads to decreased physician engagement. Misalignment between institutional mission and physician realities can contribute to distress and dissatisfaction. Well-being efforts aimed only at the individual that appear to absolve the organization from making significant change are at risk of being viewed as incomplete and insincere. Periodically reevaluating the organization's culture, values, and principles for consistency with its goals and making adjustments as needed will improve the health of the organization and its staff (Shanafelt and Noseworthy 2017).

SOCIAL SUPPORT/COMMUNITY AT WORK

Peer support has always been one of the key coping strategies engaged to process the intense and emotionally challenging experiences of caring for the medically ill. The antidote to aloneness is to create a supportive, collaborative work environment. Although prospective studies of interventions to minimize burnout are sorely needed, data support that small-group interventions that promote community (among other things) are beneficial (West et al. 2014, 2016). Team building, social events, and efforts to promote collegiality are generally well received and much appreciated (Goldman et al. 2018).

DEGREE OF MEANING DERIVED FROM WORK

Efforts that promote meaning in work are critical to minimizing burnout. Physicians who reported spending less than 20% of their time on work-related activities they find meaningful were three times more likely to experience burnout compared with those who spent more than 20% of their time on meaningful work-related activities (Shanafelt et al. 2009). Loss of meaning in work manifests in the low personal accomplishment and reduced self-efficacy component of burnout.

Physician Heal Thyself?

Given the importance of addressing burnout at both the individual and systemic levels, it might be reasonable to expect that physicians with burnout would "heal themselves." However, as we know, physicians are reluctant to seek help. This resistance to treatment must be acknowledged and addressed if any strategy designed to combat burnout is to be successful.

Barriers to Accessing Care

In a study of medical interns, Guille et al. (2010) reported that of interns who met criteria for depression by exceeding a threshold of 10 on the Patient Health Questionnaire–9, 8% were in therapy, approximately 7% reported being in combined psychotherapy and psychopharmacology treatment, and just over 85% admitted to pursuing no treatment at all. Although illness can exist without impairment, untreated illness is more likely than not to progress to include impairment. Multiple studies (e.g., Aaronson et al. 2018; Guille et al. 2010) describe a relatively consistent set of perceived barriers to resident physicians accessing care. The most common factors include time (and lack thereof), preference for self-management, lack of convenient access, confidentiality and related need to find a provider outside one's institution, concern for impact on career, stigma and related concerns for what other would think, cost, and belief that treatment doesn't work. Some of these barriers are described in more detail in the following sections.

TIME

With work-hour demands contributing to fatigue and burnout, and the ACGME limiting duty hours to 80 hours per week and keeping track of duty hour violations, there is a reality to the resident's perception that they have little time for self-care. The 80-hour work week, frequently rotating schedules, unpredictability of postcall days, and invariable unexpected clinical emergencies when trying to leave are not often in synchrony with the regular office hours of the private practitioner. However, with the increasing awareness of the impact of burnout and depression on patient care, patient safety, and physician turnover and risk for suicide, creating time for physician healthcare within the 80-hour work week has become a priority. The ACGME attempted to alleviate this barrier in 2017 with revised "Common Program Requirements" (Section VI.C, pp. 22–23; available at www.acgme.org/Portals/0/PFAssets/ProgramRequirements/CPRs_2017-07-01.pdf) mandating that programs facilitate residents being able to attend their own doctor appointments (including mental health). On-site mental health services also serve to minimize travel time and facilitate trainees accessing care.

CONFIDENTIALITY, CONCERN FOR CAREER, AND STIGMA

Stigma and fear of disciplinary action are powerful disincentives to seeking care. Physicians may feel shame about being ill, and psychiatric illness may be even more stigmatizing. They fear being seen as weak or dependent or fear that their colleagues will view the depressed resident or resident with burnout as providing inferior care. They believe this will impact their ability to collaborate or receive patient referrals. Ironically, it is often the depressed trainee who expresses greater stigma against physicians with mental illness (Schwenk et al. 2010). For example, depressed (compared with not depressed) medical students are more likely to believe that applications for residency from depressed students would be less competitive (Schwenk et al. 2010). Regardless, fears of lack of confidentiality loom large, impeding access to care. This fear interacts with the increasing reality of hacks and breaches in "secure" electronic information becoming more common. The reality, of course, as previously stated, is that untreated burnout and depression impair clinical performance. Suboptimal patient care and patient care attitudes and self-perceived and actual rates of medical errors will be more likely to negatively impact residency and fellowship opportunities than will known treatments for burnout. Department chairs, program directors, faculty, and chief residents can directly target this concern by providing education to decrease stigma and eliminate this barrier to treatment.

COST

Recent parity laws have improved insurance coverage, but at least in some states, insurance coverage for mental health remains inadequate, with high deductibles, significant copays, or limited, if any, out-of-network reimbursements. Medical centers are trying to accommodate the cost issue by supporting workforce health and safety or employee assistance programs or by developing their own internal staff mental health services.

BELIEF THAT TREATMENT DOES NOT WORK

On the list of barriers to accessing treatment is the belief among some that treatment does not work. Although there is a constant search for even more effective psychotherapeutic and psychopharmacological treatments, there are evidence-based treatment approaches for depression, anxiety, and other psychiatric/psychological diagnoses. Although individual approaches for addressing burnout are less evidenced based, stress-reduction and mindfulness techniques (e.g., meditation, yoga) and small-group discussions to promote community, connectedness, and meaning (West et al. 2014, 2016, 2018) have demonstrated benefit. As mental health professionals, it is incumbent on us to address this concern by educating our colleagues about treatment effectiveness so that we can eliminate this barrier to treatment.

Protective Factors

Having extensively described the vulnerabilities and contributors to burnout, I now briefly examine more positive and preventative approaches to minimizing burnout.

VIGNETTE 2: THE RESILIENT PSYCHIATRY RESIDENT

You are the postgraduate year-1 resident in the psychiatric emergency department and are very stressed. You do not feel very confident about your ability to assess safety or risk for violence and get very nervous in high-adrenaline situations. During the month, there are some challenging cases, but you talk the details over with the attending physician. You work well with the nurses and have good rapport with security. At the end of your day, you feel overwhelmed and exhausted but think you have learned a lot and helped patients. You and your coresidents are experiencing some stressful times working so closely together, but you also feel you are bonding a lot too.

RESILIENCE

One major strategy to limit the impairment associated with burnout is to enhance resilience. *Resilience* is the capacity to bounce back, to withstand hardship, and to repair oneself. It is positive adaptation in the face of stress or disruptive change. A more formal definition is "the process of adapting well in the face of adversity, trauma, tragedy, threats and even significant sources of stress—such as family and relationship problems, serious health problems or workplace or financial stress" (American Psychological Association Help Center, as quoted in Southwick and Charney 2012, p. 7). The resident in Vignette 2 acknowledges her anxiety about evaluating suicidal ideation and works with the attending physician to make a plan. She values a positive relationship with the nurses and security—the people whom she will need to help her manage the agitated patient. Resilient individuals combine both an optimism and realism that allows them to confront the reality they face, along with the knowledge and confidence that they will prevail. Early in her training, the resident actively faced her fears, recruited her supports, and shared the challenges of her experience with colleagues. She ended her day overwhelmed but not frustrated. Resilience keeps denial in check.

Realism manifests by objectively confronting the challenging situation. Consider another example: "I made a serious medication error. I made a mistake. There will be significant consequences." This may be the correct assessment. On the other hand, one should have the attitude and the confidence to say, "But I will prevail. I'm in a tough spot, but I will prevail." That is the optimistic outlook that buttresses resilience and staves off burnout.

MINDFULNESS/MEDITATION

Mindfulness and other stress-reduction techniques may be useful in reducing burnout, or at least elements of burnout. A meta-analysis by West et al. (2016) suggested that mindfulness interventions may have little effect on total burnout but provide significantly greater benefit over other intervention strategies in the reduction of two of the core components of burnout—emotional exhaustion and depersonalization.

CHANGING THE ORGANIZATIONAL CULTURE

As described in the section "Organizational Risk Factors for Burnout," many of the drivers of burnout, if redirected, can promote physician engagement and a thriving work environment. Along with changes to the culture of the house of medicine, promoting the importance of self-care and devaluing "putting the needs of others ahead of ourselves at all costs" might minimize the development of burnout. Numerous initiatives have been described, for example, Code Lavender (see Davidson et al. 2017) and online wellness/burnout dashboards. In addition, recommendations (Shanafelt et al. 2019a) and details about major systemic approaches at the Mayo Clinic (Shanafelt and Noseworthy 2017), WellMD Center at the Stanford University School of Medicine (https://wellmd.stanford.edu), and Johns Hopkins University (http://wellness.som.jhu.edu) are readily available.

Treatment Approaches for the Individual Physician With Burnout

As should be apparent, evidence-based treatment approaches to physician burnout are a fertile area for research. Local interventions should begin with psychoeducation and awareness about the features of burnout, its prevalence, and its consequences. Individual approaches can include resilience building, mindfulness training, perspective taking, and cognitive-behavioral approaches including cognitive reappraisal (Epstein and Privitera 2016). Efforts to restore meaning and purpose are likely to increase job satisfaction. Restructuring work hours, building breaks into the day, and promoting good sleep hygiene or a brief vacation, if feasible, could also be considered. As with most conditions, early intervention allows for maximum flexibility in treatment approach and minimization of the impact on professional and personal spheres. Addressing known barriers to accessing treatment should be part of any intervention strategy. Burnout is associated with increased stigma (Dyrbye et al. 2015) and concerns for impact on career, thus ensuring confidentiality is essential. Given that the differential of burnout includes stress, trauma, major depression, and possible personality issues, the evaluation of the physician should occur in a private, professional setting.

Conclusion

Whether burnout is an "expectable response" to the "common stressor" of medical practice or a psychiatric illness anchoring one end of the depression spectrum, it is associated with demonstrable adverse personal and professional consequences for the physician. Impairment can be subtle but exists on a continuum and can change over time. In some forms, the sequelae may not be readily observable to the physician or his or her colleagues, but multiple studies document burnout's effects on patient care and attitudes. If not attended to, burnout and its associated impairment can progress, with unfortunate outcomes for patient safety and physician well-being. Awareness of individual and work environment vulnerabilities is the first step in addressing the burnout epidemic. Recognition of the shared responsibility for the emotional health of the staff and the health of the organization by concurrently implementing individually directed and systemic interventions to promote work engagement is just what the doctor ordered.

KEY POINTS

- Critical to the process of becoming a physician is a strong desire to make a significant contribution to other people experiencing distress, along with the ability to tolerate the emotional demands of providing services to them.

- It is the very desire to help those in distress that serves, at least in part, as a vulnerability to burnout.

- Studies support that burnout has a measurable impact on patient care and physicians' attitudes toward patients.

- Both burnout and impairment exist on a continuum.

- Physicians may share a common set of personality traits, including being high-achieving, perfectionistic, and compulsive, that can be both adaptive, contributing to excellent patient care, and maladaptive, contributing to the development of burnout.

- Burnout is an individual's response to systemic issues in their professional environment, thus addressing the problem of physician burnout must be a shared responsibility of both the individual physicians and the organization in which they work.

References

Aaronson AL, Backes K, Agarwal G, et al: Mental health during residency training: assessing the barriers to seeking care. Acad Psychiatry 42(4):469–472, 2018 29450842

American Psychiatric Association: Diagnostic and Statistical Manual of Mental Disorders, 5th Edition. Arlington, VA, American Psychiatric Association, 2013

Bianchi R, Schonfeld IS: Defining physician burnout, and differentiating between burnout and depression–I. Mayo Clin Proc 92(9):1455, 2017 28870363

Bianchi R, Schonfeld IS, Laurent E: Physician burnout is better conceptualised as depression. Lancet 389(10077):1397–1398, 2017 28402821

Davidson JE, Graham P, Montross-Thomas L, et al: Code Lavender: cultivating intentional acts of kindness in response to stressful work situations. Explore (NY) 13(3):181–185, 2017 28668136

Dyrbye LN, Eacker A, Durning SJ, et al: The impact of stigma and personal experiences on the help-seeking behaviors of medical students with burnout. Acad Med 90(7):961–969, 2015 25650824

Epstein RM, Privitera MR: Doing something about physician burnout. Lancet 388(10057):2216–2217, 2016 27692468

Fahrenkopf AM, Sectish TC, Barger LK, et al: Rates of medication errors among depressed and burnt out residents: prospective cohort study. BMJ 336(7642):488–491, 2008 18258931

Federation of State Medical Boards: Policy on Physician Impairment. Washington, DC, Federation of State Medical Boards, 2011

Firth H, McIntee J, McKeown P, et al: Burnout and professional depression: related concepts? J Adv Nurs 11(6):633–641, 1986 3641852

Gabbard GO: The role of compulsiveness in the normal physician. JAMA 254(20):2926–2929, 1985 4057513

Gazelle G, Liebschutz JM, Riess H: Physician burnout: coaching a way out. J Gen Intern Med 30(4):508–513, 2015 25527340

Goldman ML, Bernstein CA, Konopasek L, et al: An intervention framework for institutions to meet new ACGME Common Program Requirements for physician well-being. Acad Psychiatry 42(4):542–547, 2018 29470799

Guille C, Speller H, Laff R, et al: Utilization and barriers to mental health services among depressed medical interns: a prospective multisite study. J Grad Med Educ 2(2):210–214, 2010 21975622

Gunderson DC: Women in medicine. Colorado Physician Health Program News 5(1):2, 11–13, 2006

Karaoglu N, Pekcan S, Durduran Y, et al: A sample of paediatric residents' loneliness-anxiety-depression-burnout and job satisfaction with probable affecting factors. J Pak Med Assoc 65(2):183–191, 2015 25842556

Krakowski AJ: Stress and the practice of medicine. II. Stressors, stresses, and strains. Psychother Psychosom 38(1):11–23, 1982 7146259

Leiter MP, Durup J: The discriminant validity of burnout and depression. Anxiety Stress Coping 7:357–373, 1994

Maslach C, Leiter MP: Understanding the burnout experience: recent research and its implications for psychiatry. World Psychiatry 15(2):103–111, 2016 27265691

Maslach C, Leiter MP: New insights into burnout and health care: strategies for improving civility and alleviating burnout. Med Teach 39(2):160–163, 2017 27841065

Melnick ER, Powsner SM, Shanafelt TD: In reply defining physician burnout, and differentiating between burnout and depression. Mayo Clin Proc 92(9):1456–1458, 2017 28870365

Myers MF, Gabbard GO: The Physician as Patient. Washington, DC, American Psychiatric Publishing, 2008

Pitt E, Rosenthal MM, Gay TL, et al: Mental health services for residents: more important than ever. Acad Med 79(9):840–844, 2004 15326006

Rogers E, Polonijo AN, Carpiano RM: Getting by with a little help from friends and colleagues: testing how residents' social support networks affect loneliness and burnout. Can Fam Physician 62(11):e677–e683, 2016 28661887

Schwenk TL, Davis L, Wimsatt LA: Depression, stigma, and suicidal ideation in medical students. JAMA 304(11):1181–1190, 2010 20841531

Shanafelt TD, Noseworthy JH: Executive leadership and physician well-being: nine organizational strategies to promote engagement and reduce burnout. Mayo Clin Proc 92(1):129–146, 2017 27871627

Shanafelt TD, Bradley KA, Wipf JE, et al: Burnout and self-reported patient care in an internal medicine residency program. Ann Intern Med 136(5):358–367, 2002 11874308

Shanafelt TD, West CP, Sloan JA, et al: Career fit and burnout among academic faculty. Arch Intern Med 169(10):990–995, 2009 19468093

Shanafelt TD, Boone S, Tan L, et al: Burnout and satisfaction with work-life balance among US physicians relative to the general US population. Arch Intern Med 172(18):1377–1385, 2012 22911330

Shanafelt TD, Gorringe G, Menaker R, et al: Impact of organizational leadership on physician burnout and satisfaction. Mayo Clin Proc 90(4):432–440, 2015a 25796117

Shanafelt TD, Hasan O, Dyrbye LN, et al: Changes in burnout and satisfaction with work-life balance in physicians and the general US working population between 2011 and 2014. Mayo Clin Proc 90(12):1600–1613, 2015b 26653297

Shanafelt TD, Mungo M, Schmitgen J, et al: Longitudinal study evaluating the association between physician burnout and changes in professional work effort. Mayo Clin Proc 91(4):422–431, 2016 27046522

Shanafelt T, Trockel M, Ripp J, et al: Building a program on well-being: key design considerations to meet the unique needs of each organization. Acad Med 94(2):156–161, 2019a 30134268

Shanafelt TD, West CP, Sinsky C et al: Changes in burnout and satisfaction with work-life integration in physicians and the general US working population between 2011 and 2017. Mayo Clin Proc Feb 13, 2019b 30803733 [Epub ahead of print]

Southwick SM, Charney DS: Resilience: The Science of Mastering Life's Greatest Challenges. New York, Cambridge University Press, 2012

West CP, Dyrbye LN, Rabatin JT, et al: Intervention to promote physician well-being, job satisfaction, and professionalism: a randomized clinical trial. JAMA Intern Med 174(4):527–533, 2014 24515493

West CP, Dyrbye LN, Erwin PJ, et al: Interventions to prevent and reduce physician burnout: a systematic review and meta-analysis. Lancet 388(10057):2272–2281, 2016 27692469

West CP, Dyrbye LN, Shanafelt TD: Physician burnout: contributors, consequences and solutions. J Intern Med 283(6):516–529, 2018 29505159

Williams ES, Konrad TR, Scheckler WE, et al: Understanding physicians' intentions to withdraw from practice: the role of job satisfaction, job stress, mental and physical health. Health Care Manage Rev 26(1):7–19, 2001 11233355

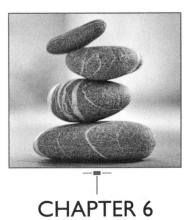

CHAPTER 6

PHYSICIAN DEPRESSION AND SUICIDE

Claudia Zimmermann, M.A., M.Sc. (Oxon)

Kenneth Thau, M.D.

Eva Schernhammer, M.D., Dr.P.H., M.Phil.

Does the choice to become a doctor increase your suicide risk? Sadly, it would seem the answer is yes. Physicians are among those professions with the highest suicide rates (Roberts et al. 2013), and although some obvious occupational hazards quickly come to mind—namely, stress and confrontation with suffering and death—there are many facets to this somber phenomenon that continue to bewilder the observer. One is the inherent paradox that the healing profession is failing to heal its own members: "That a professional caregiver can fall ill and not receive adequate care and support, despite being surrounded by other caregivers, begs for a thoughtful assessment to determine why it happens at all" (Legha 2012, p. 241). This is particularly worrisome considering that physicians tend to live healthier and longer lives than other professionals (Frank et al. 2000).

A better understanding of physician suicide is essential to lower the number of what are ultimately preventable deaths. Nonetheless, suicide is the last stop on a road that is typically paved by other mental health problems, and depression is one of the most prominent issues that is also closely connected to a perceived surge in physician burnout. A closer look at epidemiological data on prevalence as well as risk and protective factors for physician depression and suicide may shed some light on the scope of the problem, before looking at prevention strategies designed to improve a largely hidden mental health plight.

Connection Between Burnout and Depression

Burnout is characterized by an array of symptoms that share some overlap with the clinical picture of depression. However, DSM-5 (American Psychiatric Association 2013) does not list formal diagnostic criteria for burnout, which is partly due to a prevailing uncertainty regarding the status of burnout as either an autonomous diagnosis or a subtype of depressive disorder (Bianchi et al. 2015). Although most researchers agree on the importance of distinguishing between the two concepts, there is no consensus on the kind of burnout classification that would be most useful in this regard (see, e.g., the exchange between Bianchi and Schonfeld 2017 and Melnick et al. 2017). It has also been criticized that there is some variability in the conceptualization of burnout (Bianchi et al. 2017), which impedes systematic research on the distinction between burnout and depression and lowers the reliability of assessments for burnout prevalence in various medical fields.

Interestingly, the World Health Organization (WHO) takes a different approach and includes burnout in the International Classification of Diseases (ICD) but not in the section of mental disorders. In ICD-10, burnout is classified rather vaguely as "a state of vital exhaustion" in the unspecific category of "problem related to life-management difficulty" (World Health Organization 2016). This will change for ICD-11, in which burnout will be listed under "problems associated with employment or unemployment," as a syndrome "resulting from chronic workplace stress that has not been successfully managed" (World Health Organization 2018). The much more detailed definition also includes the explicit indication that the concept of burnout should only be used in an occupational context and not for other areas of life. With this classification, burnout is regarded as an occupational phenomenon, not a medical condition.

Even though there is no real clarity regarding the exact nature of the relationship between burnout and depression, there is no doubt that both conditions have a serious impact on the mental and physical health of those affected and can progress to a point where the individual can no longer function in personal or professional capacities. DSM-5 lists depressed mood and anhedonia as the two main symptoms of major depressive disorder, in addition to changes in weight, sleep, psychomotorics, reduced energy, feelings of worthlessness or guilt, trouble concentrating, and suicidal ideation. The three main dimensions of burnout are commonly categorized as emotional exhaustion, depersonalization, and a reduced sense of personal accomplishment (Maslach et al. 1997). Burnout tends to be tied to a specific situation, primarily job related, and there is evidence that people who have burnout (but not depression) are still able to enjoy activities in their personal life to a greater extent and show fewer physiological changes (Toker and Biron 2012). Depression is usually a more pervasive global state and persists independently of any specific context. Data from a Swedish twin study suggest that major depressive disorder is more influenced by genetics, whereas unique environmental factors appear to influence burnout to a higher extent (Mather et al. 2016).

The more severe forms of burnout are often accompanied by depression, and people with burnout also appear to have a higher risk of developing depression later on (Ahola et al. 2005). It has also been suggested that physicians in particular might be more willing to accept a diagnosis of burnout rather than depression (DeCaporale-Ryan et al. 2017). The stigma that unfortunately still surrounds the latter tends to emphasize individual shortcomings as the cause of this condition; with burnout, however, the focus shifts more toward the working conditions that contributed to its development. If it is true that there is actual reluctance among physicians to accept a diagnosis of depression, it would certainly warrant concern, because burnout and depression are thought to require different treatments for symptoms to improve.

Depression Among Physicians

There have been many studies on the subject of depression among medical students, but the available data can be difficult to compare because of various methods of assessing depression, even when validated screening instruments are being used. A recent systematic review conducted by Rotenstein et al. (2016) looked at an impressive selection of 195 studies and found that their estimates for the prevalence of depression or depressive symptoms among medical students ranged from 1.4% to 73.5%. When the evidence was pooled in a meta-analysis, the summary prevalence was calculated to be 27.2% (95% confidence interval (CI) = 24.7%–29.9%). Another systematic review (Mata et al. 2015) focused on medical residents, and the combined results of 54 studies suggest a prevalence rate of 28.8% (95% CI = 25.3%–32.5%). The range of prevalence estimates from individual studies was not quite as wide but was still substantial (between 20.9% and 43.2%). Secondary analysis of the longitudinal studies revealed quite a drastic surge for the first year of residency, during which depression levels went up by a median of 15.8%, followed by a more gradual increase in the following years. Many factors influence the provision of medical training in different institutions, thus creating vastly different educational environments that may directly affect depressive symptoms in trainees and explain some of the variability in prevalence rates. However, both reviews found no statistically significant difference between prevalence estimates based on studies from the United States and studies conducted elsewhere. It is also noteworthy that because of the variety of screening tools and reported cutoff points, the prevalence estimates from both reviews include results for actual clinical depression as well as depressive symptoms that put the individual at risk for clinical depression. Still, it seems reasonable to conclude that these prevalence rates are higher than those of the general population between 18 years and 39 years of age in the United States, of which an estimated 7.4% report moderate to severe depressive symptoms (Pratt and Brody 2014), based on assessment with the Patient Health Questionnaire–9 (PHQ-9).

These results are particularly alarming considering that there is some evidence that students enter medical school with mental health profiles that are similar to or better than those of other college graduates (Brazeau et al. 2014). If this is correct, there is good reason to assume that the process of medical training contributes to the development of higher than average depression prevalence later on. Although it is generally accepted that medical school and residency are stressful and challenging learning experiences designed to prepare trainees for a professional life that comes with many personal sacrifices, it is paramount to consider potential detrimental effects on the physicians' mental health. When the demands of medical education result in considerable trainee impairment, the consequences are not limited to their personal quality of life but also include worse outcomes in patient care. A study by Fahrenkopf et al. (2008) showed that depressed residents had a rate of medication errors six times higher than their nondepressed peers.

A longitudinal study from Norway repeatedly screened the 1993/1994 graduates of all Norwegian medical schools ($N=631$) for severe depressive symptoms over the course of 15 years (Støen Grotmol et al. 2013). Their prevalence rate, based on the General Health Questionnaire–28 (GHQ-28), was highest during the last year of medical school (T1, 13.7%), followed by a significant decrease 1 year after graduation, after which the rate stayed more or less the same for the rest of the study period (7.2% at the last follow-up 15 years later, T5). Similar to the systematic reviews for medical students and residents, this study did not detect a significant gender difference in depression prevalence. This does not correspond with depression in the global general population, where women's rates are considerably higher than men's (World Health Organization 2017). There is some evidence that depression prevalence in the general population varies during the adult life span, with higher rates during early adulthood followed by a decline, but only when other risk factors are statistically controlled (Jorm 2000). This might be true for physicians as well, but because of a shortage of prospective studies, it is unclear whether this tendency is caused by the aging process or a cohort effect. If it is the latter, then it could be that the higher rate of depressive symptoms among the current younger cohorts of physicians will also be observable as they age.

Unfortunately, we do not have as much data on depression levels among fully trained physicians because their professional circumstances vary greatly and, as a population, they are more difficult to study than medical trainees. One study used the Center for Epidemiological Studies Depression Scale (CES-D) to assess the mental health of 706 alumni from a Japanese medical school (mean age, 37.5 years) and found that 28% (men 26%, women 34%) showed symptoms of depression (Tomioka et al. 2011). Another Japanese study screened a national sample of 3,862 physicians (mean age, ~50.0 years) with the Quick Inventory of Depressive Symptomatology—Self-Report (QIDS-SR), resulting in a considerably lower depression prevalence of 8.3% for the male and 10.5% for the female respondents (Wada et al. 2010). A survey among 1,488 physicians (mean age, 37.4 years) from northeastern China revealed a staggering prevalence of depressive symptoms in 65.3%, based on CES-D scores (Wang et al. 2010). Another study conducted with 616 village doctors (mean age, 46.2 years) from eastern China (Gu et al. 2017) estimated their prevalence rate of depressive symptoms at 27.4%, again based on CES-D scores. Data from 2,641 physicians in public hospitals (mean age, 39.8 years) of southern China (Gong et al. 2014) showed that 28.1% displayed mild depressive symptoms according to the Zung Self-Rating Depression Scale (SDS).

Variability in depression prevalence can also be observed in Western countries: a survey of 423 Dutch hospital physicians (mean age, 41 years) from one medical center (Ruitenburg et al. 2012) used the Brief Symptom Inventory, and 29% screened positive for depression (residents had a slightly higher rate of 31%, other doctors 27%). A nationwide study of 7,926 British physicians (mean age, ~46.7 years) found a prevalence rate of 10.8% using the PHQ-9 (Bourne et al. 2015). Their American colleagues were tested with the same instrument in a study of 1,154 physicians from Michigan (mean age, 50 years), with similar results of 11.3% (Schwenk et al. 2008). Results from the Canadian Physician Health Study revealed that 23.2% of the 3,213 physicians (mean age, ~49.8 years) reportedly felt "sad, blue, or depressed for 2 weeks or more in a row" in the year before the survey, and 20.8% reported having had a 2-week period of anhedonia (Compton and Frank 2011).

Not all of these studies reported results stratified by gender, and where they do, the difference is mostly not significant, even though the depression rates of female doctors are higher in all but one case. This may account for some of the variability because the proportion of female study participants varied (from 22% to 58%). However, the expected effect (higher share of female physicians equals higher depression prevalence) was not consistent across studies. Cross-cultural differences in depression rates can also be assumed to play a role, because many international studies looking at the general population have shown that prevalence differs between countries and regions

(Kessler and Bromet 2013). This holds true even when assessment instrument and study design are the same across countries, as with the World Mental Health Survey Initiative by the WHO. As an example, their estimates for the prevalence of a major depressive episode within the past 12 months ranged from 2.2% (Japan) to 10.4% (Brazil) in 18 countries from every continent (Kessler et al. 2010). These differences do not simply indicate how often depression actually occurs in various cultural contexts, they also seem to reflect diverse severity thresholds in reporting depressive symptoms. A cross-national WHO study showed that depressed people from countries with the highest depression prevalence rates reported the lowest levels of impairment from their depression, in contrast with depressed people from countries with the lowest prevalence rates, who in turn reported the highest degree of impairment (Simon et al. 2002). This would imply that people who have equally severe depressive symptoms might still respond differently to the same question regarding the intensity of said symptoms simply because they measure their own experience against perceived societal standards.

As we can see, it is difficult to summarize the available evidence, and there are some weaknesses to consider. Almost all of these studies used self-administered questionnaires that were distributed by mail or electronically, and many had low response rates. This could be a potential source of bias, for example, if depressed doctors were less (or more) likely to participate compared with those without mental health problems. Similar to the studies that were analyzed in the reviews of medical students and residents, different assessment instruments were used, and the cutoff points used to calculate prevalence rates often correspond with different levels of severity in depressive symptoms (which can vary from mild to severe). Aside from self-reported prevalence rates, depression levels can also be assessed by looking at antidepressant use, although there are not much data on physicians in particular. A Finnish study (Buscariolli et al. 2018) found that male health professionals had a slightly higher rate of antidepressant purchase (31%) compared with other occupations (24%), but this was not the case for females (35% for female health professionals vs. 34% for other occupations).

Although it is difficult to estimate the prevalence of clinically significant depressive disorder among physicians and compare it to the general population, we can safely assume that those with subthreshold depression are at a substantially higher risk of developing major depressive disorder; a review of prospective studies concerning the general population showed that this was a consistent finding, even though the heterogeneity across studies prevented a meta-analysis of the increase in incidence (Cuijpers and Smit 2004). It has also been established that the course of major depressive disorder is characterized by a fluctuation of symptoms along a continuum of intensity (Judd and Akiskal 2000), which emphasizes the importance of longitudinal studies looking at lifetime prevalence of depression.

A long-term prospective study of 1,190 male medical students who graduated from Johns Hopkins University between 1948 and 1964 found that the cumulative incidence of self-reported clinical depression was 12% at the 40-year follow-up (Ford et al. 1998). This rate is similar to the male general population at the time, for which the lifetime prevalence of major depressive disorder was estimated at 12.7% based on data from the 1992 National Comorbidity Survey (Blazer et al. 1994). Data from the 4,501 respondents of the Women Physicians' Health Study, which included medical graduates from 1950 to 1989, suggest a self-reported prevalence rate for depression of 19.5% (Frank and Dingle 1999). Although this is considerably higher than the rate among male physicians, it is again fairly similar to the estimated lifetime prevalence of major depressive disorder for the female general population, which is 21.3% (Blazer et al. 1994). Obviously, these estimates are based on older data, so the situation could have changed in the meantime.

More recent data (Hasin et al. 2018) suggest a higher estimate of 20.6% for the lifetime prevalence of major depressive disorder in the U.S. general population (men 14.7%, women 26.1%), so the seemingly high depression rates among physicians in the more recent cross-sectional studies could still be in line with general rates.

In summary, there is convincing evidence that medical students and residents have depression to a higher extent than the general population. The picture is not quite as clear for fully trained physicians, although many individual studies report elevated rates of depressive symptoms, which may well indicate that doctors as a professional group carry a higher burden of impairment caused by depressive symptoms. The consequences should not be underestimated—depression in physicians has been associated with more medical errors and worse outcomes in patient care, disruptive professional conduct (Brown et al. 2009), and a negative impact on doctor-patient relationships (Bright and Krahn 2011). On a personal level, depression causes a diminished quality of life, loss of relationships, and a higher risk of serious physical conditions, such as coronary artery disease (Ford et al. 1998). Finally, depression sometimes ends in death; it is the most common mental disorder in people who commit suicide (Bertolote and Fleischmann 2002).

Suicide Among Physicians

According to estimations by the WHO, there were about 804,000 suicides worldwide in the year 2012, which amounts to an age-adjusted suicide rate of 11.4 per 100,000 population (15.0 for males and 8.0 for females). About 43,400 suicides were reported in the United States, resulting in a slightly higher suicide rate of 12.1 and a much more pronounced gender difference (19.4 for males and 5.2 for females). This alarming number also constitutes a 24% increase compared with the suicide rate for the year 2000 (Saxena et al. 2014).

The healing profession seems to have a long-standing history of higher suicide rates, although the extent of this phenomenon remains contended. Early comments on the high incidence of suicide among American physi-

cians date back to the late nineteenth century (Legha 2012), and the first editorial on this topic by the *Journal of the American Medical Association* was
issued in 1903. Back in those days, the medical profession was less regulated
and institutionalized, and many physicians worked in trying circumstances
with little compensation in the way of prestige and financial rewards. Interestingly, this rather challenging environment was considered to be a per-
fectly sufficient explanation for the high number of physician suicides: "That
more do not do this we think speaks well for the profession, both here and
elsewhere" (JAMA 1903, p. 263). This changed drastically during the twentieth century, when the main focus was not the environment but the individual
physician. The search for personal characteristics that could provide explanations for an increased suicide risk among physicians follows the development of a new professional identity that fostered the ideal of the infallible,
all-knowing experts whose personal qualities not only enabled them to serve
in this highly challenging profession but set them apart from "ordinary" people and common mental health problems. At best, physician suicides were
treated with silence; at worst, they were seen as indicators of personal weakness, irresponsibility, and preexisting negative character traits, retrospec-
tively proving that someone was not "cut out" to succeed in a demanding
professional environment like medicine.

A change of perspective began to take place in the 1960s and 1970s,
when the discourse surrounding physician suicide started to take into account a wider range of factors, among them the lack of support for struggling
physicians by a medical culture that was essentially in denial about the vulnerability of its members. A report from the American Medical Association
(AMA) in 1973, aptly titled "The Sick Physician," set the tone for a new paradigm in dealing with mental health problems among physicians (Council
on Mental Health 1973). Treatable health problems such as alcoholism and
drug dependence were recognized as important risk factors for suicidality,
and the focus shifted toward providing support and rehabilitation for those
affected, together with an emphasis on more research and awareness. Precisely 30 years later, the AMA issued a consensus statement on depression
and suicide in physicians, with further-developed recommendations on how
to approach this persisting problem on an individual and institutional level
(Center et al. 2003).

What do we know about the prevalence of suicide among physicians? A
meta-analysis of 25 studies from Europe and North America (Schernhammer and Colditz 2004) suggested a slightly increased suicide rate for male
doctors when compared with the general population (overall suicide rate ratio of 1.41; 95% CI = 1.21–1.65), and a considerably higher suicide rate for female doctors (2.27; 95% CI = 1.90–2.73). New studies that were published
after 2003 paint a more varied picture. Yaghmour et al. (2017) analyzed data
from all residents in Accreditation Council for Graduate Medical Education–accredited programs from 2000 to 2014 and calculated a suicide rate
that was lower when compared with the age- and gender-matched general

population, both for male and female residents. Nonetheless, suicide was the second leading cause of death (after neoplastic disease), and a comparison of age groups revealed increased suicide rates in older cohorts, which reached higher levels than those of the general population. Higher age in physicians seems to be an important risk factor, because other studies observed similar trends (Gold et al. 2013; Hem et al. 2005).

A study from Brazil for the state of Sao Paolo (Palhares-Alves et al. 2015) looked at physician suicides between 2000 and 2009 and found rates comparable with the general population, although suicides of female physicians were slightly overrepresented. Evidence from Queensland, Australia, for the time period of 1990–2007 (Kõlves and De Leo 2013) showed a lower suicide rate for male doctors compared with the general population (suicide rate ratio 0.69; 95% CI=0.43–1.09) but a higher rate for female doctors (1.74; 95% CI=0.76–3.78). The findings of a Norwegian study (Hem et al. 2005) based on data from 1960 to 2000 suggested an elevated suicide rate for both male and female physicians, but they also reported a statistically significant decrease in the suicide rate of male physicians over the last observed decade. Although the suicide rate for female physicians also decreased over the entire time span, it was still twice as high as in the general population. An American cohort study from 1948 to 1998 (Torre et al. 2005) found that physicians had significantly lower all-cause mortality rates but considerably elevated suicide mortality, more so for women than men.

In summary, the available evidence appears to confirm the notion of a higher suicide risk for physicians, especially among female doctors and older age cohorts. When looking at the relationship between gender and suicide, the global numbers suggest a male-to-female ratio of roughly 2:1 in the general population, which can be much higher for individual countries like the United States, where the number of suicides by men in 2012 was almost four times as high as those by women (Saxena et al. 2014). However, this does not seem to be the case for physicians, where the higher suicide rate of female doctors (compared with the female general population) indicates that their suicide incidence is almost up to the level of their male colleagues (Reimer et al. 2005). One explanation for this phenomenon is the choice of suicide method: women in the general population tend to use less lethal means than men, but this is not true of female physicians, who also have access to potent medicinal drugs and knowledge about lethal dosages. An Australian study (Milner et al. 2017) based on mortality data from 2001 to 2012 showed that people who work in professions that grant them access to high-risk suicide means (e.g., firearms for police forces or drugs for medical care personnel) used these so-called hard suicide methods more frequently, which results in higher overall suicide rates. It was also observed that this particularly affected the female suicide rate in these professions, who had a higher elevation than men when compared with other professionals without access to effective suicide methods. In fact, it seems like the rate of suicide attempts is actually lower among physicians than among the general population. However, because physicians have more knowledge than the average person about how to effectively end a life, their attempts are more likely to result in death (Kuhn and Flanagan 2017).

It is also interesting to look at the characteristics of those physicians who took their own lives in comparison with those who died by suicide within the general population. Data from the National Violent Death Reporting System for 2003 to 2008 from 16 American states (Gold et al. 2013) suggested that physician suicides were significantly less likely to be preceded by the death of a close friend or family member, whereas a professional problem (e.g., tensions with coworkers, poor performance reviews, increased pressure, feared layoff as well as job loss and difficulty finding a new one) was more common than in others who died by suicide. Interestingly, physicians seemed to have higher rates of known mental health disorders, but toxicology testing revealed that they were not more likely to have ingested antidepressant medication. However, they had a dramatically higher likelihood of testing positive for barbiturates, benzodiazepines, and antipsychotics, to an extent where it is difficult to distinguish whether their use was intended to be therapeutic or toxic (or to lower inhibitions). This is one reason why many have speculated that the number of physician suicides is actually higher than suggested by statistics, because it can be assumed that quite a few physician suicides are misclassified as accidental poisonings. While this might be due to the uncertainty regarding intentions for drug use, it is also possible that the stigma that still surrounds suicide in the medical community could result in the intentional misrepresentation of a suicide as an accident (Reimer et al. 2005).

Depression and Suicide Among Psychiatrists

It has long been claimed that psychiatry as a specialty carries a relatively high burden of both depression and suicide. With regard to depression and other mental health disorders, evidence from the past decades mostly seems to support this assumption, although the significance of study results is often compromised by small sample sizes. In an early U.S. study of 111 female physicians (Welner et al. 1979), the 22 psychiatrists reported a drastically higher lifetime prevalence of depressive symptoms compared with other medical specialties (73% vs. 46%). A Scottish study compared 39 psychiatrists with a group of 149 surgeons and other physicians and found that the psychiatrists reported significantly higher levels of emotional exhaustion and depression (Deary et al. 1996). A Finnish national survey of 3,133 physicians (Korkeila et al. 2003) showed that the 170 psychiatrists had a significantly higher rate of depression during the past 12 months than their colleagues (14% vs. 8%) as well as a higher prevalence of suicidal thoughts (37% vs. 22%).

On the basis of these results, it is not possible to tell if psychiatry as a specialty causes higher depression rates or whether individuals with preexisting depressive tendencies are more inclined to choose this field for their profession. This question has attracted attention for quite a while, and in the second half of the twentieth century the second option seems to have prevailed: "quite a few young physicians choose psychiatry as their specialty due to their unconscious needs and conflicts, seeking solutions to their own unconscious problems" (Braun 1973, p. 81). A large study of 4,501 female physicians (again from the Women Physicians' Health Study) tried to shed some light on the matter by exploring the characteristics of their subject group. In addition to significantly higher rates of depression, they found that female psychiatrists were more likely than other female physicians to report a personal or family history of psychiatric disorders as well as a family history of sexual abuse, domestic violence, or eating disorders (although the differences were small). Although this could be indicative of a slightly higher predisposition toward mental health problems, the authors also point out that this might be due to the presumably better abilities of psychiatrists in identifying these conditions. Either way, it would seem like the answer to this question is more complex and quite possibly a combination of the two explanations, because "the practice of psychiatry can be isolating and has unique stressors involving great emotional and empathic requirements of the psychiatrist" (Frank et al. 2001, p. 211).

The hypothesis that psychiatrists are more prone to mental illness because of their personal characteristics is closely connected to the debate about psychiatrists' suicide rate. Decades ago, it seemed somewhat well established that psychiatry loses a higher share of doctors to suicide, but the studies that supported this conclusion were mostly based on the analysis of obituaries and have since been deemed methodologically limited (Center et al. 2003). Even at the time, the debate surrounding psychiatrist suicides was criticized because it included "numerous statements that psychiatrists have a greater liability to mental disturbance. This has been done before it has been established that psychiatrists have the highest [suicide] rate.... It is an injustice to the majority of psychiatrists to have the results of a few questionably designed studies generalized onto the whole profession" (Rosen 1973, p. 246). The fact that the supposedly higher suicide rate of psychiatrists received this much attention needs to be placed in the context of psychiatry as a developing field of medicine that was still subjected to criticism (Legha 2012). The emphasis on high rates of suicidality in psychiatry at a time when suicides were predominantly perceived as a sad consequence of individual frailty can be seen as part of the dynamic in marginalizing the scientific merit of psychiatry: "Psychiatrists, after all, should know how to preserve a healthy state of mind" (von Brauchitsch 1976, p. 40).

In fact, the evidence was and continues to be ambivalent: a review of the existing literature in the late 1970s found no evidence that the suicide rate of psychiatrists was higher than in other medical specialties or even the general population (Bergman 1979), whereas a U.S. study looking at physician deaths from 1967 to 1972 found that the suicide rate of psychiatrists was twice as high as expected (Rich and Pitts 1980). Several newer studies have also found that psychiatrists are among those whose specialties are particularly affected by high suicide rates (Hawton et al. 2001; Torre et al. 2005); only a few studies did not (Arnetz et al. 1987). More evidence based on greater sample sizes is needed to allow for an informed discussion on the potential implications of high suicide rates among psychiatrists.

Risk and Protective Factors

Depression is one of the main risk factors for suicide. Thus, both depression and suicide are influenced by many shared risk and protective factors. There are a good deal of data on biological, cognitive, and social risk factors of depression (Dobson and Dozois 2008). The most prominent ones include family history of mental illness, chronic physical or mental disorders (including substance abuse disorders), major life changes and stress, lack of social support, low socioeconomic status, sleep disorders, and certain medications. Risk factors for depression have also been shown to vary across the lifespan (Schaakxs et al. 2017) and gender (Karger 2014). Other specific suicide risk factors are general hopelessness, professional failures, and family problems, as well as shame and humiliation (Goldsmith et al. 2002). Although these risk factors apply universally, the strength of their influence (especially on suicide) varies depending on cultural contexts.

In addition to these general risk factors, there are other influences that specifically affect physicians as a group, both on an individual level and with regard to their professional activity, and may have an impact on their depression risk. A Canadian study found that a high proportion of physicians identify with the Type A personality, which is characterized by perfectionism, competitiveness, anxiety, and high goal orientation (Lemaire and Wallace 2014). This could increase their tendency toward excessive self-criticism, a known risk factor of depression, and exacerbate the fear of making mistakes, another potent stressor (Firth-Cozens 1998). With regard to work-related risk factors, there are the obvious emotional demands of practicing medicine, which often means having to cope with intense suffering and death. Professional relationships, while often rewarding, can also increase risk. Complaints, unrealistic expectations, and aggressive behavior on the patient side put pressure on physicians (Edwards et al. 2002), similar to conflicts, bullying, and competition on the colleague side (Garelick and Fagin 2004).

Other occupational risk factors include a heavy workload that often comes with little control over working hours and shift structure, which commonly results in depression risk factors such as sleep deprivation and social isolation (Firth-Cozens and Cording 2004). Additionally, doctors generally have easier access to prescription drugs and possess knowledge of their effects. This facilitates the development of substance abuse disorder, a significant risk factor for depression and suicide and a widespread problem among physicians (Merlo and Gold 2008). There is also evidence to suggest that risk factors regarding personality and work environment do not merely add up but interact in specific ways; for example, some personality characteristics such as neuroticism predict greater stress and emotional exhaustion among physicians (McManus et al. 2004). However, a study of mental health personnel found that organizational characteristics were still the better predictors of exhaustion compared with individual characteristics (Thomsen et al. 1999).

There is less evidence on influences that protect against depression and suicide. In general, social support is one of the most well-known protective factors, because a high connectedness with family and friends helps one to cope with a multitude of negative life events and stressors. This is also thought to be the reason why marriage has been shown to lower suicide risk. Other protective factors include religious beliefs, coping skills, and restricted access to lethal means (Goldsmith et al. 2002). For those who have mental health conditions, adequate treatment has also been identified as a major protective factor against suicide (Mann 2002), one that holds particular relevance for physicians. Several authors have written on the subject of barriers to mental health treatment (Bright and Krahn 2011; Guille et al. 2010) and listed a complex array of problems. Doctors (especially in early career stages) appear to have a low propensity to seek help because of lack of time and access, worries about confidentiality, stigma, cost, and fear of documentation on their academic record (Hu et al. 2012). Concerns regarding job prospects and medical licensing are not unfounded, and the licensing policies of many medical boards regarding impairment due to mental health problems have been heavily criticized (Center et al. 2003).

Prevention and Intervention Initiatives

When it comes to acting on the existing knowledge in order to improve the lives of struggling or at-risk physicians, it is essential to design interventions that take the specific needs and challenges of their situations into account, especially the fact that doctors are often handicapped in seeking help for their mental health problems. The good news is that the many recent appeals to confront the problem of depression and suicide among physicians (Center et al. 2003; Khan et al. 2015) have not gone unnoticed, although the first official call for action by the AMA already dates back to 1973: "Educational programs should be developed for the medical student and the physician in training, emphasizing their high vulnerability to psychiatric disorders, alcoholism, and drug dependence" (Council on Mental Health 1973, p. 648). Several universities and hospitals have begun to implement and evaluate various programs, and the following section contains just a selection of notable initiatives.

One landmark program in this regard is the suicide prevention and depression awareness program launched in 2009 at the University of California (UC)–San Diego (Moutier et al. 2012). The integrative approach focused on providing education on the subject as well as screening, assessment, and referral to treatment when needed. Aimed at trainees and faculty alike, the goal—in addition to raising awareness and preventing suicides—was to destigmatize the process of help seeking. A recent report (Zisook et al. 2016) stated that during the initial 5 years, more than 4,400 people of all target groups were invited to complete the screening, with response rates between 17% (residents and fellows) and 33% (students). The depression prevalence varied between 7% (faculty) and 10% (residents and fellows), and overall about 10% of respondents were classified as at-risk for suicide. Alarmingly, only 17% of them were taking antidepressant medication, and psychotherapy or counseling was even less prevalent (12%), so the need for further assessment and treatment referrals is obvious. A replication of the program at University of California, Davis, in 2013 had an even lower response rate of 8%, although a follow-up with a small number of respondents revealed symptom improvement and a desire for the program to continue (Haskins et al. 2016). The web-based screening tool used at both sites was developed by the American Foundation for Suicide Prevention (2018) to foster the use of mental health services before the emergence of a crisis and is available for implementation in any medical organization.

It makes sense to emphasize prevention efforts for medical trainees, not just because they carry a high burden regarding depression but also because investments in their self-care skills and habits is likely to pay off for decades to come. As a population, they are more easily reached and have not yet fully internalized the potentially problematic aspects of medical culture. Khan et al. (2015, p. 848) called for further action regarding the incorporation of mental health aspects into medical training, stating that "mental health and wellness education should begin as early as medical school orientation," and some training institutions have shown initiative in this regard. The medical faculty of Heidelberg University in Germany tried peer-led stress prevention seminars in the first year of medical school, which received positive ratings by the attending students and were consequently integrated into the medical curriculum (Bugaj et al. 2016). At the Medical University of Graz, Austria, the newly structured "Peer2Peer" program offers an elective course on psychosocial crisis intervention and stress management, combined with further lectures and workshops and a consultation service providing peer support in crises and psychosocial stress situations (Vajda 2016). Peer-led counseling is considered a particularly low-threshold approach, which not only makes it easier for students to reach out but also strengthens the perception that their peer group is an active stakeholder in their mental well-being.

The fact that programs based on voluntary participation are generally afflicted with low response rates has led to calls for more binding methods of engaging target groups (Batra et al. 2018). Sofka et al. (2018) reported on a universal well-being assessment for interns and residents at West Virginia University who could only "opt out" if they did not wish to attend. The intervention included a "wellness day" without work duties in combination with an evaluation by a therapist, who helped them to create a tailored "wellness plan." Overall, 93% of eligible candidates participated, and evaluation results indicated that they found it convenient and reported a higher likelihood of using these services in the future. Comprehensive programs with more than one component also seem to help with increasing the utilization of mental health services; Ey et al. (2016) reported that a well-being program providing counseling, psychiatric evaluation, and wellness workshops for residents and faculty at the Oregon Health and Science University was monitored for 10 years, with an increase in uptake from 5% to 25% of eligible trainees. Faculty utilization had far lower growth rates (from 6% to 8%). Another comprehensive program that has been around since 2005 is the Vanderbilt Medical Student Wellness Program, consisting of faculty mentoring, a student wellness committee, and a curriculum adjunct focused on the personal growth of students. Anecdotal evidence suggests that it is well received, with almost every first- or second-year student involved in at least two components (Drolet and Rodgers 2010).

However, because most of these programs are rather new, there are not much data on their effectiveness. A systematic review on the association between learning environment interventions and medical student well-being examined 28 studies and found limited evidence that some specific interventions improved students' mental health status, which could be due to the fact that most of the available data were of rather poor quality with respect to study design, sample size, and intervention comparators (Wasson et al. 2016). Evaluations of prevention initiatives among trained physicians are even sparser. A systematic review on methods for the prevention and reduction of burnout among physicians found that clinically relevant reduction of burnout symptoms can be achieved by organizational strategies as well as approaches that are focused on the individual (West et al. 2016). However, no single intervention distinguished itself with regard to effectiveness, so it remains uncertain which programs provide the greatest value for organizations or physicians. There is also little knowledge on how to integrate organizational and individual-focused strategies and about variability in intervention effectiveness for specific groups of physicians.

Another avenue that shows some promise is the web-based delivery of interventions to improve mental health, because they can circumvent some hindrances that prevent physicians from seeking help, namely, confidentiality issues, stigma, and lack of time. In a systematic review by Pospos et al. (2018), the results of a search for effective methods to alleviate stress and improve mental health (cognitive-behavioral therapy, meditation, mindfulness, breathing, and relaxation techniques) were used to select general web-based or mobile applications that delivered said methods and were deemed useful for healthcare professionals. One of them, a web-based program for cognitive-behavioral therapy, was tested in a randomized clinical trial with the objective of reducing suicidal ideation in medical interns. Encouragingly, the intervention group was significantly less likely to endorse suicidal ideation compared with the control subjects (Guille et al. 2015).

There is some evidence that physicians prefer peer support to institution-alized programs or mental health professionals; this was implemented in the form of a one-on-one peer support program at Brigham and Women's Hospital in 2009 (Hu et al. 2012). It was one of the first of its kind and has inspired many similar programs. Again, the advantages of this approach are not limited to any immediate beneficial effects for the participating physicians but include the potential to shape the medical community "away from a culture of invulnerability, isolation, and shame and toward a culture that truly values a sense of shared organizational responsibility for clinician well-being and patient safety" (Shapiro and Galowitz 2016, p. 1200).

Conclusion

Promoting mental health among physicians is an important step in the right direction, even though we are still a long way from universal, standardized programs tested for efficacy. Even though improvements in stress or depression scores are a laudable achievement, at the end of the day we also want to see a reduction in the number of physician suicides. For this purpose, more research is needed on the specific needs and challenges of physicians throughout their career and in various professional circumstances. We also do not know enough about protective factors or what contributes to the resilience of those physicians who are exposed to several risk factors but manage to keep their psychological distress at bay.

However, more research and more interventions are unlikely to solve the problem, especially with regard to suicide. If we assume that the work environment of physicians is systematically putting them at risk, then we also need to consider structural aspects in healthcare and look at the big picture, the future development of institutionalized medicine. One of the problematic issues surrounding physician suicides concerns the difficulty of noticing when someone has depression; stress, fatigue, sleep disturbance, a less active social life, and occasional irritability are not generally seen as symptoms that warrant concern but as the everyday characteristics of being a doctor. The challenge of figuring out an often precariously small difference between what is normal and what constitutes a serious health risk is placed on the affected physicians and their surroundings, but the responsibility for the situation at large is shared by many stakeholders who could also play a part in improving it.

Society in general seems to be moving toward greater openness and acceptance regarding mental health problems, and there has been some progress in addressing physician depression and suicide within the medical community and beyond, as evidenced by a recent documentary on suicide among young physicians called *Do No Harm* (Symon 2018). Still, there is more to be done. The temptation to revert to silence and neglect a painful topic is still alive and well today, and persisting change requires an ongoing effort. After all, one piece of advice regarding physician suicide from 1903 still holds true today: "It is not a bad thing to be reminded of unpleasant facts, if by such reminders any influence whatever is exerted toward doing away with the evils that exist" (JAMA 1903, p. 264).

KEY POINTS

- Rates of depression among medical students and residents are higher than in the general population, and depression levels among fully trained physicians might be elevated as well.

- Compared with the general population, suicide rate seems slightly higher among male physicians and significantly higher among female physicians.

- There is some evidence for higher depression rates among psychiatrists compared with other medical specialties, but more data are needed to confirm a potentially elevated suicide rate.

- Physicians as a professional group are affected by additional risk factors for depression and suicide, both on an individual and organizational level.

- It can be difficult for physicians to seek help for mental health problems because of several barriers that affect them professionally.

- More research is needed on protective factors for depression and suicide among physicians.

- There are promising prevention strategies to promote mental health among physicians, especially during medical training, but more evidence on their effectiveness is needed.

References

Ahola K, Honkonen T, Isometsä E, et al: The relationship between job-related burnout and depressive disorders—results from the Finnish Health 2000 Study. J Affect Disord 88(1):55–62, 2005 16038984

American Foundation for Suicide Prevention: Interactive Screening Program. New York, American Foundation for Suicide Prevention, 2018. Available at: https://afsp.org/our-work/interactive-screening-program. Accessed August 8, 2018.

American Psychiatric Association: Diagnostic and Statistical Manual of Mental Disorders, 5th Edition. Arlington, VA, American Psychiatric Association, 2013

Arnetz BB, Hörte LG, Hedberg A, et al: Suicide patterns among physicians related to other academics as well as to the general population: results from a national long-term prospective study. Acta Psychiatr Scand 75(2):139–143, 1987 3494382

Batra M, McPhillips H, Shugerman R: Improving resident use of mental health resources: it's time for an opt-out strategy to address physician burnout and depression (commentary). J Grad Med Educ 10(1):67–69, 2018 29467976

Bergman J: The suicide rate among psychiatrists revisited. Suicide Life Threat Behav 9(4):219–226, 1979 516127

Bertolote JM, Fleischmann A: Suicide and psychiatric diagnosis: a worldwide perspective. World Psychiatry 1(3):181–185, 2002 16946849

Bianchi R, Schonfeld IS: Defining physician burnout, and differentiating between burnout and depression-I. Mayo Clin Proc 92(9):1455, 2017 28870363

Bianchi R, Schonfeld IS, Laurent E: Burnout-depression overlap: a review. Clin Psychol Rev 36:28–41, 2015 25638755

Bianchi R, Schonfeld IS, Laurent E: Biological research on burnout-depression overlap: long-standing limitations and on-going reflections. Neurosci Biobehav Rev 83:238–239, 2017 29079491

Blazer DG, Kessler RC, McGonagle KA, et al: The prevalence and distribution of major depression in a national community sample: the National Comorbidity Survey. Am J Psychiatry 151(7):979–986, 1994 8010383

Bourne T, Wynants L, Peters M, et al: The impact of complaints procedures on the welfare, health and clinical practise of 7926 doctors in the UK: a cross-sectional survey. BMJ Open 5(1):e006687–e006687, 2015 25592686

Braun M: Suicide in psychiatrists. JAMA 223(1):81, 1973 4739104

Brazeau CMLR, Shanafelt T, Durning SJ, et al: Distress among matriculating medical students relative to the general population. Acad Med 89(11):1520–1525, 2014 25250752

Bright RP, Krahn L: Depression and suicide among physicians. Curr Psychiatr 10(4):16–30, 2011

Brown SD, Goske MJ, Johnson CM: Beyond substance abuse: stress, burnout, and depression as causes of physician impairment and disruptive behavior. J Am Coll Radiol 6(7):479–485, 2009 19560063

Bugaj TJ, Mücksch C, Schmid C, et al: Peer-led stress prevention seminars in the first year of medical school—a project report. GMS J Med Educ 33(1):Doc3, 2016 26958651

Buscariolli A, Kouvonen A, Kokkinen L, et al: Human service work, gender and antidepressant use: a nationwide register-based 19-year follow-up of 752 683 women and men. Occup Environ Med 75(6):401–406, 2018 29374096

Center C, Davis M, Detre T, et al: Confronting depression and suicide in physicians: a consensus statement. JAMA 289(23):3161–3166, 2003 12813122

Compton MT, Frank E: Mental health concerns among Canadian physicians: results from the 2007–2008 Canadian Physician Health Study. Compr Psychiatry 52(5):542–547, 2011 21129737

Council on Mental Health: The sick physician. Impairment by psychiatric disorders, including alcoholism and drug dependence. JAMA 223(6):684–687, 1973 4739202

Cuijpers P, Smit F: Subthreshold depression as a risk indicator for major depressive disorder: a systematic review of prospective studies. Acta Psychiatr Scand 109(5):325–331, 2004 15049768

Deary IJ, Agius RM, Sadler A: Personality and stress in consultant psychiatrists. Int J Soc Psychiatry 42(2):112–123, 1996 8811395

DeCaporale-Ryan L, Sakran JV, Grant SB, et al: The undiagnosed pandemic: burnout and depression within the surgical community. Curr Probl Surg 54(9):453–502, 2017 29073980

Dobson KS, Dozois DJA: Risk Factors in Depression. Cambridge, MA, Academic Press, 2008

Drolet BC, Rodgers S: A comprehensive medical student wellness program—design and implementation at Vanderbilt School of Medicine. Acad Med 85(1):103–110, 2010 20042835

Edwards N, Kornacki MJ, Silversin J: Unhappy doctors: what are the causes and what can be done? BMJ 324(7341):835–838, 2002 11934779

Ey S, Moffit M, Kinzie JM, Brunett PH: Feasibility of a comprehensive wellness and suicide prevention program: a decade of caring for physicians in training and practice. J Grad Med Educ 8(5):747–753, 2016 28018541

Fahrenkopf AM, Sectish TC, Barger LK, et al: Rates of medication errors among depressed and burnt out residents: prospective cohort study. BMJ 336(7642):488–491, 2008 18258931

Firth-Cozens J: Individual and organizational predictors of depression in general practitioners. Br J Gen Pract 48(435):1647–1651, 1998 10071396

Firth-Cozens J, Cording H: What matters more in patient care? Giving doctors shorter hours of work or a good night's sleep? Qual Saf Health Care 13(3):165–166, 2004 15175481

Ford DE, Mead LA, Chang PP, et al: Depression is a risk factor for coronary artery disease in men: the precursors study. Arch Intern Med 158(13):1422–1426, 1998 9665350

Frank E, Dingle AD: Self-reported depression and suicide attempts among U.S. women physicians. Am J Psychiatry 156(12):1887–1894, 1999 10588401

Frank E, Biola H, Burnett CA: Mortality rates and causes among U.S. physicians. Am J Prev Med 19(3):155–159, 2000 11020591

Frank E, Boswell L, Dickstein L, et al: Characteristics of female psychiatrists. Am J Psychiatry 158(2):205–212, 2001 11156802

Garelick A, Fagin L: Doctor to doctor: getting on with colleagues. Adv Psychiatr Treat 10(3):225–232, 2004

Gold KJ, Sen A, Schwenk TL: Details on suicide among US physicians: data from the National Violent Death Reporting System. Gen Hosp Psychiatry 35(1):45–49, 2013 23123101

Goldsmith SK, Pellmar TC, Kleinman AM, et al: Reducing Suicide: A National Imperative. Washington, DC, National Academies Press, 2002

Gong Y, Han T, Chen W, et al: Prevalence of anxiety and depressive symptoms and related risk factors among physicians in China: a cross-sectional study. PLoS One 9(7):e103242, 2014 25050618

Gu L-X, Chu J, Qi Z-B, et al: Depressive symptoms and correlates among village doctors in China. Asian J Psychiatr 28:188–192, 2017 28711838

Guille C, Speller H, Laff R, et al: Utilization and barriers to mental health services among depressed medical interns: a prospective multisite study. J Grad Med Educ 2(2):210–214, 2010 21975622

Guille C, Zhao Z, Krystal J, et al: Web-based cognitive behavioral therapy intervention for the prevention of suicidal ideation in medical interns: a randomized clinical trial. JAMA Psychiatry 72(12):1192–1198, 2015 26535958

Hasin DS, Sarvet AL, Meyers JL et al: Epidemiology of adult DSM-5 major depressive disorder and its specifiers in the United States. JAMA Psychiatry 75(4):336–346, 2018 29450462

Haskins J, Carson JG, Chang CH, et al: The suicide prevention, depression awareness, and clinical engagement program for faculty and residents at the University of California, Davis Health System. Acad Psychiatry 40(1):23–29, 2016 26063680

Hawton K, Clements A, Sakarovitch C, et al: Suicide in doctors: a study of risk according to gender, seniority and specialty in medical practitioners in England and Wales, 1979–1995. J Epidemiol Community Health 55(5):296–300, 2001 11297646

Hem E, Haldorsen T, Aasland OG, et al: Suicide rates according to education with a particular focus on physicians in Norway 1960–2000. Psychol Med 35(6):873–880, 2005 15997607

Hu Y-Y, Fix ML, Hevelone ND, et al: Physicians' needs in coping with emotional stressors: the case for peer support. Arch Surg 147(3):212–217, 2012 22106247

JAMA: Suicides of physicians and the reasons. JAMA 41(4):263–264, 1903

Jorm AF: Does old age reduce the risk of anxiety and depression? A review of epidemiological studies across the adult life span. Psychol Med 30(1):11–22, 2000 10722172

Judd LL, Akiskal HS: Delineating the longitudinal structure of depressive illness: beyond clinical subtypes and duration thresholds. Pharmacopsychiatry 33(1):3–7, 2000 10721877

Karger A: Geschlechtsspezifische Aspekte bei depressiven Erkrankungen. Bundesgesundheitsblatt 57(9):1092–1098, 2014

Kessler RC, Birnbaum HG, Shahly V, et al: Age differences in the prevalence and co-morbidity of DSM-IV major depressive episodes: results from the WHO World Mental Health Survey Initiative. Depress Anxiety 27(4):351–364, 2010 20037917

Kessler RC, Bromet EJ: The epidemiology of depression across cultures. Annu Rev Public Health 34:119–138, 2013 23514317

Khan R, Lin JS, Mata DA: Addressing depression and suicide among physician trainees. JAMA Psychiatry 72(8):848, 2015 26107398

Kõlves K, De Leo D: Suicide in medical doctors and nurses: an analysis of the Queensland Suicide Register. J Nerv Ment Dis 201(11):987–990, 2013 24177487

Korkeila JA, Töyry S, Kumpulainen K, et al: Burnout and self-perceived health among Finnish psychiatrists and child psychiatrists: a national survey. Scand J Public Health 31(2):85–91, 2003 12745757

Kuhn CM, Flanagan EM: Prendre soin de soi, un impératif professionnel: l'épuisement professionnel, la dépression et le suicide chez les médecins. Can J Anaesth 64(2):158–168, 2017 27910035

Legha RK: A history of physician suicide in America. J Med Humanit 33(4):219–244, 2012 22872527

Lemaire JB, Wallace JE: How physicians identify with predetermined personalities and links to perceived performance and wellness outcomes: a cross-sectional study. BMC Health Serv Res 14:616, 2014 25471536

Mann JJ: A current perspective of suicide and attempted suicide. Ann Intern Med 136(4):302–311, 2002 11848728

Maslach C, Jackson SE, Leiter MP: The Maslach Burnout Inventory, 3rd edition, in Evaluating Stress: A Book of Resources. Lanham, MD, Scarecrow Education, 1997, pp 191–218

Mata DA, Ramos MA, Bansal N, et al: Prevalence of depression and depressive symptoms among resident physicians: a systematic review and meta-analysis. JAMA 314(22):2373–2383, 2015 26647259

Mather L, Blom V, Bergström G, et al: An underlying common factor, influenced by genetics and unique environment, explains the covariation between major depressive disorder, generalized anxiety disorder, and burnout: a Swedish twin study. Twin Res Hum Genet 19(6):619–627, 2016 27620693

McManus IC, Keeling A, Paice E: Stress, burnout and doctors' attitudes to work are determined by personality and learning style: a twelve year longitudinal study of UK medical graduates. BMC Med 2:29, 2004 15317650

Melnick ER, Powsner SM, Shanafelt TD: In reply defining physician burnout, and differentiating between burnout and depression. Mayo Clin Proc 92(9):1456–1458, 2017 28870365

Merlo LJ, Gold MS: Prescription opioid abuse and dependence among physicians: hypotheses and treatment. Harv Rev Psychiatry 16(3):181–194, 2008 18569039

Milner A, Witt K, Maheen H, et al: Access to means of suicide, occupation and the risk of suicide: a national study over 12 years of coronial data. BMC Psychiatry 17(1):125, 2017 28376757

Moutier C, Norcross W, Jong P, et al: The suicide prevention and depression awareness program at the University of California, San Diego School of Medicine. Acad Med 87(3):320–326, 2012 22373625

Palhares-Alves HN, Palhares DM, Laranjeira R, et al: Suicide among physicians in the state of São Paulo, Brazil, across one decade. Br J Psychiatry 37(2):146–149, 2015 26083813

Pospos S, Young IT, Downs N, et al: Web-based tools and mobile applications to mitigate burnout, depression, and suicidality among healthcare students and professionals: a systematic review. Acad Psychiatry 42(1):109–120, 2018 29256033

Pratt LA, Brody DJ: Depression in the U.S. household population, 2009–2012. NCHS Data Brief (172):1–8, 2014 25470183

Reimer C, Trinkaus S, Jurkat HB: Suicidal tendencies of physicians—an overview. Psychiatr Prax 32(8):381–385, 2005 16308801

Rich CL, Pitts FN Jr: Suicide by psychiatrists: a study of medical specialists among 18,730 consecutive physician deaths during a five-year period, 1967–72. J Clin Psychiatry 41(8):261–263, 1980 7400103

Roberts SE, Jaremin B, Lloyd K: High-risk occupations for suicide. Psychol Med 43(6):1231–1240, 2013 23098158

Rosen DH: Suicide rates among psychiatrists. JAMA 224(2):246–247, 1973 4739503

Rotenstein LS, Ramos MA, Torre M, et al: Prevalence of depression, depressive symptoms, and suicidal ideation among medical students: a systematic review and meta-analysis. JAMA 316(21):2214–2236, 2016 27923088

Ruitenburg MM, Frings-Dresen MH, Sluiter JK: The prevalence of common mental disorders among hospital physicians and their association with self-reported work ability: a cross-sectional study. BMC Health Serv Res 12:292–298, 2012 22938170

Saxena S, Krug EG, Chestnov O (eds): Preventing suicide: A global imperative. Geneva, Switzerland, World Health Organization, 2014

Schaakxs R, Comijs HC, van der Mast RC, et al: Risk factors for depression: differential across age? Am J Geriatr Psychiatry 25(9):966–977, 2017 28529007

Schernhammer ES, Colditz GA: Suicide rates among physicians: a quantitative and gender assessment (meta-analysis). Am J Psychiatry 161(12):2295–2302, 2004 15569903

Schwenk TL, Gorenflo DW, Leja LM: A survey on the impact of being depressed on the professional status and mental health care of physicians. J Clin Psychiatry 69(4):617–620, 2008 18426258

Shapiro J, Galowitz P: Peer support for clinicians: a programmatic approach. Acad Med 91(9):1200–1204, 2016 27355784

Simon GE, Goldberg DP, Von Korff M, et al: Understanding cross-national differences in depression prevalence. Psychol Med 32(4):585–594, 2002 12102373

Sofka S, Grey C, Lerfald N, et al: Implementing a universal well-being assessment to mitigate barriers to resident utilization of mental health resources. J Grad Med Educ 10(1):63–66, 2018 29467975

Støen Grotmol K, Gude T, Moum T, et al: Risk factors at medical school for later severe depression: a 15-year longitudinal, nationwide study (NORDOC). J Affect Disord 146(1):106–111, 2013 23017539

Symon R: Do No Harm: Exposing the Hippocratic Hoax (film). Los Angeles, CA, Symon Productions, 2018. Available at: http://donoharmfilm.com. Accessed August 8, 2018.

Thomsen S, Soares J, Nolan P, et al: Feelings of professional fulfilment and exhaustion in mental health personnel: the importance of organisational and individual factors. Psychother Psychosom 68(3):157–164, 1999 10224515

Toker S, Biron M: Job burnout and depression: unraveling their temporal relationship and considering the role of physical activity. J Appl Psychol 97(3):699–710, 2012 22229693

Tomioka K, Morita N, Saeki K, et al: Working hours, occupational stress and depression among physicians. Occup Med (Lond) 61(3):163–170, 2011 21383384

Torre DM, Wang N-Y, Meoni LA, et al: Suicide compared to other causes of mortality in physicians. Suicide Life Threat Behav 35(2):146–153, 2005 15843332

Vajda C: "Peer2Peer"—a university program for knowledge transfer and consultation in dealing with psychosocial crises in med-school and medical career. GMS J Med Educ 33(4):Doc52, 2016 27579352

von Brauchitsch H: The physician's suicide revisited. J Nerv Ment Dis 162(1):40–45, 1976 1245848

Wada K, Yoshikawa T, Goto T, et al: National survey of the association of depressive symptoms with the number of off duty and on-call, and sleep hours among physicians working in Japanese hospitals: a cross sectional study. BMC Public Health 10:127, 2010 20222990

Wang J-N, Sun W, Chi T-S, et al: Prevalence and associated factors of depressive symptoms among Chinese doctors: a cross-sectional survey. Int Arch Occup Environ Health 83(8):905–911, 2010 20112108

Wasson LT, Cusmano A, Meli L, et al: Association between learning environment interventions and medical student well-being: a systematic review. JAMA 316(21):2237–2252, 2016 27923091

Welner A, Marten S, Wochnick E, et al: Psychiatric disorders among professional women. Arch Gen Psychiatry 36(2):169–173, 1979 420538

West CP, Dyrbye LN, Erwin PJ, et al: Interventions to prevent and reduce physician burnout: a systematic review and meta-analysis. Lancet 388(10057):2272–2281, 2016 27692469

World Health Organization: Z73.0 Burn-out, in International Statistical Classification of Diseases and Related Health Problems, 10th Revision, ICD-10:Version 2016. Geneva, Switzerland, World Health Organization, 2016. Available at: https://icd.who.int/browse10/2016/en. Accessed June 3, 2019.

World Health Organization: Depression and Other Common Mental Disorders: Global Health Estimates. Geneva, Switzerland, World Health Organization, 2017

World Health Organization: QD85 Burn-out, in International Statistical Classification of Diseases and Related Health Problems for Mortality and Morbidity Statistics, ICD-11-MMS, 2018 Version, 11th Revision. Geneva, Switzerland, World Health Organization, 2018. Available at: https://icd.who.int/browse11/l-m/en. Accessed June 3, 2019.

Yaghmour NA, Brigham TP, Richter T, et al: Causes of death of residents in ACGME-accredited programs 2000 through 2014: implications for the learning environment. Acad Med 92(7):976–983, 2017 28514230

Zisook S, Young I, Doran N, et al: Suicidal ideation among students and physicians at a U.S. medical school: a healer education, assessment and referral (HEAR) program report. Omega (Westport) 74:35–61, 2016

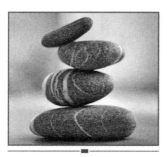

PART III

ENVIRONMENTAL FACTORS
LEADING
TO BURNOUT

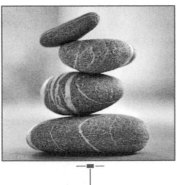

CHAPTER 7

U.S. PHYSICIANS AND WORK-HOME CONFLICT

Sheila LoboPrabhu, M.D.

H. Steven Moffic, M.D.

Physicians often struggle with maintaining a balance between their work life and home responsibilities. Those in the medical profession are characterized by a substantial and intense work commitment. Physicians now report facing a high workload along with low autonomy and job control. Balancing work and home life presents unique challenges for physicians because of long work hours and the ethical priority of patient care. In recent times, changes in society and the practice of medicine have added new challenges such as more female physicians, more two-physician marriages, and the business control of medical practice. For younger physicians, medicine may be less of a calling than in the past and more of a job. In addition, physicians' residency training often coincides with the family founding life stage, potentially leading to high levels of work-family conflict (Fuss et al. 2008).

The meaning of work-life balance is different for every person depending on their life view, career and home aspirations, psychological makeup, and their ability to tolerate the joys and challenges of daily life (Mattock 2015). One definition of *work-life balance* is that it focuses on satisfaction with work and the ability to have a happy life away from work (Alexander and Ballou 2018). As burnout has risen to epidemic levels in physicians, so has dissatisfaction with work-life balance. Although work-life balance is unique for each physician, satisfaction in both areas requires adequate emotional investment and realization of important personal meaning. There is a need for research trials and studies of new interventions to improve work-life balance.

Work-home interference and work-family conflict have been defined as a form of inter-role conflict in which role pressures from the work and family domains are mutually incompatible so that participation in one role is made more difficult by participation in another role (Greenhaus and Beutell 1985). Work-family conflict occurs when experiences in one role interfere with meeting the requirements and achieving effectiveness in the other role (Edwards and Rothbard 2000).

Prior research indicates that in a good marriage, the job does not come first (Kafry and Pines 1980). As a lawyer preparing for a difficult trial described, "It is very important to me to know that I can come home at night and be with someone I love who loves and appreciates me. It keeps intolerable things in perspective" (Pines and Aronson 1988, p. 210). In the other direction, problematic marriages can have a very harmful effect on work, as described by a computer consultant who said, "Now that my marriage is on the rocks, the tension is draining all my creative energy. And being creative is essential to my work" (Pines and Aronson 1988, p. 210).

Traditionally, physicians were thought to have a particular challenge with work-home balance, hence the assumption that one was "married to medicine" because of the unending needs of patients. Most often, that applied to the male physician. Currently, as more female physicians have entered the field, and because younger physicians may have different motivations for becoming a physician, a change may be occurring.

Even so, recent research substantiates that the level of physician dissatisfaction with work-life balance corresponds to the level of burnout, about 40% for each in the year 2012 (Shanafelt et al. 2012). Moreover, measures of both burnout and work-life balance in physicians indicated a deterioration from 2011 to 2014, although that was not so for workers in general (Shanafelt et al. 2015). At its worst, this increase in physician burnout and work-home conflict may contribute to the high rate of physician suicide (Wible 2017).

Physician wellness is a complex, multifaceted concept that encompasses physicians' physical, mental, and emotional health and well-being (Wallace et al. 2009). Research shows that physicians' stress, fatigue, burnout, depression, and general psychological distress negatively affect healthcare systems and patient care (Fahrenkopf et al. 2008; Shanafelt et al. 2005). It is therefore extremely important for physicians to pay attention to their own physical and emotional well-being not only for their own sake but also to provide safe and effective patient care.

It is important to address work-home conflict and its role in adversely affecting physicians' health and wellness. In this chapter, we explore issues of work-life balance and work-home conflict and how they can be a potential cause of physician burnout.

Role Conflict

Role conflict occurs when there are incompatible demands placed on a person, such that compliance with both would be difficult. Excessive demands can be made on the physician both at work and at home.

At work, demands can vary according to physician specialty, academic versus private practice, work settings, work timings, and patient volume. Excessive workplace demands predispose a physician to experiencing role conflict because time limitations prevent the physician from also being able to adequately meet home and family demands. For example, high divorce rates and significant stress are experienced by families of academic surgeons because it is well known that these physicians experience heavy demands on their time and physical energy (Fabri et al. 1989). General internists, who face the heavy demands of frontline care, have higher rates of burnout and lower satisfaction with work-life balance than most specialties. When hospitalists and outpatient general internists were compared, burnout was common in both groups, although the hospitalists were more satisfied with work-life balance because they were more likely than the internists to agree that their work schedule leaves enough time for personal life and family (Roberts et al. 2014). When family medicine residents were asked what their greatest fear or concern is about pursuing a career in academic family medicine, 31% stated "lack of readiness or mentorship" and the second most common response was "work-life balance and burnout" at 17% (Lin et al. 2018).

At home, some examples of stressors likely to create role conflict between work roles and home roles are marriage, pregnancy, childbirth, and caregiving. Demerouti et al. (2012) noted that life stages partly determine career development and therefore the specific working conditions (job demands and job resources) and family conditions (family demands and family resources) that individuals experience at different times in their work life. Work-family conflict occurs when there is dissonance between work and home demands. Young adults experience high inter-role conflict and low facilitation because of high demands and low resources in both life domains, whereas older adults experience the opposite pattern—that is, low conflict and high facilitation because of low demands and high resources in both domains. Individuals in middle adulthood experience high work-family conflict but also high family-work facilitation because of high job demands and resources in both life domains. Integrating life and career stage perspectives and the experience of work-family interface is very practical because it provides a mechanism to make informed decisions about the need for and benefits of work-family programs.

The prevalence of female physicians has been increasing and now equals that of men in medical school. Women are at particular risk for role conflict during the childbearing and caregiving years. Both physical issues (the burden of maternity and childbearing being borne disproportionately by women) and societal expectations (women are more often primary caregivers of the ill and elderly than men) result in heavier home demands on female physicians (Eek and Axmon 2015).

Effects of Work-Home Conflict on the Physician

Work-life conflict can impact both a physician's work and home life.

WORK LIFE

Work-home conflict can have enormous impact on a physician's work performance, resulting in greater risk of medical errors (West et al. 2009), physician distress (West et al. 2011), burnout (Dyrbye and Shanafelt 2011), sickness absenteeism from work (Clays et al. 2009; Jansen et al. 2006), and physician career decisions that affect the adequacy of the physician workforce (Dyrbye et al. 2012). In a study about the mental health of hospital consultants, high job stress was associated with poor mental health; high job satisfaction protects consultants' mental health against the harmful effects of job stress (Taylor et al. 2005).

HOME LIFE

Work-home conflict can also affect a physician's home life. Unequal distribution of home duties along with a heavy total workload has been suggested as an explanation of why women tend to report negative work-home balance to a higher degree than men (Eek and Axmon 2015). However, an imbalance between work and home responsibilities has been associated with suboptimal health in both women and men (Blom et al. 2014; Eek and Axmon 2015). Common issues important to physicians in their home lives are the quality of the relationship with their spouse or significant other and satisfaction in being a parent. In a study in southern California measuring marital and parental satisfaction among 656 male and female married physicians, about half the physicians reported marital satisfaction (63% of male physicians and 45% of female physicians). Two factors were associated with high marital satisfaction: a supportive spouse (odds ratio (OR) 10.37) and role conflict (OR 0.61). Major factors associated with parental satisfaction of married physicians with children were a supportive spouse (OR 2.24), role conflict

(OR 0.35), salaried practice setting (OR 2.14), marriage to a spouse working as a professional (OR 2.14), and marriage to a spouse working as a home-maker (OR 2.33). The number of hours worked was not found to be related to either satisfaction score but rather to an intervening variable: role conflict (Warde et al. 1999). This suggests that although physicians often work long hours, it is not the work hours themselves that affect physician satisfaction. The more detrimental factor than hours worked is the experience of role conflict by the physician. This suggests that when there are incompatible de-mands placed on the physician such that success at work and in home life at the same time is difficult, then physician satisfaction decreases.

CAREER CHOICES

Some of the effects of role conflict on career choices made because of home stressors are discussed in the following subsections.

Childbirth

The Spillover-Crossover Model is used in psychological research to examine the impact of the work domain on the home domain and, consequently, the transference of work-related emotions from the employee to others at home, particularly the partner (Bakker et al. 2009). Spillover effects apply to situa-tions in which there is inter-role conflict. That is, involvement in a work role may impose strain on the family role (work spillover to home). Similarly, ex-cessive home responsibilities can result in home spillover to work by creat-ing strain and time constraints at work. Because people have a limited, fixed amount of resources (e.g., energy, time), problems and compromise in the quality of their work life and home life may arise when different roles draw on these same resources. Grice et al. (2008) found that work-family conflict negatively impacts women's health after childbirth. The ability to change work hours and to take work home were associated with increased home spillover to work (with the negative consequence of the physician's home life interfering with work responsibilities). The ability to take time off was asso-ciated with decreased job spillover to home and therefore less stress for the physician and her family.

Career Changes and Reduction in Hours

In a study about gender differences in resources and negotiation among highly motivated physician-scientists, Holliday et al. (2015) noted a gender gap: female researchers had less access to research space and equipment than male researchers. Also, women were more likely to have asked for a re-duction in clinical hours (24.1% women vs. 19.3% men) and to have raised concerns about unfair treatment (50.2% women vs. 38.2% men). In a study about career changes made by physicians for the sake of their marriage or children, the findings were that more female than male physicians and more younger than older female and male physicians experienced at least moderate levels of role conflict. Younger female and male physicians did not differ in their rates of making a career change for the sake of their marriage, but female physicians from both age cohorts were more likely than male physicians to have made career changes for their children. The most common type of career change made by physicians for marriage or children was a decrease in work hours (Warde et al. 1996).

Career Progress for Women

In a national survey of 862 women in academic medicine, Levinson et al. (1989) found that it is possible for women to combine motherhood with a fulfilling career in academic medicine, but it is difficult to accomplish, and most women (78%) believe that motherhood slows the progress of their careers. Of the study subjects, 72% took no time off before labor and delivery, and 83% were back at work within 12 weeks. In another study by Bering et al. (2018), 801 female physicians were surveyed. The survey showed that 64% of female physicians defer important life decisions in pursuit of their medical career, 86% reported waiting to have children, and 22% reported waiting to get married. In the nondeferring group, 85% of women would choose medicine again as a career, but only 71% of women in the deferment group would do so. Physicians who would choose medicine again stated reasons such as career satisfaction, positive patient interactions, and intellectual stimulation. Those who would not choose medicine again reported poor work-life balance, decreasing job satisfaction, and insurance or administrative burden.

Female leadership in medicine is disproportionately small, likely due to the obstacles to combining work and family (Wietsma 2014). Recently, female medical graduates slightly outnumbered male medical graduates at the time of graduation from medical school. Yet women who enter academic medicine have been less likely to be promoted than men or to serve in leadership positions (Nonnemaker 2000). Some of the barriers to career development include sporadic focus on career advancement, time-consuming child care, women's tendency toward understatement, and the responsibilities of caring for a family (Figueroa 2016). The Institute of Medicine, in its landmark publication *Beyond Bias and Barriers: Fulfilling the Potential of Women in Academic Science and Engineering* (Institute of Medicine et al. 2006), explained why women are underrepresented in academic medicine.

Academic Physicians

In a study of early-career physician researchers who received K08 or K23 National Institutes of Health awards between 2006 and 2009, 74% of physicians responded to the survey, and 1,049 respondents were academic physicians. Women were more likely than men to have domestic partners who were employed full-time (85.6% vs. 44.9%). Among married or partnered respondents with children, women spent 8.5 hours a week more than men on domestic activities. In the subgroup with spouses or domestic partners who were employed full-time, women were more likely to take time off during disruptions of childcare arrangements than men (42.6% vs. 12.4%). Most men's spouses or domestic partners were not employed full-time, which contrasted sharply with the experience of women (Jagsi et al. 2013).

MEDICAL MARRIAGES

A 2004 survey of 603 members of the American Medical Association Alliance (physicians' spouses) indicated high levels of marital adjustment and overall satisfaction with work-life balance. Wives' marital adjustment was affected by the age of the oldest child, their husband's work hours, and wives' work outside the home (Sotile and Sotile 2004).

In 2013, Shanafelt et al. surveyed 1,644 spouses/partners of physicians, and 891 responded. They reported generally high satisfaction with their relationships. The mean time spent with their physician partner each day appeared to be a dominant factor associated with relationship satisfaction and outweighed any specific characteristic of the physician's practice, including specialty, practice setting, and work hours.

A landmark study in 1987 by Gabbard, Menninger, and Coyne showed that, contrary to expectations, the number of hours a physician spends at work did not affect marital satisfaction (Gabbard et al. 1987). Instead, the main conflicts in medical marriages were differences in partners' need for intimacy, perception of problems in the relationship and in each other, and communication styles of the partners. Lack of time because of practice demands seemed to be a complaint serving the function of externalizing conflicts in the marriage onto factors outside the marriage. Shortly after, in 1990, Spendlove et al. studied 116 resident physicians, 106 new attorneys, and the spouses of both groups. They found no differences in marital adjustment between resident physicians and attorneys or between the two spouse groups. In general, the spouses had higher marital adjustment scores than the professionals, and female professionals scored higher than male professionals. The two most important factors associated with adjustment were perceived level of emotional support from one's spouse for one's career and the level of such support given to one's spouse for their career.

In a 2008 American College of Surgeons survey, 7,905 surgeons responded to the survey (Dyrbye et al. 2010). Surgeons whose domestic partner was a physician were younger, newer to practice, and more likely to delay having children and to believe that childrearing had slowed their career advancement. The surgeons were less likely to believe that they had enough time for their personal and family life compared with their colleagues whose domestic partner was a working nonphysician or who were at home and not engaged in outside employment. Surgeons in dual-physician relationships more often experienced a recent career conflict with their domestic partner and a work-home conflict than surgeons whose domestic partners were working nonphysicians. Surgeons whose domestic partner was another surgeon faced even greater challenges in these areas. Surgeons who married or were partnered with another physician were more likely to be depressed and have low quality of life because of their mental health than surgeons whose domestic partners were at home.

In 2009, an appreciative inquiry survey of 25 physicians (10 from dual-physician and 15 from single-physician relationships) showed that four main themes emerged during the qualitative interviews: spouses rely on mutual support in their relationship, spouses recognize the important roles of each family member, spouses share values, and spouses acknowledge the benefit of being a physician to the couple's relationship. These findings show that physicians can identify strategies to navigate the difficult aspects of their lives (Perlman et al. 2015).

PSYCHOLOGICAL FACTORS

When discussing work-home conflict, it is also important to consider why some physicians may experience work-home conflict as more stressful than others. Some examples of individual psychological factors that may play a role include self-esteem, personality traits, and the physician's personal history. There is a strong association between job performance–based self-esteem and work-home conflict (Innstrand et al. 2010). Therefore, individual vulnerability (job performance–based self-esteem) contributes to the explanation of work-home conflict.

Hahn and Dormann (2013) examined the roles of partners and children for employees' psychological detachment from work when they are off work. Employees' and their partners' work-home segmentation preference was associated with employees' psychological detachment from work during their time off. The relationship between partners' work-home segmentation preference and employees' psychological detachment was weaker when there were children in the home. Both employees' and their partners' psychological detachment contributed to employees' well-being. This study showed that physicians' ability to "leave work at the workplace" and engage in psychological detachment from work during their time off can contribute to their well-being.

Work-Home Conflict and Burnout

The four life quadrants in individuals' lives can be considered: career, family, friends, and self (Figueroa 2016). Physicians must place different emphasis on different life quadrants at different life stages to maintain successful work-home balance.

Many physicians are at risk of excessive focus on patient care and other work, given its time-consuming and complex demands. Clark et al. (2014) studied 340 working adults and examined the mechanisms through which workaholism and work engagement impact work-home conflict and enrichment, respectively. They studied the mediating role of positive and negative emotions (e.g., joviality, guilt) in the relationship between workaholism, work engagement, and work-home outcomes. Results showed that positive emotions (particularly joviality and self-assurance) mediate the relationship between work engagement and work-home enrichment. Negative emotions (particularly anxiety, anger, and disappointment) were found to mediate the relationship between workaholism and work-home conflict. Grol et al. (1985) noted that positive feelings about work experienced by general practitioners correlated with more openness to patients, more attention to psychosocial aspects of care, and greater rates of referrals to specialists. However, practitioners' negative feelings correlated with a higher prescription rate and with giving little explanation of treatment to patients. This shows that the way work is experienced by general practitioners correlates with the quality of care that they provide.

Factors negatively affecting work-life balance for physicians are higher number of hours worked (Dyrbye et al. 2012), having to use an electronic health record (Alexander and Ballou 2018), heavy workload, and working under pressure (Mache et al. 2015). Protective factors are age (likely due to better coping strategies based on longer job experience) (Thomas 2009); job flexibility such as working part-time, childcare accommodation, and maternity leave (Demerouti et al. 2001); social support received; and maintaining a sense of community (Mache et al. 2015). In a study of 7,288 physician survey responders from all specialties from the American Physician Masterfile, Dyrbye et al. (2014) noted that work-home conflict within the previous 3 weeks was commonly reported by physicians and their employed partners (44.3% and 55.7%, respectively). Greater work hours for physicians and their employed partners were independently associated with work-home conflict (OR 1.31 and 1.23 for each additional 10 hours worked, respectively). Physicians and partners who had experienced a recent work-home conflict were more likely to have symptoms of burnout (47.1% vs. 26.6% for physicians with and without work-home conflict and 42.4% vs. 23.8% for partners with and without work-home conflict).

In a study about self-reported patient care by 155 emergency physicians, Lu et al. (2015) found that 57.1% of physicians reported burnout, which can be one of the causes of negative feelings. As mentioned in previous chapters, burnout is often considered to be a syndrome of emotional exhaustion, depersonalization, and a sense of low personal accomplishment. High rates of burnout can negatively impact the quality of patient care and result in medication errors, job turnover, absenteeism, low morale, and deterioration of physician health (Dewa et al. 2014; Halbesleben and Rathert 2008). In a study of 960 physicians who answered a mailed survey, measures of burnout strongly predicted career satisfaction or dissatisfaction. The strongest predictor of satisfactory work-life balance and lower rates of burnout was having some control over schedule and hours worked. Physician gender, age, and specialty were not found to be strong independent predictors of career satisfaction, work-life balance, or burnout (Keeton et al. 2007). This national physician survey suggested that physicians can struggle with work-life balance and yet remain highly satisfied with their career (male physicians' rate of reporting of high satisfaction was 79% and female physicians' rate was 76%).

Researchers Arnold Bakker and Evangelia Demerouti developed the Job Demands-Resources Model of employee well-being (Demerouti et al. 2001). The model lists working conditions in two categories: job demands and job resources. *Job demands* are physical or emotional stressors at work such as time pressures, heavy workload, stressful working environment, role ambiguity, emotionally tiring work, and poor relationships. *Job resources* (job positives) are physical, social, and organizational factors that help the employee achieve goals and reduce stress. They include autonomy, strong work relationships, opportunities for advancement, coaching and mentoring, and learning and development. The Job Demands-Resources Model states that when job demands are high and job positives are low, stress and burnout are common. However, good job positives can offset the effects of extreme job demands, and they can encourage motivation and engagement.

Factors associated with burnout are work-home conflict, number of hours worked, nights on call per week, academic rank, and annual income (Dyrbye et al. 2012). Dyrbye et al. (2011a, 2011b) showed that work-home conflicts play a role in burnout and career satisfaction for both male and female physicians. It is notable that not only the presence of work-home conflicts but also how the most recent work-home conflict was resolved was an independent predictor of burnout and career satisfaction for both male and female physicians.

Personality traits such as perfectionism, an exaggerated sense of responsibility, and performance anxiety can also predispose individuals to physician burnout (Oreskovich and Anderson 2013).

Medical staff burnout leads to frequent changes of jobs, withdrawal from medical practice, sickness absenteeism, and conflicts in family life. This suggests that not only does work-home conflict lead to burnout but also that burnout can lead to conflicts in family life. There is therefore a two-way relationship between work-home conflict and burnout.

Another issue to consider is depression in physicians. Nitzsche et al. (2013) studied employees' positive and negative work-home interactions and their association with depressive symptoms and noted that positive work-home interactions were associated with fewer depressive symptoms, and negative work-home interactions were associated with more depressive symptoms. This study has important implications for the prevention of depression in employees in high-stress jobs, such as physicians. It notes the importance of developing strategies aimed at reducing conflict between work and personal life and promoting a positive exchange between these two domains.

Managing Work-Home Conflict

For most people, a cornerstone for well-being is the maintenance of a balanced life (Yellowlees 2018). Whether working long, hard hours or not, there is still an opportunity to balance work, relationships, and other interests. Given the epidemic rate of burnout in physicians, it is crucial to address the aspect of burnout that relates to the individual physician, even if most of the causes of burnout are organizational and related to the workplace system. In this section, we examine which interventions and management strategies can reduce work-home conflict among physicians and thereby reduce vulnerability to burnout.

LEVELS OF INTERVENTION

As burnout started to rise in the general workplace before it did so in medical workplaces, some prevention and mitigation strategies emerged (Pines and Aronson 1988). These were based on the premise that the interaction can go in both directions: burnout at work can spill over to one's personal life, and problems in one's personal life can spill over into work. Conflict between one's work and personal life can affect the relationship with a spouse or partner; conflict can stem from time management issues, meeting the emotional needs of one another, integrating mutual expectations, and determining if there is enough agreement with respective value systems.

Work-home conflict often differs with life stages (Demerouti et al. 2012). For instance, in early adulthood, high demands and low resources are common in both life spheres. Expecting and recognizing these stages can help in making informed decisions about intervention.

Interventions for addressing work-life conflict and subsequent burnout can be discussed as 1) individual and 2) organizational strategies. The interventions for the individual can be examined further by 1) addressing work factors and 2) addressing home factors.

Individual Interventions

Addressing work factors.   The meaning of work-life balance is different for every person (Mattock 2015). Work-life balance should first be addressed in medical school, then later during residency, and throughout a physician's professional life. Addressing work factors such as the need for physicians to engage in self-care at work (e.g., maintaining adequate nutrition and hydration, controlling the caffeine intake that one uses to counteract sleep deprivation) can have important and lasting effects on physicians' well-being and help mitigate the risk of burnout (Brandt 2017). Common strategies to maintain wellness and prevent burnout include building downtime in one's schedule, eliminating unnecessary activities, prioritizing errands, being physically active, and relaxing intermittently. Increasing clerical burden is one of the biggest causes of burnout in medicine. Time-motion studies show that for every 1 hour physicians spend with patients, they spend 1–2 more hours finishing notes, documenting phone calls, ordering tests, reviewing results, responding to patient requests, prescribing medications, and communicating with staff. Most of this work is not reimbursed. Instead it is done as "work after work" at night, on weekends, and even on vacation (Wright and Katz 2018). In addition to the organizational interventions needed to help physicians manage their workday more effectively, more attention paid by each individual physician to effective time management of their busy schedule can result in improved quality of work and home life for physicians.

Addressing home factors.   Physicians also need to pay attention to time management on the individual level and allocate time for activities that are relaxing and rewarding in their home lives. Interestingly, when both partners have careers in the same field, mutual benefit was common (Nye and Hoffman 1963). On the other hand, dual-career marriages face difficult choices regarding whose career comes first (Shanafelt et al. 2013). One intervention for time conflict is for both partners to list their work and home demands side by side and to examine and discuss each other's lists periodically. Spouses and partners of U.S. physicians in a national study by Shanafelt et al. (2013) reported that the amount of time spent with their physician partners each day appears to be a dominant factor associated with relationship satisfaction and overshadows any professional characteristic of the physician's practice including specialty area, practice setting, and work hours. Some of the resiliency found in medical (dual-physician) marriages has been attributed to maintaining flexibility, successfully managing conflict, and making time for communication and intimacy amid demanding careers (Perlman et al. 2015).

A majority of surgeons, who traditionally worked very long hours, felt that their work schedule precluded enough time for personal and family life (Raja and Stein 2014). No wonder that surgeons had a divorce rate of 33% even after being married 30 years. Given the assumption that work and life will never be equal for surgeons, one intervention recommends a work-life budget that needs to be individualized. The steps in creating this budget would include identifying how time is spent now, setting goals to identify long-term objectives, and tracking results. Because the balance is a dynamic one, intermittent review is necessary.

When outside intervention is needed for conflict in couples or families of physicians, formal couples therapy or family therapy is one option. In addition, when available, burnout workshops can be helpful. Such workshops can be done at a workplace or with other couples. The goals of such workshops may include discussion of the concept of burnout, identification of causative stresses, identification of what is under one's control, and development of coping tools.

For those in the caring professions such as teachers, counselors, and health professionals, some specific issues seem to influence work-home conflicts and balance. One common risk for professionals in caring professions is the tendency to provide one-way caring (Skovholt 2001). Partners and friends can be attracted to them because of their caring attitude. An overall self-care strategy focuses on being careful about limiting the number of one-way caring relationships in their personal lives.

Organizational Interventions

At the organizational level, attempts to intervene and manage problems with work-life conflict and burnout have emerged. For instance, a study of family medicine physicians demonstrated that just being aware of work-life balance can be beneficial. Adding simple work-life mindfulness activities provides further benefits (Fortney et al. 2013). Mindfulness-based stress reduction training has five major themes: awareness of thoughts, emotions, bodily sensations, and behavior; increased self-reflection; acceptance and nonjudgment; increased resilience; and relating to others (Verweij et al. 2018).

An initiative by the University of Colorado named Ambulatory Process Excellence (APEX) had medical assistants gather data, reconcile medications, set the agenda for patient visits, and identify opportunities for preventive care. The medical assistant shared this information with the physician or provider and remained in the room to document the visit. Within 6 months after launching APEX, burnout rates among clinicians dropped from 53% to 13%, the rates of preventive patient screenings rose sharply, and practice efficiency improved by three extra patients per doctor per day. The program was cost neutral and yet very successful in terms of physician and patient satisfaction rates (Wright and Katz 2018).

Work management techniques to prevent negative spillover to home life include the Results Only Work Environment (ROWE) initiative (Moen et al. 2013). Designed by two individuals in a human resources department, this initiative encourages supervisors and employees to focus on results and not just time spent on the job. It aims to shift organizational culture so that all employees can control the time, timing, and location of their work in order to maximize productivity while maintaining employee satisfaction and wellness. The key point is for employees to have as much control over their work as practically possible.

Creating flexible work arrangements after childbirth can also have a positive effect on physician satisfaction. Vanek and Vanek (2001) surveyed two community-based private practice groups with a combined 13-years of experience with job sharing and found that a majority of respondents rated job sharing as successful, and most wanted it to continue. Job sharers derived considerable personal benefit from the arrangement and had significantly more positive attitudes toward work than full-time physicians. Job sharing appeared to have little impact on practice parameters.

Specific subgroups of physicians may have greater challenges for avoiding or reducing work-home balance. One such group is female physicians (McMurray et al. 2000). Bering et al. (2018) reported that 64% of female physicians defer important life decisions in pursuit of their medical career. Proposed solutions included support from colleagues and significant others for balancing work and home life. Finding the right job fit is very important. Alternatively, for some women physicians, the assumption that they are not as committed to work as men can cause stress. One female psychiatrist who continued to work while pregnant at week 39 recommended (Budde 2018) the following:

- Providing adequate leave time for residents having children, not only biological mothers but also adoptive parents, same-sex male couples, and birth fathers
- Not assuming that family issues are women's issues
- Reducing male physician harassment of female physicians

Besides what the statistical studies in work-home interaction tell us, individual narratives can portray the challenges in greater depth and variety and with emotionality. One recent physician personal narrative used the metaphor of being "fracked to the core" to explain her journey to get "beyond burnout" (Humikowski 2018). One pediatrician raised the question of whether chasing after work-life balance actually produced more frustration than satisfaction (Schwingshackl 2014). He was reminded of the entrance gate at the Auschwitz concentration camp, which displayed the words "Arbeit macht frei" (work sets you free) and recommended a new approach, which is to try to integrate, rather than separate, all daily activities. Instead of work-life balance, he reframed the question as a life-nature-universe balance. This means, paraphrasing the writer John Irving, "finding a way of life we love and having the courage to live it." Another physician, a plastic surgeon, recommended an honest assessment of what gives one joy in all aspects of life (Bajaj 2018). The joy might come from relationships at work and home, running in the morning with one's dogs, and getting enough sleep.

PSYCHIATRIST WORK-HOME CONFLICT

One might assume that psychiatrists would be better than other physicians at work-home balance because psychiatry makes one more aware of oneself, and perhaps less judgmental, and broadens one's perspective. On the other hand, the necessity for draining emotional and empathic connections with patients may lessen emotional availability in one's home life. One might also assume that psychiatric knowledge about people, relationships, and child development would make for a better home life. However, imposing intrusive psychiatric interpretations onto relationships with loved ones and children may be distancing and demeaning.

Such mixed effects of being a psychiatrist seemed to play out in the children of psychiatrists. Exploring the popular assumption that children of psychiatrists tended to be "crazy" kids, one well-known study answered with a qualified "yes" (Maeder 1989). Interviewing scores of psychiatrists, the investigator found tendencies to be too intrusive in the children's inner lives with interpretations. If a psychiatrist's office was at home, there was fear of violating taboos and competition with patients for attention and love. The result was more "neurotic" adults. Spouses could feel analyzed more than loved.

In the later revisiting of this topic after psychiatry became more biologically oriented, the American Psychiatric Association started to hold an annual workshop on "Children of Psychiatrists" (Dickstein 2016). The adult children of one of this chapter's authors, H.S.M., were invited to the workshop a few years ago and jokingly said that the only psychiatric advice they got was "Don't think about it" from their psychiatrist father. In general, hearing from the children seemed to be inspiring, reassuring, and challenging to the psychiatrist parents present.

Given that the knowledge of psychiatrists can be applied to all aspects of life, might that lead psychiatrists to be more interested in life outside of work (Moffic 2012)? That can lead to more depth in the appreciation of sports, movies, and politics. That may be so, but it is often countered by some degree of isolation. Members of the public fear they will be analyzed by the psychiatrist or, alternatively, want to divulge everything about themselves for a quick consultation. That is why many psychiatrists, when they first meet someone new, do not divulge that they are psychiatrists.

As psychiatrists tend to be more of a blank screen in their work and because confidentiality is so crucial, they tend to write less about their own challenges in work-home balance. Psychiatrists' narratives about themselves are much less common than those of other physicians. One psychiatrist did write about when she was becoming burned out and turned that into a bridge between work and home by setting up a blog called "Freud & Fashion.... Because It's Stylish to Talk About Mental Health, Especially How We Maintain Our Own." Taking this type of public exposure further, Dr. David Goldbloom, a Canadian psychiatrist, writes in his recent bestselling book about a week in his practice (Goldbloom and Bryden 2016). He self-discloses and integrates his life events into a discussion about his professional work in order to emphasize the intersection between the lives of psychiatrists and patients.

Conclusion

Historically, work-home conflict has been a unique challenge for physicians. There may be an ethical contribution to that problem. Although the American Psychiatric Association's *Principles of Medical Ethics* conveys an ethical responsibility to patients, colleagues, society, and oneself in the preamble, there is no mention of an ethical responsibility to care for loved ones (American Psychiatric Association 2013). Providing stable care for loved ones at home can result in a healthy home life and therefore result in peace of mind for the physician. Yet maintaining physician wellness by maintaining a healthy and happy work life and home life is imperative for physicians to continue to provide safe and effective patient care. Reciprocal caring between physicians and their families is a big contributor to physician wellness and therefore to safe patient care. Given the lack of a formalized ethical prioritization of home life, physicians should consider taking a personal work-home ethical oath, as suggested by the authors of this chapter, such as, "I will put the patient first when I am practicing medicine, but put the needs of my loved ones and myself first when I am not practicing medicine."

Marriages between two physicians are especially vulnerable because long work hours and patient needs often leave inadequate time for spouses and a home life. Enough mutual emotional support between spouses helps to mitigate conflict. Finding time for other home-life interests is difficult, yet important, because outside interests may mitigate the detrimental effects of burnout.

Added to these traditional work-life challenges for physicians are the current changes in society and medicine. Female physicians may have unique work-life balance problems if they are also the primary caregiver of children or elderly family members. In medicine, big corporate business has changed the nature of practice so that physicians have less control over their practices, resulting in an increase in workplace burnout. This epidemic rate of burnout can cause home life to become a more important source of meaning and positive support. Yet, on the other hand, home life can become the target of displaced anger at the work obstacles to fulfilling a sense of calling. How younger physicians view a medical career may also produce new home-life concerns and adaptations.

Most, though not all, of the interventions and management of work-home conflicts tend to rely on common sense and be anecdotal. As more attention is paid to physician burnout, there is increasingly more research and innovation, including even reframing the problem and how to combine work and home in new ways. Chapter 13, "Role of Health System Innovation in Preventing Psychiatrist Burnout," contains more information on healthcare systems' innovations to prevent physician burnout. The nature of being a psychiatrist can also add unique considerations to reducing work-home conflict.

KEY POINTS

- Work-home conflict is a unique challenge for physicians because of long work hours and the ethical priority of patient care.
- As burnout has risen to epidemic levels in physicians, so has dissatisfaction with work-life balance.

- Although work-life balance is unique for each physician, satisfaction in both areas requires adequate emotional investment and realization of important personal meaning.

- Changes in society and the practice of medicine have added new challenges to work-life balance, such as the increase in female physicians, more two-physician marriages, and the business control of medical practice.

- For younger physicians, medicine may be less of a calling than in the past and more of a job.

- Psychiatrists seem to have some unique work-home life considerations because of specialized knowledge and expertise in personal psychology, which can be used for benefit or harm.

- There is a need for research trials and studies of new interventions to improve work-home balance.

- Given the lack of a formalized ethical prioritization of home life, physicians should consider taking a personal work-home ethical oath to personally strive to maintain daily work-life balance.

References

Alexander AG, Ballou KA: Work-life balance, burnout, and the electronic health record. Am J Med 131(8):857–858, 2018 29608876

American Psychiatric Association: The Principles of Medical Ethics, With Annotations Especially Applicable to Psychiatry. Arlington, VA, American Psychiatric Association, 2013

Bajaj AK: Work/life balance: it is just plain hard. Ann Plast Surg 80(5S suppl 5):S245–S246, 2018 29596086

Bakker AB, Demerouti E, Burke R: Workaholism and relationship quality: a spillover-crossover perspective. J Occup Health Psychol 14(1):23–33, 2009 19210044

Bering J, Pflibsen L, Eno C, et al: Deferred personal life decisions of women physicians. J Womens Health (Larchmt) 27(5):584–589, 2018 29634448

Blom V, Sverke M, Bodin L, et al: Work-home interference and burnout: a study based on Swedish twins. J Occup Environ Med 56(4):361–366, 2014 24709761

Brandt ML: Sustaining a career in surgery. Am J Surg 214(4):707–714, 2017 28693842

Budde K: Babies and burnout: should being a mom mean giving up ambition? Psychiatric News, Feb 22, 2018

Clark MA, Michel JS, Stevens GW, et al: Workaholism, work engagement and work-home outcomes: exploring the mediating role of positive and negative emotions. Stress Health 30(4):287–300, 2014 23913863

Clays E, Kittel F, Godin I, et al: Measures of work-family conflict predict sickness absence from work. J Occup Environ Med 51(8):879–886, 2009 19667836

Demerouti E, Bakker AB, Nachreiner F, et al: The Job Demands-Resources Model of burnout. J Appl Psychol 86(3):499–512, 2001 11419809

Demerouti E, Peeters MC, van der Heijden BI: Work-family interface from a life and career stage perspective: the role of demands and resources. Int J Psychol 47(4):241–258, 2012 22793870

Dewa CS, Loong D, Bonato S, et al: How does burnout affect physician productivity? A systematic literature review. BMC Health Serv Res 14:325, 2014 25066375

Dickstein LJ: Children of psychiatrists revisited. Psychiatric News. June 28, 2016

Dyrbye LN, Shanafelt TD: Physician burnout: a potential threat to successful health care reform. JAMA 305(19):2009–2010, 2011 21586718

Dyrbye LN, Shanafelt TD, Balch CM, et al: Physicians married or partnered to physicians: a comparative study in the American College of Surgeons. J Am Coll Surg 211(5):663–671, 2010 21035046

Dyrbye LN, Shanafelt TD, Balch CM, et al: Relationship between work-home conflicts and burnout among American surgeons: a comparison by sex. Arch Surg 146(2):211–217, 2011a 21339435

Dyrbye LN, West CP, Satele D, et al: Work/home conflict and burnout among academic internal medicine physicians. Arch Intern Med 171(13):1207–1209, 2011b 21747018

Dyrbye LN, Freischlag J, Kaups KL, et al: Work-home conflicts have a substantial impact on career decisions that affect the adequacy of the surgical workforce. Arch Surg 147(10):933–939, 2012 23117833

Dyrbye LN, Sotile W, Boone S, et al: A survey of U.S. physicians and their partners regarding the impact of work-home conflict. J Gen Intern Med 29(1):155–161, 2014 24043567

Edwards JR, Rothbard NP: Mechanisms linking work and family: clarifying the relationship between work and family constructs. Acad Manage Rev 25(1):178–199, 2000

Eek F, Axmon A: Gender inequality at home is associated with poorer health for women. Scand J Public Health 43(2):176–182, 2015 25504654

Fabri PJ, McDaniel MD, Gaskill HV 3rd, et al: Great expectations: stress and the medical family. 1987 Committee on Issues, Association for Academic Surgery. J Surg Res 47(5):379–382, 1989 2811353

Fahrenkopf AM, Sectish TC, Barger LK, et al: Rates of medication errors among depressed and burnt out residents: prospective cohort study. BMJ 336(7642):488–491, 2008 18258931

Figueroa M: Work-life balance does not mean an equal balance. Front Pediatr 4(18):18, 2016 27014668

Fortney L, Luchterhand C, Zakletskaia L, et al: Abbreviated mindfulness intervention for job satisfaction, quality of life, and compassion in primary care clinicians: a pilot study. Ann Fam Med 11(5):412–420, 2013 24019272

Fuss I, Nübling M, Hasselhorn HM, et al: Working conditions and work-family conflict in German hospital physicians: psychosocial and organisational predictors and consequences. BMC Public Health 8:353, 2008 18840296

Gabbard GO, Menninger RW, Coyne L: Sources of conflict in the medical marriage. Am J Psychiatry 144(5):567–572, 1987 3578565

Goldbloom DS, Bryden P: How Can I Help? A Week in My Life as a Psychiatrist. New York, Simon and Schuster, 2016

Greenhaus JH, Beutell NJ: Sources of conflict between work and family roles. Acad Manage Rev 10(1):76–88, 1985

Grice MM, McGovern PM, Alexander BH: Flexible work arrangements and work-family conflict after childbirth. Occup Med (Lond) 58(7):468–474, 2008 18667390

Grol R, Mokkink H, Smits A, et al: Work satisfaction of general practitioners and the quality of patient care. Fam Pract 2(3):128–135, 1985 4043602

Hahn VC, Dormann C: The role of partners and children for employees' psychological detachment from work and well-being. J Appl Psychol 98(1):26–36, 2013 23106684

Halbesleben JR, Rathert C: Linking physician burnout and patient outcomes: exploring the dyadic relationship between physicians and patients. Health Care Manage Rev 33(1):29–39, 2008 18091442

Holliday E, Griffith KA, De Castro R, et al: Gender differences in resources and negotiation among highly motivated physician-scientists. J Gen Intern Med 30(4):401–407, 2015 25112462

Humikowski CA: Beyond burnout. JAMA 320(4):343–344, 2018 30043069

Innstrand ST, Langballe EM, Espnes GA, et al: Personal vulnerability and work-home interaction: the effect of job performance-based self-esteem on work/home conflict and facilitation. Scand J Psychol 51(6):480–487, 2010 20338010

Institute of Medicine, National Academy of Sciences, National Academy of Engineering, et al: Beyond Bias and Barriers: Fulfilling the Potential of Women in Academic Science and Engineering. Washington, DC, National Academies Press, 2006

Jagsi R, Griffith KA, Stewart A, et al: Gender differences in salary in a recent cohort of early career physician-researchers. Acad Med 88(11):1689–1699, 2013 24072109

Jansen NW, Kant IJ, van Amelsvoort LG, et al: Work-family conflict as a risk factor for sickness absence. Occup Environ Med 63(7):488–494, 2006 16698806

Kafry D, Pines A: The experience of tedium in life and work. Hum Relat 33(7):477–503, 1980

Keeton K, Fenner DE, Johnson TR, et al: Predictors of physician career satisfaction, work-life balance, and burnout. Obstet Gynecol 109(4):949–955, 2007 17400859

Levinson W, Tolle SW, Lewis C: Women in academic medicine. Combining career and family. N Engl J Med 321(22):1511–1517, 1989 2811971

Lin S, Nguyen C, Walters E, et al: Residents' perspectives on careers in academic medicine: obstacles and opportunities. Fam Med 50(3):204–211, 2018 29537463

Lu DW, Dresden S, McCloskey C, et al: Impact of burnout on self-reported patient care among emergency physicians. West J Emerg Med 16(7):996–1001, 2015 26759643

Mache S. Bernberg M, Vitzthum K, et al: Managing work-family conflict in the medical profession: working conditions and individual resources as related factors. BMJ Open 5(4):e006871, 2015 25941177

Maeder T: Children of Psychiatrists and Other Psychotherapists. New York, Harper and Row, 1989

Mattock SL: Leadership and work-life balance. J Trauma Nurs 22(6):306–307, 2015 26574942

McMurray JE, Linzer M, Konrad TR, et al: The work lives of women physicians: results from the physician work life study. J Gen Intern Med 15(6):372–380, 2000 10886471

Moen P, Fan W, Kelly EL: Team-level flexibility, work-home spillover, and health behavior. Soc Sci Med 84:69–79, 2013 23517706

Moffic HS: Once a psychiatrist, always a psychiatrist? Psychiatric Times, July 25, 2012

Nitzsche A, Jung J, Pfaff H, et al: Employees' negative and positive work-home interaction and their association with depressive symptoms. Am J Ind Med 56(5):590–598, 2013 22996944

Nonnemaker L: Women physicians in academic medicine: new insights from cohort studies. N Engl J Med 342(6):399–405, 2000 10666431

Nye FI, Hoffman LW (eds): The Employed Mother in America. Chicago, IL, Rand McNally, 1963

Oreskovich M, Anderson J: Physician personalities and burnout. Bulletin of the American College of Surgeons, June 1, 2013. Available at: http://bulletin.facs.org/2013/06/personalities-and-burnout/#.WzQcbMuWzIU. Accessed June 27, 2018.

Perlman RL, Ross PT, Lypson ML: Having it all: medicine and a family. Mayo Clin Proc 90(6):713–715, 2015 26046406

Pines A, Aronson E: Career Burnout: Causes and Cures. New York, Free Press, 1988

Raja S, Stein SL: Work-life balance: history, costs, and budgeting for balance. Clin Colon Rectal Surg 27(2):71–74, 2014 25067921

Roberts DL, Shanafelt TD, Dyrbye LN, et al: A national comparison of burnout and work-life balance among internal medicine hospitalists and outpatient general internists. J Hosp Med 9(3):176–181, 2014 24435981

Schwingshackl A: The fallacy of chasing after work-life balance. Front Pediatr 2:26, 2014 24745004

Shanafelt TD, West C, Zhao X, et al: Relationship between increased personal well-being and enhanced empathy among internal medicine residents. J Gen Intern Med 20(7):559–564, 2005 16050855

Shanafelt TD, Boone S, Tan L, et al: Burnout and satisfaction with work-life balance among US physicians relative to the general US population. Arch Intern Med 172(18):1377–1385, 2012 22911330

Shanafelt TD, Boone SL, Dyrbye LN, et al: The medical marriage: a national survey of the spouses/partners of US physicians. Mayo Clin Proc 88(3):216–225, 2013 23489448

Shanafelt TD, Hasan O, Dyrbye LN, et al: Changes in burnout and satisfaction with work-life balance in physicians and the general US working population between 2011 and 2014. Mayo Clin Proc 90(12):1600–1613, 2015 26653297

Skovholt TM: The Resilient Practitioner: Burnout Prevention and Self-Care Strategies for Counselors, Therapists, Teachers, and Health Professionals. Boston, MA, Allyn and Bacon, 2001

Sotile WM, Sotile MO: Physicians' wives evaluate their marriages, their husbands, and life in medicine: results of the AMA-Alliance Medical Marriage Survey. Bull Menninger Clin 68(1):39–59, 2004 15113033

Spendlove DC, Reed BD, Whitman N, et al: Marital adjustment among housestaff and new attorneys. Acad Med 65(9):599–603, 1990 2400480

Taylor C, Graham J, Potts HW, et al: Changes in mental health of UK hospital consultants since the mid-1990s. Lancet 366(9487):742–744, 2005 16125591

Thomas KW: Intrinsic Motivation at Work: What Really Drives Employee Engagement. San Francisco, CA, Bernett Koehler, 2009

Vanek EP, Vanek JA: Job sharing as an employment alternative in group medical practice. Med Group Manage J 48(3):20–24, 2001 11383405

Verweij H, van Ravesteijn H, van Hooff MLM, et al: Does mindfulness training enhance the professional development of residents? A qualitative study. Acad Med 93(9):1335–1340, 2018 29697426

Wallace JE, Lemaire JB, Ghali WA: Physician wellness: a missing quality indicator. Lancet 374(9702):1714–1721, 2009 19914516

Warde C, Allen W, Gelberg L: Physician role conflict and resulting career changes. Gender and generational differences. J Gen Intern Med 11(12):729–735, 1996 9016419

Warde CM, Moonesinghe K, Allen W, et al: Marital and parental satisfaction of married physicians with children. J Gen Intern Med 14(3):157–165, 1999 10203621

West CP, Tan AD, Habermann TM, et al: Association of resident fatigue and distress with perceived medical errors. JAMA 302(12):1294–1300, 2009 19773564

West CP, Shanafelt TD, Kolars JC: Quality of life, burnout, educational debt, and medical knowledge among internal medicine residents. JAMA 306(9):952–960, 2011 21900135

Wible P: Physician Suicide Letters. Eugene, OR, Pam Wible, M.D., 2017

Wietsma AC: Barriers to success for female physicians in academic medicine. J Community Hosp Intern Med Perspect July 31, 2014 25147633 Epub

Wright AA, Katz IT: Beyond burnout: redesigning care to restore meaning and sanity for physicians. N Engl J Med 378(4):309–311, 2018 29365301

Yellowlees P: Addressing physician health and well-being is patient safety issue. Psychiatric News, June 14, 2018

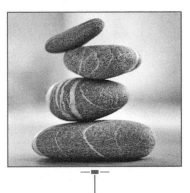

CHAPTER 8

ELECTRONIC HEALTH RECORDS AND PHYSICIAN BURNOUT

Stewart Babbott, M.D., FACP

Philip J. Kroth, M.D., M.Sc.

Since the enactment of the American Recovery and Reinvestment Act (ARRA) and the Health Information Technology for Economic and Clinical Health (HITECH) Act in 2009, the rate of adoption of health information technologies (HITs), including the electronic health record (EHR), has significantly increased. These federal acts defined the "meaningful use" programs that provided more than $30 billion in funding for incentive payments to individual physicians and healthcare organizations for adopting EHRs with certain prescribed functionalities. Today, the majority of U.S. physicians use EHRs in most clinical settings. Despite the potential of this technology to improve the quality, efficiency, and the costs of healthcare, many physicians believe that these promises have not been realized and that EHRs are a significant cause of increasing stress and burnout in the medical profession.

In addition to the many administrative and documentation tasks, many physicians believe that the presence of the EHR in the clinical setting interferes with the doctor-patient relationship because physicians pay more attention to the computer screen than the patient sitting in the exam room. These technologies have had unintended consequences on the physician-patient relationship as well as the job satisfaction of physicians. Verghese (2008, p. 2749) coined the term "iPatient," saying "What is tragic about tending to the iPatient is that it can't begin to compare with the joy, excitement, intellectual pleasure, pride, disappointment and lessons in humility that trainees [and practicing physicians] might experience by learning from the real patient's body examined at the bedside."

Rosenthal and Verghese (2016, p. 1814) amplified the importance of finding—and, if needed, rediscovering—meaning in our work. Speaking of the hospital setting, they noted the changes in practice and technology as well as the disconnect between the patient and physician: "The majority of what we define as 'work' takes place away from the patient, in work rooms and on computers."

In keeping the focus on patients and their care, Kommer (2018) noted how EHRs do not facilitate documentation of the patient's narrative, insights into the patient, and clinical reasoning for their care. It is these and other tensions that challenge physicians. In this chapter, we describe the profound way in which the adoption of modern health information and communications technologies causes increased stress and burnout of their users.

Rise of Electronic Health Record Adoption

Figure 8–1 shows the adoption rates of EHRs from surveys conducted by the Office of the National Coordinator for Health Information Technology (ONC) of "basic systems" and "certified systems" from 2008 to 2015. The ONC defines a basic EHR as one that includes patient demographics, problem lists, medication lists, lab results, radiology reports, and computerized provider order entry for medications, as well as results management in the form of reports for viewing radiology, lab, and diagnostic test results. A certified EHR is one that meets the technological capability, functionality, and security requirements specified by the Department of Health and Human Services.

The originally touted benefits of EHRs included interoperability between systems of care, computerized decision support that would drive quality and efficiency improvements, and access to patient data for better population health. Despite widespread adoption, many of these benefits are yet to be realized. Halamka and Tripathi (2017, p. 907) noted, "burdensome requirements imposed costs on providers and vendors without offering sustained benefit. These deficiencies were manifested in five key areas: usability, workflow, innovation, interoperability, and patient engagement."

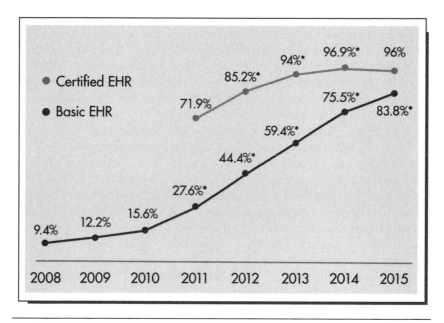

FIGURE 8–1.   Electronic health record (EHR) adoption rates by U.S. physicians.

*Significantly different from previous year ($p<0.05$).

Source.   Reprinted from JaWanna H, Pylylpchuk Y, Searcy T, et al.: "Adoption of Electronic Health Record Systems Among U.S. Non-Federal Acute Care Hospitals: 2008–2015." *ONC Data Brief,* no. 35, May 2016, Figure 1. Available at: https://dashboard.healthit.gov/evaluations/data-briefs/non-federal-acute-care-hospital-ehr-adoption-2008-2015.php. Accessed November 7, 2018.

The rise of EHR adoption is a proxy for a more profound change in the entire practice environment.

EHRs are extremely disruptive technologies. They divert the focus off the patient and onto the computer screen, allow tasks to be shifted onto the physician, and increase the cognitive load during the documentation process. The mere presence of an EHR in the exam room changes the "doctor-patient" dynamic to a "doctor-patient-computer" dynamic. Indeed, in a recent study, the majority of physicians report that maintaining eye contact with the patient has become much more difficult when an EHR is involved (Kroth et al. 2018).

During the paper era, the original purpose of the chart was primarily for documentation of care. The presence of the EHR has facilitated expansion to include other purposes, many of which are beyond the immediate care of the patient. For example, the billing function is now inextricably linked to the form of the encounter or procedure note, increasing note length and complexity. Centers for Medicare and Medicaid Services and other agencies now require the electronic reporting of a raft of quality metrics, and researchers want to mine patient data for new discoveries. These added purposes of the patient record usually require structured text, and the physician's role has been expanded to include entry of an increasing amount of required structured data. EHRs have also enabled new functions that old paper records systems could not perform such as e-prescribing. This has facilitated a shifting of more task burdens onto physicians who have to know where to route a prescription when they are e-prescribing. In and of itself, this is not a substantial additional burden, but when performed multiple times per day and accompanied by multiple other EHR-related processes that also increase task load, the total increased task burden on physician EHR users is significant.

The adoption of the EHR did not come with additional time in physicians' schedules to accommodate the new data entry and task burdens. This causes what has been termed "self-acceleration" or "hyperwork," where the only option open to workers asked to do more during the same time interval without any additional support is to try to speed up or work harder (Viviers et al. 2008). It is similar to workers on an assembly line that is sped up to produce more cars per hour without giving the workers additional support, better tools, or retooling of the line. The faster line may work for a time, but eventually, the rate of quality defects will increase as will the rate of workers' burnout.

Prevalence of Physician Burnout

The physician burnout rate not only is significantly higher than the burnout rate of the general working U.S. population but is also significantly increasing while the rate for the general population is flat (Shanafelt et al. 2015). A national sample of U.S. physicians surveyed in 2014 using the Maslach Burnout Inventory (Maslach et al. 1996) to measure physician burnout levels showed that 54.4% of physicians noted at least one symptom of burnout. This percentage increased from a similar survey performed in 2011 that showed 45.5% of physicians reporting at least one symptom of burnout. The general working U.S. population surveyed at the same time showed a burnout rate of 28% in both 2011 and 2014.

There were substantially different rates of burnout reported by specialty groups, with rates greater in "front-line specialties" such as family medicine, internal medicine, and emergency medicine. Burnout rates were also greater in midcareer physicians. Psychiatry had 40.7% of psychiatrists reporting burnout in 2011 and significantly more (47.6%) reporting burnout in 2014. Both of these are less than the mean burnout rate for physicians in general.

Linzer et al. (2016) studied academic general internal medicine physicians and found that 67% reported high stress, 38% reported burnout, 57% described too much EHR home time, 49% noted low work control, 58% reported very busy or chaotic workplaces, and 62% reported high documentation time pressure. High stress and poor work control were significantly associated with burnout.

Measuring Burnout and Why Burnout Matters

Measuring burnout, stress, and satisfaction is essential to effect change. One resource is the National Academy of Medicine Action Collaborative on Clinician Well-Being and Resilience (https://nam.edu/initiatives/clinician-resilience-and-well-being), which has a tool kit and other materials on physician burnout.

There is a growing literature highlighting how physician burnout can have negative consequences on the health of physicians and for their practice organizations (Shanafelt and Noseworthy 2017; Wallace et al. 2009). Physician burnout can negatively impact physicians' personal relationships and mental health and can be associated with increased alcohol and substance abuse.

Burnout increases physician turnover, which in turn is very costly to practice groups and to health systems. Costs of increased turnover include more recruitment costs, lost revenue and additional cross-coverage costs during recruitment, decreased billing while new physicians learn a new practice, and the costs to the practice group and to the patients because of lost continuity. Estimated physician replacement costs are between $500,000 and $1,000,000 per physician who leaves the practice (Shanafelt et al. 2017).

There are direct links between burnout and the career plans of U.S. physicians. Sinsky et al. (2017) showed that independent predictors of intent to reduce clinical work hours or leave practice included burnout, dissatisfaction with work-life integration, and dissatisfaction with the EHR. One in five physicians in this study reported that it was likely or definite that they would reduce their clinical hours in the next 12 months. More striking was that 27% reported they would likely or definitely leave their current practice position in the next 24 months. Statistically significant independent predictors of intent to reduce clinical work hours and leave current practice included burnout (odds ratio [OR} 1.81), dissatisfaction with work-life integration (OR 1.65), and dissatisfaction with the EHR (OR 1.44). Reducing physician burnout is clearly an important goal in maintaining a healthy and adequately sized physician workforce.

Electronic Health Records and Practice Factors

PRACTICE ENVIRONMENT CHANGES AND RELATIONSHIP TO THE ELECTRONIC HEALTH RECORD

The practice environment is continually changing, and often in profound ways. In 2009, Wallace and colleagues noted rapid changes in medicine, such as increased patient care demands, remuneration issues, growing bureaucracy with medical practice, increased accountability, conflict between the needs of the organization and patients, and decreased physician autonomy. Friedberg et al. (2013) also noted fluctuating reimbursement, new care delivery models, and more widespread use of EHRs.

Highlighting these pressures, Linzer et al. (2009) reported on physician reactions and care quality related to working conditions in primary care. They found that more than half of physicians reported time pressure during clinic visits, and 48% noted that their work pace was chaotic. Twenty-six percent reported burnout, and 78% reported low control over their work. Adverse workflow (time pressure and chaotic environments), low work control, and unfavorable organizational culture were strongly associated with low physician satisfaction, high stress, burnout, and intent to leave practice.

We noted in the section "Rise of Electronic Health Record Adoption" how the EHR has enabled the patient record to have more purposes than just continuity of care and how many of the new purposes have significantly increased the task burden on physicians. This issue, combined with how EHRs take physician focus away from the patient, are in a sense the perfect storm for increasing stress and burnout in the practice environment. Zulman et al. (2016), in an article titled "Evolutionary Pressures on the Electronic Health Record: Caring for Complexity," noted that care is increasingly complex. Specifically, the content of care, processes of care, reporting of outcomes, and particularly coordination of care have greatly increased. In all this, the patients, their stories, and the context of their care can get lost. Zulman et al. call for the design of EHRs that reduce physicians' documentation burden and for the reduction of billing, coding, and other tangential functions.

SPECIFIC STUDIES ON THE ELECTRONIC HEALTH RECORD AND PHYSICIAN RESPONSES

In 2014, Babbott and colleagues analyzed the relationship between EHR functionality levels and burnout. They identified three levels of EHR functionality (low, moderate, and high) based on the number of EHR functions available. Compared with the low-functionality group, there were higher stress and lower satisfaction scores among the moderate group. Physicians in the high-functionality group reported lower satisfaction compared with the low-functionality group. For the time pressure measure (time needed/time scheduled), only the high-functionality group reported time pressure associated with more burnout, dissatisfaction, and intent to leave practice. These findings suggest that 1) as EHRs gain functionality levels and become more complex, physician stress will increase and job satisfaction will decrease, and 2) for EHRs with moderate numbers of functions, physicians may rely on paper or other systems that add to time and administrative burdens.

In 2013, Friedberg and colleagues addressed factors affecting physician satisfaction. Regarding EHRs, physicians liked the remote access to patient information and that EHRs show the potential to improve care. However, physicians faced a number of challenges: poor EHR usability, time-consuming data entry, interference with face-to-face patient care, inefficient and less fulfilling work content, inability to exchange health information between EHR products, degradation of clinical documentation (specifically, using templated notes), and the high costs of implementation.

Shanafelt et al. (2016) assessed EHR use and the relationship between physician burnout and job satisfaction. The mean responses for physicians who used EHRs showed that only 36% were satisfied or very satisfied, with approximately 33% of psychiatrists noting this level of satisfaction. Regarding the same satisfaction measures for clerical burden, the mean was only 37% of physicians (43% of psychiatrists). Those physicians who used patient portals, EHRs, and computerized physician order entry (CPOE) had lower satisfaction with clerical burden and higher rates of burnout. In a multivariable analysis, physicians using CPOE had approximately 30% higher risk of burnout after adjusting for other factors. Shanafelt et al. (2016, p. 844) concluded, "Physicians who used EHRs or CPOE were at higher risk for burnout regardless of whether they were or were not satisfied with their EHR or CPOE."

CLERICAL BURDEN

Sinsky et al. (2016) reported on allocation of physician time in ambulatory practice for four specialties (family medicine, internal medicine, cardiology, and orthopedics) in four states. They used a direct-observation method and physician diaries to assess clerical burden. Looking at work activities during office hours, they found that physicians spent 33% of their time on direct clinical face time and 49% on EHR and desk work. Of the 49.2%, 38.5% was spent on documentation and review tasks, 6.3% on test results, 2.4% on medications, and 2% on other orders. The remaining time was spent on personal breaks, transit time, and other tasks. They found that for every hour physicians provided in direct clinical face-to-face time with patients, nearly 2 additional hours were spent on EHR and desk work within the workday, and another 1–2 hours of personal time each night were spent doing additional computer or other clerical work.

Arndt et al. (2017) used EHR event logs to assess family physicians' time in the EHR during and after scheduled work hours. In an 8 A.M.–6 P.M. work day, these physicians spent 4.5 hours in the EHR and the remainder on non-EHR-related activities. They spent an additional 1.4 hours per day working at home, equating to a total workday of 11.4 hours. Two-thirds of EHR time was spent in clerical or in-box work. The authors reinforced the point that both the number and variety of clinical tasks has increased and that the EHR is not the whole story. They suggested addressing documentation support, order entry, asynchronous patient care (care not in the presence of the patient), and communication as promising areas for practice redesign.

In 2018, Kroth and colleagues conducted physician focus groups at three institutions with different commercial EHRs to determine what design features are associated with physician stress and burnout. Almost all participants had multiple criticisms of current EHR design and reported many unintended consequences of HIT and EHR use. These included 1) excessive data entry requirements, 2) inefficiently designed user interfaces, 3) insufficient health information exchange from outside institutions, 4) information overload, and 5) interference with the patient-physician relationship as factors associated with EHR use, and as well as 6) ergonomic problems due to traditional clinical architecture poorly retrofitted with HIT equipment.

PSYCHIATRY-SPECIFIC VIEWS AND LITERATURE

As noted earlier, psychiatrists have reported less burnout, less satisfaction with EHRs in general, and greater satisfaction related to their amount of clerical burden when compared with the reported mean satisfaction for all specialties (Shanafelt et al. 2015). It is likely that the same forces driving increased complexity in EHRs such as quality improvement, cost reduction, and billing no doubt affect psychiatrists as well. Domaney et al. (2018) reported a pilot study of psychiatry residents and faculty looking at EHR use and burnout. Using the Maslach Burnout Inventory (Maslach et al. 1996), Domaney et al. (2018, p. 650) noted emotional exhaustion correlated with hours spent on the EHR outside of work, total EHR time, and hours reviewing EHR notes. Interestingly, "the magnitude of the correlation between EHR use and emotional exhaustion was stronger than those for current clinical service hours of exercise, amount of sleep or hours spent on enjoyable activities."

PRACTICE FACTORS: THE DOCTOR-PATIENT-COMPUTER RELATIONSHIP

The fact that the computer screen directly competes for eye contact and disrupts the doctor-patient relationship is one of the most troublesome EHR design elements that physicians report as challenging (Kroth et al. 2018). Toll (2012, p. 2498) noted that the physician's full focus on the patient during the encounter is a "simple act of caring [which] creates a connection between two human beings...now the computer has entered this timeless dynamic as a third player." The use of the computer has changed how we practice, "pick and click according to the EHRs' pathways, rather than by following the patterns of learning and thinking we have internalized over years of training and practice...and, this takes time."

Alkureishi et al. (2016) performed a systematic review of the impact of EHR use on the patient-physician relationship and communication. Studies addressing physician focus noted negative communication behaviors with EHR use, including interrupted patient and doctor speech patterns, increased gaze shifts, episodes of multitasking, and low rates of sharing the computer screen with patients. However, for patient perceptions, the majority of studies reported no change in overall patient satisfaction, communication, or the patient-doctor relationship.

Lee et al. (2016) interviewed 108 patients on their positive and negative impressions of the EHR use by physicians. Overall, 90% of patients were satisfied with physician EHR use and 59% noted that the computer had a positive effect on their relationship; 85% of patients' perceptions of EHR use were positive, mostly around aspects of clinical care. Of the negative perceptions, most were around communications functions and physical focus. One possible explanation is that patients value the enhanced communication that EHRs can offer (e.g., patient portals, email). However, physicians often feel there can be an additional time burden if enough time is not built into their workday to support using these newer patient communication channels and meeting newer patient expectations for rapid responses to their electronic messages.

One approach to enhance communication is to ensure that the clinical space is designed for optimal patient-physician interaction. This can involve two screens, a movable screen or tablet depending on the exam room layout. Another approach is to bring the computer into the conversation to help with patient understanding of clinical information and to provide an opportunity for education. Setting expectations for doctor-patient communication in the clinical encounter and the uses of EHRs can be helpful. This can include a mix of direct face-to-face interaction, leaving the computer aside initially, and then more directed screen focus as data are reviewed and tasks are performed. Similarly, it is important to set expectations for how the patient and the physician will interact electronically outside the exam room. This includes the types of messages, responses, and response time expectations. Lee et al. (2016) noted that many physicians are already trained in these techniques, and they proposed a curriculum to meet these needs.

Models for Burnout and Sustainability

The EHR and issues of burnout have many possible etiologies, including personal, practice, and organizational factors. The following three models show how these factors relate to each other and help the psychiatrist frame observations or concerns in larger contexts. By the end of this chapter, you should be able to use these models in your conversations with stakeholders and practice leaders in defining approaches, gathering data, and developing initiatives to address burnout.

MINIMIZING ERROR, MAXIMIZING OUTCOME (MEMO) STUDY MODEL

Linzer et al. (2009) addressed the impact of organizational climate on physicians and their patients. In this study, work conditions such as poor organizational culture, time pressure, chaotic work pace, and lack of work control were strongly associated with adverse physician reactions (Figure 8–2). As we consider the EHR, each of the listed work conditions could be related to the EHR itself or to how it is implemented and used. For example, when a new EHR is adopted, practice structure might change with how patients flow through the practice; workflow may be subject to increased time pressure; job characteristics can change, accompanied by less control; and the organizational culture may change with the new needs of the EHR and related policies. Physicians' reactions to the EHR can vary.

RECIPROCITY OF WELLNESS MODEL OF PHYSICIAN WELL-BEING

The Reciprocity of Wellness Model of Physician Well-Being (Bohman et al. 2017) has three reciprocal domains of physician well-being: 1) personal resilience, 2) efficiency of practice, and 3) culture of wellness. These three factors are equal in importance, and each reciprocally influences the others (Figure 8–3). Regarding the EHR, this model can suggest a balance for physicians to be resilient in their work with the technology, for the practice to be efficient and provide support, and for the culture of wellness in recognizing that the EHR itself and the requisite changes in practice are significant stressors for the physicians and all team members. Benefits of this model are in recognizing that physicians have a role in modulating and addressing some personal factors and responses, that the practice and the administrators have roles in ensuring efficiency of the practice system, and all stakeholders, including those in management, have roles in developing and sustaining a culture of wellness.

MAYO CLINIC MODEL FOR KEY DRIVERS OF BURNOUT AND ENGAGEMENT

The Mayo Clinic Model for Key Drivers of Burnout and Engagement by Shanafelt and Noseworthy (2017) highlights seven "driver dimensions" that are key to addressing engagement and decreasing burnout (Figure 8–4).

This model considers factors at the individual, practice, organization, and national levels and reinforces what other models have shown: there are multiple stakeholders, responses, approaches, and actions, and all have roles (Figure 8–5). This model specifically highlights two higher levels: 1) the organization in which the physician may practice and 2) the national advocacy or health policy level. Although many physicians can feel that advocacy or action at these higher levels is difficult or nearly impossible at the individual or practice levels, it is encouraging that much work continues by national professional organizations, such as the American Medical Association (AMA) and the National Academy of Medicine (NAM).

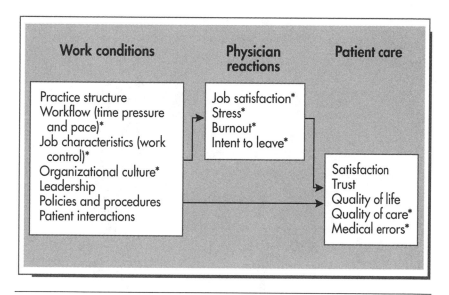

FIGURE 8–2. Minimizing Error, Maximizing Outcome study conceptual model.

*Related to hypotheses for the current topic.

Source. From *Annals of Internal Medicine,* Linzer M, Manwell LB, Williams ES, et al: "Working Conditions in Primary Care: Physician Reactions and Care Quality." 151(1):28–36, W6–9. Copyright © 2009 American College of Physicians. All Rights Reserved. Reprinted with the permission of American College of Physicians, Inc.

SYNTHESIS OF THE MODELS AND HOW TO CONSIDER THEM IN THE SETTING OF THE ELECTRONIC HEALTH RECORD

These models, taken individually or in combination, help to place the physician, their practice, and their organization in a larger context. Because stakeholders can feel overwhelmed, it can be hard to "know where you are" or how to "get started." These models can facilitate that process. Very importantly, these models can help physicians and their business leaders to have a common understanding—whether or not they agree—on how to envision the issues around physician well-being, stress, burnout, and intent to leave and where to target interventions. All these models underscore how the EHR and related technologies are inextricably linked to a variety of other factors such as governmental policy, clinic process, technology design, and physician culture.

1. The *Minimizing Error, Maximizing Outcome (MEMO) Model* offers specifics on practice factors, reactions by physicians, and outcomes. This reaches

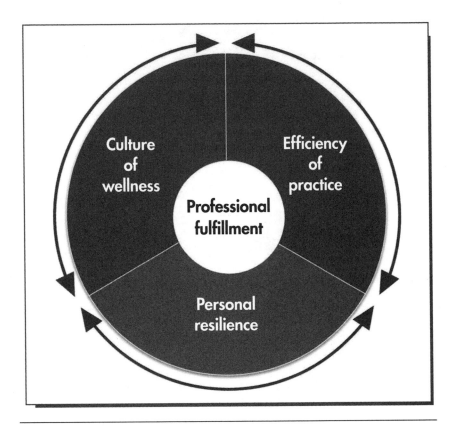

FIGURE 8–3.   Stanford Model for Physician Well-Being.

Culture of wellness = organizational work environment, values and behaviors that pro-mote self-care, personal and professional growth, and compassion for ourselves, our colleagues, and our patients; efficiency of practice = workplace systems, processes, and practices that promote safety, quality, effectiveness, positive patient and colleague in-teractions, and work-life balance; personal resilience = individual skills, behaviors, and attitudes that contribute to physical, emotional, and professional well-being.

Source.   Reprinted from Bohman B, Dyrbye L, Sinsky CA: "Physician Well-Being: The Reciprocity of Practice Efficiency, Culture of Wellness, and Personal Resilience." NEJM Catalyst, August 7, 2017. Property of Stanford University, Stanford, Califor-nia. Copyright © 2016. Used with permission.

the clinical levels very specifically and therefore provides more ways in which one can understand elements of the practice and address them.

2. The *Reciprocity Model* offers three linked and reciprocal key compo-nents for which stakeholders can acknowledge their roles in physician well-being. Related to the EHR, there is a role for physician resilience in the face of increasing demands. However, there is a limit to this expecta-tion. The domains of efficiency of practice—which can be fully function-

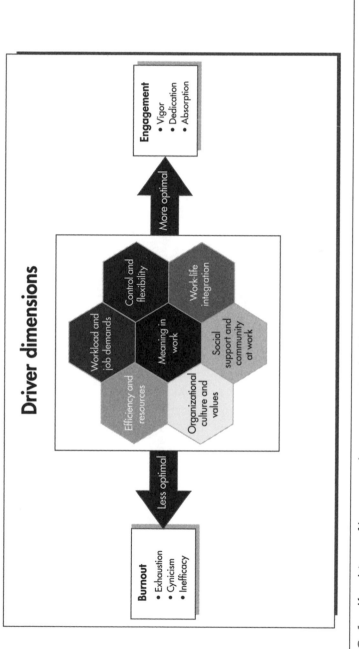

Driver dimensions

- Workload and job demands
- Control and flexibility
- Efficiency and resources
- Meaning in work
- Work-life integration
- Organizational culture and values
- Social support and community at work

Less optimal

More optimal

Burnout
- Exhaustion
- Cynicism
- Inefficacy

Engagement
- Vigor
- Dedication
- Absorption

FIGURE 8–4. Key drivers of burnout and engagement in physicians.

Source. Reprinted from *Mayo Clinic Proceedings*, 92(1), Shanafelt TD, Noseworthy JH, "Executive Leadership and Physician Well-Being: Nine Organizational Strategies to Promote Engagement and Reduce Burnout," pp. 129–146, Copyright 2017, with permission from Elsevier.

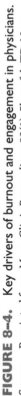

Drivers of burnout and engagement in physicians	Individual factors	Work unit factors	Organization factors	National factors

Workload and job demands	• Specialty
	• Practice location
	• Decision to increase work to increase income
		• Productivity expectations
		• Team structure
		• Efficiency
		• Use of allied health professionals
			• Productivity targets
			• Method of compensation
			  - Salary
			  - Productivity based
			• Payer mix
				• Structure reimbursement
				  - Medicare/Medicaid
				  - Bundled payments
				  - Documentation requirements

Efficiency and resources	• Experience
	• Ability to prioritize
	• Personal efficiency
	• Organizational skills
	• Willingness to delegate
	• Ability to say "no"
		• Availability of support staff and their experience
		• Patient check-in efficiency/process
		• Use of scribes
		• Team huddles
		• Use of allied health professionals
			• Integration of care
			• Use of patient portal
			• Institutional efficiency:
			  - EHR
			  - Appointment system
			  - Ordering systems
			• How regulations interpreted and applied
				• Integration of care
				• Requirements for:
				  - Electronic prescribing
				  - Medication reconciliation
				  - Meaningful use of EHR
				• Certification agency facility regulations (JCAHO)
				• Precertifications for tests/treatments

Meaning in work	• Self-awareness of most personally meaningful aspect of work
	• Ability to shape career to focus on interests
	• Doctor–patient relationships
	• Personal recognition of positive events at work
		• Match of work to talents and interests of individuals
		• Opportunities for involvement
		  - Education
		  - Research
		  - Leadership
			• Organizational culture
			• Practice environment
			• Opportunities for professional development
				• Evolving supervisory role of physicians (potentially less direct patient contact)
				• Reduced funding
				  - Research
				  - Education
				• Regulations that increase clerical work

	Individual	Work unit	Organization	National
Culture and values	• Personal values • Professional values • Level of altruism • Moral compass/ethics • Commitment to organization	• Behavior of work unit leader • Work unit norms and expectations • Equity/fairness	• Organization's mission - Service/quality vs profit • Organization's values • Behavior of senior leaders • Communication/ messaging • Organizational norms and expectations • Just culture	• System of coverage for uninsured • Structure reimbursement - What is rewarded • Regulations
Control and flexibility	• Personality • Assertiveness • Intentionality	• Degree of flexibility: - Control of physician calendars - Clinic start/end times - Vacation scheduling - Call schedule	• Scheduling system • Policies • Affiliations that restrict referrals • Rigid application practice guidelines	• Precertifications for tests/ treatments • Insurance networks that restrict referrals • Practice guidelines
Social support and community at work	• Personality traits • Length of service • Relationship-building skills	• Collegiality in practice environment • Physical configuration of work unit space • Social gatherings to promote community • Team structure	• Collegiality across the organization • Physician lounge • Strategies to build community • Social gatherings	• Support and community created by medical/specialty societies
Work-life integration	• Priorities and values • Personal characteristics - Spouse/partner - Children/dependents - Health issues	• Call schedule • Structure night/weekend coverage • Cross-coverage for time away • Expectations/role models	• Vacation policies • Sick/medical leave • Policies - Part-time work - Flexible scheduling • Expectations/role models	• Requirements for: - Maintenance certification - Licensing • Regulations that increase clerical work

FIGURE 8–5. Drivers of burnout and engagement with examples of individual, work unit, organization, and national factors that influence each driver.

EHR = electronic health record; JCAHO = Joint Commission on Accreditation of Healthcare Organizations (now known as The Joint Commission). *Source.* Reprinted from *Mayo Clinic Proceedings,* 92(1), Shanafelt TD, Noseworthy JH, "Executive Leadership and Physician Well-Being: Nine Organizational Strategies to Promote Engagement and Reduce Burnout," pp. 129–146, Copyright 2017, with permission from Elsevier.

ing EHRs, support for EHR use, and well-supported and efficient practice models—are directly and equally linked. So too is the culture of wellness, which requires communication, teamwork, shared understanding, and supportive leadership.

3. The *Mayo Clinic Key Drivers Model* offers four levels of focus (individual, practice, organization, and national levels) and more detail on drivers of burnout and satisfaction. For EHRs specifically, the model shows how each of the levels can have roles in addressing EHR and practice issues. Importantly, this shows how national organizations and large practice organizations can play roles in advocacy.

Interventions and Approaches

Calls for collaboration to reduce EHR-related stress include the collaboration of the vendor as well as regulatory and payment organizations. As the literature suggests and the models highlight, there are many practice issues that can relate directly or indirectly to the EHR and clinical practice. Measurements of well-being, stress, and burnout are essential in defining issues and assessing program outcomes. A number of tools based on the specific measurement goals are available (Dyrbye et al. 2018; Linzer et al. 2015b; Maslach et al. 1996). In the subsections that follow, we explore five approaches for individual, practice, organization, national policy, and vendor/institutional liaison engagement.

INDIVIDUAL APPROACHES

There are measures that individual physicians can take to help mitigate the stress induced by EHR use and reduce their chances of burnout. Individual resiliency can help mitigate a significant portion of the stress caused by EHR use. Exercise, resiliency training, setting clear work-life boundaries, talking with colleagues, and eating a healthy diet are all helpful coping strategies reported by physicians struggling with EHR-related stress (Kroth et al. 2018).

A number of approaches include mindfulness and mindfulness-based stress reduction (Beckman et al. 2012; Epstein and Krasner 2013; Krasner et al. 2009). In a study using semistructured interviews of 200 German physicians about approaches to fostering resilience, Zwack and Schweitzer (2013) noted three dimensions on how to foster resilience: 1) job-related gratification derived from treatment interactions; 2) practices such as leisure-time activities, self-demarcation, limitation of working hours, and continuous professional development; and 3) attitudes such as acceptance of professional and personal boundaries, a focus on positive aspects of work, and personal reflexivity.

Although physicians may bemoan taking EHR training, some physicians report a positive effect on EHR-related stress when they make the time for periodic EHR retraining. Some clinics have formalized reoccurring meetings during protected time where physicians and other clinic staff share helpful "tricks and hints" approaches to working more efficiently with the EHR and with the clinic process. This kind of group activity can also provide a venue for physicians and clinic staff to vent frustrations and brainstorm possible solutions. Stevens et al. (2017) described designing individualized EHR learning plans for clinicians. The authors used direct observation and EHR use logs to design specific learning plans to meet the needs of individual clinicians. Specialty professional societies and national organizations such as the AMA (see StepsForward, available at https://www.stepsforward.org/modules/physician-burnout) and the NAM (Dyrbye et al. 2018) offer support for individuals and practices.

PRACTICE-LEVEL APPROACHES

In 2013, Sinsky and colleagues studied 23 high-functioning practices, looking at innovations that could facilitate joy in practice and mitigate physician burnout. They noted problems such as "great amounts of time spent documenting and complying with administrative and regulatory requirements," for which innovations noted were scribing, assistant order entry, and standardized prescription renewal. They found another problem to be "computerized technology that pushes more work to the physician," for which innovations included in-basket management by designated team members and verbal messaging between team members (p. 274).

Linzer et al. (2014) proposed "10 bold steps" to prevent burnout. They noted that institutional metrics, work conditions, career development, and self-care were integral to preventing burnout. Regarding the EHR, they emphasized the importance of the following practice approaches: increasing visit length, including "desktop slots" (time dedicated in the clinical schedule to address patient care issues such as calls, labs, and refills), measuring workloads, and creating an organizational dashboard to monitor and continuously measure these variables. These practice approaches address physician concerns about work expectations, workload, and adequate time and support for practice and the use of EHRs in general. These approaches have some applicability to psychiatric practice as well.

The Healthy Work Place study reported that practice-level interventions, such as improved communication, collaboration on workflow redesign, and quality-improvement projects directed at physician concerns, were able to improve burnout, dissatisfaction, and retention (Linzer et al. 2015b). In addition, scribing, assistant order entry, and standardized prescription renewal are practice-based innovations thought to be helpful in reducing physician burnout and increasing the joy of practice (Sinsky et al. 2013). As mentioned previously, EHR technology has facilitated task shifting of existing (and newly EHR-created) tasks onto physicians. System-level interventions that either provide support to physicians to accomplish the added tasks or to shift the added physician tasks to other clinic personnel are helpful.

Calls for change from the platform of practice to these higher organizational levels include those of Linzer et al. (2015a), who call for the "end of the 15–20 minute primary care visit." The authors begin their article with an aphorism: "We can do it fast, we can do it well, we can do it cheap. Pick two." Linzer et al. note that, given the time pressures of the office visit, it is very difficult to meet all three measures of providing quick, good-quality, and low-cost healthcare all at the same time, and they discuss problems experienced by patients and primary care providers. They highlight changes in practice, increase in tasks, fee for service models of care, and EHRs and suggest approaches to address these critical issues, including practice redesign (local or practice level) and advocacy for payment reform (national level).

ORGANIZATION-LEVEL APPROACHES

In 2008, the Institute for Healthcare Improvement defined the "Triple Aim" with these three goals: 1) improving the individual experience of care, 2) improving the health of populations, and 3) reducing the cost of healthcare. Bodenheimer and Sinsky (2014) defined the "Quadruple Aim," adding a fourth aim: *improving the work-life of healthcare providers.* They noted that the well-being of the healthcare team is a prerequisite for the Triple Aim and reinforced the importance of support for highly functioning teams. From the EHR perspective, they noted the importance of team documentation for care, assistance with order entry, prescription processing, and charge capture. The fourth aim is also described as *finding joy and meaning in work* and how doing so improves the experience of providing care (Sikka et al. 2015). Sikka et al. (2015, p. 609) noted that "the precondition for restoring joy and meaning is to ensure that the workforce has physical and psychological freedom from harm, neglect and disrespect." Although the fourth aim does not specifically address EHR-related issues, if embraced by a practice, the need to discuss and address EHR issues would be inevitable.

As mentioned in the section "Measuring Burnout and Why Burnout Matters," the consequences of burnout can be costly for an organization. It is important that leadership is aware of these costs and finds objective ways to measure, monitor, and manage them. Leadership is obviously more willing to act when a process or organizational change that reduces EHR-related stress also saves the organization money. Positioning the goal of reducing physician stress in this manner sets up a "win-win" solution of sorts and is an approach that most leaders will seriously consider. In a *Health Affairs Blog* entry, "Physician Burnout Is a Public Health Crisis: A Message to Our Fellow Health Care CEOs," Noseworthy et al. (2017) noted the reasons and consequences for burnout, including the role of technology and EHRs, with an 11-point call to action that includes addressing the burden of EHR on all users, monitoring clerical burden, and enhancing team-based models of care. The NAM has a similar national call to address burnout as a threat to safe, high-quality care (Dyrbye et al. 2017).

NATIONAL POLICY APPROACHES

National professional organizations are addressing these issues, including the NAM (Dzau et al. 2018) and the many organizations that are members of well-being and advocacy initiatives. Under the auspices of the NAM, Ommaya et al. (2018) issued a position paper titled "Care-Centered Clinical Documentation in the Digital Environment: Solutions to Alleviate Burnout." A recent charter on physician well-being noted organizational commitments to well-being, including the use of quality improvement strategies to improve technology and the physician environment and to reduce administrative burden (Thomas et al. 2018).

Over the past decade, U.S. federal health policy has created an almost insatiable hunger for more data as the requirements for data reporting have increased. The most recent examples include the HITECH Act of 2009 and the Medicare Access and CHIP Reauthorization Act of 2015 (MACRA). In fact, the average length of clinical notes has essentially doubled since enactment of HITECH (Downing et al. 2018). Physicians outside the United States are more likely to report satisfaction with their EHRs, where clinical documentation is significantly smaller and contains much less information in support of billing and compliance (Downing et al. 2018). If U.S. health policy continues to increase data-reporting requirements as with HITECH and MACRA, the data entry burden on individual physicians and healthcare organizations will likely not decrease. U.S. health policy has unintentionally been a major force behind the increase in the physician documentation burden and therefore is a major contributor to the rate of physician burnout. It is clear that advocacy around reducing federal-level documentation requirements, and perhaps including required reporting on physician working conditions and burnout, is going to be essential in mitigating the burnout problem.

VENDOR/INSTITUTIONAL LIAISON APPROACHES

In addition to existing measures of well-being, stress, and burnout, new metrics have been proposed. DiAngi et al. (2017) recommend six new practice metrics to improve professional fulfillment: work after work (the time spent outside the scheduled day performing clinically related tasks), click counts, teamwork, being present, fair pay, and regulatory balance.

Most commercial EHRs capture data on how all physicians use the EHR in the form of usage logs. These logs capture down to the mouse click exactly how physicians and others are using the EHR. Healthcare systems can use the log data to identify physician users who are struggling by comparing average performance on specific task types of individual users to that of group, department, and national averages. Those who, for example, require significantly more mouse clicks or screen transitions than the average can be given special help with training or other support. Usage data can also be employed to improve the design of EHR user interfaces by reducing the average number of clicks and screen transitions for common EHR tasks such as prescription writing.

Currently, these data are typically available only to the EHR vendors and to institutional leadership. From a patient and physician standpoint, making these data more widely available would likely support efforts to better support physicians working to reduce burnout. National efforts could be created to assess and compare the efficiency of design of EHR systems for standardized tasks such as prescription writing, note creation, and patient allergy documentation. Currently, EHR vendors are not cooperating to standardize user interfaces for standardized tasks, although the aviation industry does this for flight deck design where issues of safety are involved.

An example of assessment of the work environment in which vendors have a role is provided by O'Malley et al. (2015); EHRs were assessed regarding support for primary care teamwork. In a study of practices that were part of patient-centered medical homes, they assessed practice teamwork. Positive findings for facilitating communication included instant messaging, task management software, and creation of evidence-based templates for symptom-specific data collection. However, areas of challenge included lack of integrated care management software and care plans, poor practice registry functionality, poor interoperability, and inadequate ease of tracking patient data over time. They called on vendors to address these and similar issues.

Outcomes of Interventions to Address Burnout

West et al. (2016) performed a meta-analysis of interventions to prevent and reduce physician burnout. They identified effective individual-focused strategies such as mindfulness-based approaches, stress management training, and small-group programs. Organizational approaches included duty-hour requirements and locally developed clinical work process modifications. The next steps include further assessment of which approaches are best for specific populations. On the basis of the models presented, this report addresses more of the individual and practice factors rather than the larger organizational and national advocacy approaches. All are important to advance the field of physician well-being in general and for those using EHRs in particular.

Conclusion

Physician burnout is a complex and multifaceted problem that is going to require a complex and multifaceted solution. There is no one solution that is going to solve the problem. We describe multiple levels of the U.S. healthcare system where interventions will be required in a coordinated manner if we are to solve the burnout problem. In this chapter, we focus on how EHR and other health information technologies are one of the major facets of the problem, and we propose some potential solutions.

Obviously, such a complex and many-faceted solution will not be implemented quickly and will require the active participation of those who work on all levels of our healthcare system. What is at stake is more than just the health, well-being, and efficiency of our physician workforce, it is the health and well-being of all the patients we serve.

KEY POINTS

- EHR technology deployment has proven to be extremely disruptive and is inextricably linked to changes in clinic and physician work processes, the regulatory environment, and physician culture.

- The presence of the EHR in the clinical environment has enabled the increase in the number of clerical tasks performed by physicians, including new tasks made possible only by the EHR itself; many of these tasks are for purposes beyond patient care.

- Physicians using EHRs with a high number of functions experience stress, with more time pressure to do the work compared with the time allotted for that work.

- Physicians note that they experience stress when they work with systems with electronic patient portals and those with computerized physician order entry.

- The clerical burden for physicians is significant, with one study showing that physicians spend 2 hours on computer and clerical activities for every hour of face-to-face time with a patient in the workday and then an additional 1–2 hours at night on practice activities.

- The doctor-patient-computer relationship feels more strained to the physician than to the patient; both need to acknowledge the presence and uses of technology and maintain a focus on interpersonal professional relationships.

- The Quadruple Aim, which includes physician well-being as a quality indicator, is evidence of the gradual move to recognize the role that well-being and burnout play in physicians' lives.

- Conceptual models for burnout/satisfaction and placing the EHR and practice in context can be helpful in developing the next steps for personal or organizational advocacy and change.

- The contribution to the physician burnout problem by EHR technology is a multifaceted and complex problem that is going to require solutions that address the problem at the individual physician, practice, organization, policy, and EHR vendor levels.

References

Alkureishi MA, Lee WW, Lyons M, et al: Impact of electronic medical record use on the patient-doctor relationship and communication: a systematic review. J Gen Intern Med 31(5):548–560, 2016 26786877

Arndt BG, Beasley JW, Watkinson MD, et al: Tethered to the EHR: primary care physician workload assessment using EHR event log data and time-motion observations. Ann Fam Med 15(5):419–426, 2017 28893811

Babbott S, Manwell LB, Brown R, et al: Electronic medical records and physician stress in primary care: results from the MEMO Study. J Am Med Inform Assoc 21(e1):e100–e106, 2014 24005796

Beckman HB, Wendland M, Mooney C, et al: The impact of a program in mindful communication on primary care physicians. Acad Med 87(6):815–819, 2012 22534599

Bodenheimer T, Sinsky C: From triple to quadruple aim: care of the patient requires care of the provider. Ann Fam Med 12(6):573–576, 2014 25384822

Bohman B, Dyrbye L, Sinsky CA: Physician well-being: the reciprocity of practice efficiency, culture of wellness, and personal resilience. NEJM Catalyst, August 7, 2017. Available at: https://catalyst.nejm.org/physician-well-being-efficiency-wellness-resilience. Accessed October 24, 2018.

DiAngi YT, Lee TC, Sinsky CA: Novel metrics for improving professional fulfillment. Ann Intern Med 167(10):740–741, 2017 29052698

Domaney NM, Torous J, Greenberg WE: Exploring the association between electronic health record use and burnout among psychiatry residents and faculty: a pilot survey study. Acad Psychiatry 42(5):648–652, 2018 29785625

Downing NL, Bates DW, Longhurst CA: Physician burnout in the electronic health record era: are we ignoring the real cause? Ann Intern Med 169(1):50–51, 2018 29801050

Dyrbye LN, Shanafelt TD, Sinsky CA, et al: Burnout among health care professionals: a call to explore and address this under-recognized threat to safe, high-quality care. National Academy of Medicine discussion paper. NAM Perspectives, July 5, 2017. Available at: https://nam.edu/wp-content/uploads/2017/07/Burnout-Among-Health-Care-Professionals-A-Call-to-Explore-and-Address-This-Underrecognized-Threat.pdf. Accessed October 24, 2018.

Dyrbye LN, Meyers D, Ripp J, et al: A pragmatic approach for organizations to measure health care professional well-being. National Academy of Medicine discussion paper. NAM Perpsectives, 2018. Available at: https://nam.edu/a-pragmatic-approach-for-organizations-to-measure-health-care-professional-well-being. Accessed October 1, 2018.

Dzau VJ, Kirch DG, Nasca TJ: To care is human—collectively confronting the clinician-burnout crisis. N Engl J Med 378(4):312–314, 2018 29365296

Epstein RM, Krasner MS: Physician resilience: what it means, why it matters, and how to promote it. Acad Med 88(3):301–303, 2013 23442430

Friedberg MW, Chen PG, Van Busum KR et al: Factors Affecting Physician Professional Satisfaction and Their Implications for Patient Care, Health Systems, and Health Policy. Santa Monica, CA, RAND Corp, 2013

Halamka JD, Tripathi M: The HITECH Era in retrospect. N Engl J Med 377(10):907–909, 2017 28877012

Kommer CG: Good documentation. JAMA 320(9):875–876, 2018 30193280

Krasner MS, Epstein RM, Beckman H, et al: Association of an educational program in mindful communication with burnout, empathy, and attitudes among primary care physicians. JAMA 302(12):1284–1293, 2009 19773563

Kroth PJ, Morioka-Douglas N, Veres S, et al: The electronic elephant in the room: physicians and the electronic health record. JAMA Open 1(1):49–56, 2018

Lee WW, Alkureishi MA, Ukabiala O, et al: Patient perceptions of electronic medical record use by faculty and resident physicians: a mixed methods study. J Gen Intern Med 31(11):1315–1322, 2016 27400921

Linzer M, Manwell LB, Williams ES, et al: Working conditions in primary care: physician reactions and care quality. Ann Intern Med 151(1):28–36, W6–9, 2009 19581644

Linzer M, Levine R, Meltzer D, et al: 10 bold steps to prevent burnout in general internal medicine. J Gen Intern Med 29(1):18–20, 2014 24002633

Linzer M, Bitton A, Tu SP, et al: The end of the 15–20 minute primary care visit. J Gen Intern Med 30(11):1584–1586, 2015a 25900539

Linzer M, Poplau S, Grossman E, et al: A cluster randomized trial of interventions to improve work conditions and clinician burnout in primary care: results from the Health Work Place Study (HWP). J Gen Intern Med 30(8):1105–1111, 2015b

Linzer M, Poplau S, Babbott S, et al: Worklife and wellness in academic general internal medicine: results from a national survey. J Gen Intern Med 31(9):1004–1010, 2016 27138425

Maslach C, Jackson S, Leiter M: Maslach Burnout Inventory Manual, 3rd Edition. Palo Alto, CA, Consulting Psychologists Press, 1996

Noseworthy J, Madara J, Cosgrove D, et al: Physician burnout is a public health crisis: a message to our fellow health care CEOs. Health Affairs, March 28, 2017. Available at: https://www.healthaffairs.org/do/10.1377/hblog20170328.059397/full/. Accessed October 24, 2018.

O'Malley AS, Draper K, Gourevitch R, et al: Electronic health records and support for primary care teamwork. J Am Med Inform Assoc 22(2):426–434, 2015 25627278

Ommaya AK, Cipriano PF, Hoyt DB, et al: Care-centered clinical documentation in the digital environment: solutions to alleviate burnout. National Academy of Medicine discussion paper. NAM Perspectives, January 29, 2018

Rosenthal DI, Verghese A: Meaning and the nature of physicians' work. N Engl J Med 375(19):1813–1815, 2016 27959650

Shanafelt TD, Noseworthy JH: Executive leadership and physician well-being: nine organizational strategies to promote engagement and reduce burnout. Mayo Clin Proc 92(1):129–146, 2017 27871627

Shanafelt TD, Hasan O, Dyrbye LN, et al: Changes in burnout and satisfaction with work-life balance in physicians and the general U.S. working population between 2011 and 2014. Mayo Clin Proc 90(12):1600–1613, 2015 26653297

Shanafelt TD, Dyrbye LN, Sinsky C, et al: Relationship between clerical burden and characteristics of the electronic environment with physician burnout and professional satisfaction. Mayo Clin Proc 91(7):836–848, 2016 27313121

Shanafelt T, Goh J, Sinsky C: The business case for investing in physician well-being. JAMA Intern Med 177(12):1826–1832, 2017 28973070

Sikka R, Morath JM, Leape L: The Quadruple Aim: care, health, cost and meaning in work. BMJ Qual Saf 24(10):608–610, 2015 26038586

Sinsky CA, Willard-Grace R, Schutzbank AM, et al: In search of joy in practice: a report of 23 high-functioning primary care practices. Ann Fam Med 11(3):272–278, 2013 23690328

Sinsky C, Colligan L, Li L, et al: Allocation of physician time in ambulatory practice: a time and motion study in 4 specialties. Ann Intern Med 165(11):753–760, 2016 27595430

Sinsky CA, Dyrbye LN, West CP, et al: Professional satisfaction and the career plans of US physicians. Mayo Clin Proc 92(11):1625–1635, 2017 29101932

Stevens LA, DiAngi YT, Schremp JD, et al: Designing an individualized EHR learning plan for providers. Appl Clin Inform 8(3):924–935, 2017 30027541

Thomas LR, Ripp JA, West CP: Charter on physician well-being. JAMA 319(15):1541–1542, 2018 29596592

Toll E: A piece of my mind. The cost of technology. JAMA 307(23):2497–2498, 2012 22797449

Verghese A: Culture shock—patient as icon, icon as patient. N Engl J Med 359(26):2748–2751, 2008 19109572

Viviers S, Lachance L, Maranda MF, et al: Burnout, psychological distress, and over-work: the case of Quebec's ophthalmologists. Can J Ophthalmol 43(5):535–546, 2008 18982028

Wallace JE, Lemaire JB, Ghali WA: Physician wellness: a missing quality indicator. Lancet 374(9702):1714–1721, 2009 19914516

West CP, Dyrbye LN, Erwin PJ, et al: Interventions to prevent and reduce physician burnout: a systematic review and meta-analysis. Lancet 388(10057):2272–2281, 2016 27692469

Zulman DM, Shah NH, Verghese A: Evolutionary pressures on the electronic health record: caring for complexity. JAMA 316(9):923–924, 2016 27532804

Zwack J, Schweitzer J: If every fifth physician is affected by burnout, what about the other four? Resilience strategies of experienced physicians. Acad Med 88(3):382–389, 2013 23348093

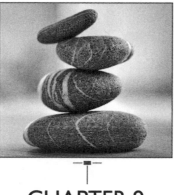

CHAPTER 9

PHYSICIAN SATISFACTION AND BURNOUT AT VARIOUS CAREER STAGES

Luis T. Sanchez, M.D.
Gary Chinman, M.D.

In this chapter, we focus on the stages of a physician's career and their relevance to personal and professional satisfaction, including their association with the burnout phenomenon. Satisfaction is gained when personal, work, and career expectations are met, contributing to well-being, happiness, and acceptance of personal/work aspirations and goals. Being satisfied can be gender, family, age, and career-stage dependent. Contributory work factors can include the right mix of responsibilities, a balanced workload, support, mentoring, career growth, and leadership opportunities. Physicians also value autonomy, a competitive income, and reasonable benefits if employed by an organization.

Psychiatrists focus their expertise on those patients affected by mental health issues and are trained to have compassion for their patients, which often involves an understanding of the life circumstances and dilemmas faced by patients. In this process of caring for others, psychiatrists may tend to ignore their own self-care and wellness, thereby putting their own health at risk. Even though psychiatrists, possibly more than other specialists, have both the opportunity and obligation for self-reflection, and have access to clinical supervision and psychotherapy, they can still be vulnerable to personal and professional stresses that contribute to burnout. They can become demoralized and devalued, experiencing the burnout symptoms of emotional exhaustion, depersonalization, and a sense of meager personal accomplishment and dissatisfaction (West et al. 2018). In addition to their own burnout, psychiatrists are often exposed to burnout in their medical colleagues and may be obligated to ensure that these colleagues seek appropriate assistance so that patients are protected and safe (Massachusetts Board of Registration in Medicine 2018).

The phenomena of physician satisfaction and burnout are not mutually exclusive but can co-occur and often do. For example, psychiatrists or doctors can feel fulfilled by their medical work, believing that their clinical interventions have meaningful and positive impact on their patients' lives, while also experiencing work fatigue related to bureaucratic, regulatory, and other demands. In these situations, the clinicians' capacity to experience gratification from the clinical improvement of their patients may also render them more vulnerable to the nonclinical requirements of their work. However, these phenomena are depicted as distinct in this chapter, although we acknowledge they can coexist.

In this chapter, we highlight career stages and their potential contributors to burnout and well-being (Table 9–1 illustrates these changes and contributors) and correlate these professional stages to Erik Erikson's (1950) stages of psychosocial development, where applicable. Family of origin, preadolescence, adolescence, high school, and college experiences have relevance to the later medical career. Vignettes that capture the career stage–related dilemmas and satisfactions associated with burnout and professional fulfillment are also included. In addition to the Eriksonian stages of development, each stage of a physician's career also seems to bring about ethical challenges (Table 9–2 illustrates these stages). One framework to consider with these ethical dilemmas regarding physician satisfaction and burnout and their potential effects on patient care follows similar stages of moral development as depicted by Kohlberg (1981). Healthcare ethics are of paramount importance to the work of physicians (American Medical Association 2016) and integral to each physician's stage of moral development and values clarification.

Physician Health

Physician health programs (PHPs) are an important resource for all physicians. Almost every state has a PHP, as do the Canadian provinces. Often

TABLE 9–1. Contributors to satisfaction and burnout

Career stage	Satisfaction	Burnout
Student/resident	Contentment with medicine as a career choice	Uncertainty about a medical career
	Enjoyment of the work	Overwhelmed by the work
	Resilience in response to stress	Anxiety/depression in response to stress
Early career	Job stability	Dissatisfaction with medicine
	Satisfaction with job choice	Dissatisfied with psychiatry
	Work-life balance	Overwhelmed by work
	Resilience	Anxiety/depression
Mid career	Work-life balance	Clinical/administrative burdens
	Sense of being productive	Cynicism about achievements, struggles
	Vibrant family/personal life	Isolation/loneliness
Senior phase	Enjoyable career	Emotional distress
	Well-being and wellness	Marital/relationship conflicts
	Financial stability	Financial problems
	Healthy relationships	Isolation/loneliness
	Productive life	Depression/substance abuse
	Planned retirement	Medical and/or cognitive impairments

thought of as programs for physicians with primarily substance use disorders, they offer additional services, including the promotion of physician health and wellness and the prevention and remediation of burnout.

It is important for psychiatrists to be aware of the functioning of PHPs as a referral source for those physicians in distress. PHPs have the mission of providing services to physicians, and often medical students, for a range of health-related illnesses, including substance use disorders, mental health issues, physical illnesses, behavioral problems, and cognitive concerns (DuPont et al. 2009a). Additionally, many programs are available to assist with addictions, including gambling, sexual, eating, and, more recently, internet addictions. Physicians are either self-referred or referred by concerned colleagues, hospitals, or medical licensing boards for an assessment and referral for treat-

TABLE 9–2.   **Stages of development**

Career stage	Erikson stage	Outcomes
Student/resident	5, Identity/confusion	"Who am I"
		Sense of self
		Establishing a work identity
Early career	6, Intimacy/isolation	Developing caring relationships
		Commitment to others
Mid career	7, Generativity/stagnation	Usefulness
		Accomplishments
		Contributions to society
Senior phase	8, Integrity/despair	Successful life
		Acceptance of self
		Wisdom

ment. Although the functioning of one PHP can vary from another, the PHP can provide a confidential setting for the physician or medical student to share stresses, concerns, and frustrations with their experience of medicine and to discuss options for assistance. PHPs are becoming more available to physicians, residency programs, clinics, and hospitals to engage physicians and trainees early on regarding issues of burnout and to provide support and services (Krall et al. 2012).

Physician Satisfaction

As in other specialties, contributors to professional and personal satisfaction include the psychiatrist's professional competence, personal self-care, and adherence to the delivery of excellent and ethical care. It is a challenge to contend with the emotional intensity of clinical illnesses while maintaining an empathic stance with neither underinvolvement nor overinvolvement. This balanced stance requires the psychiatrist to be emotionally fit, clinically competent, and unencumbered by impairments.

Psychiatrists can work in a variety of settings, which is another unique aspect separating our work from that of most other specialties. Broadly, these settings can be inpatient, outpatient, private practice, consultative, hospital based, clinic based, or administrative. This broad range of settings allows for job change if the psychiatrist becomes dissatisfied or experiences burnout.

On psychiatric inpatient units, which typically have acutely or chronically mentally ill patients, psychiatrists often provide care to those with suicidal or homicidal ideation. Also, restraint and seclusion of patients is common and accompanied by monitored adherence to rules and regulations. In addition, physicians and staff are often at risk for harm by patients.

On the opposite end of the physical infrastructure, solo private practice requires simply an office and two chairs. That apparent simplicity, however, can mask the actual complexity of private practice, which requires the practitioner to listen extremely well, interact therapeutically with the patient, accommodate to clinical improvement, and maintain critically important boundary behaviors, always with ethical professionalism. Adding to the challenge of solo private practice is the sparse opportunity for collegial support and supervision, which can contribute to isolation. This, in turn, can advance the development of burnout, boundary violations, and an overall compromised practice.

The ascendancy of the electronic health record (EHR) and its problems for practitioners are well known. Although it affords more efficient retrieval of information and improves collaboration with other providers, it can also contribute to the expansion of work hours by requiring practitioners to finish clinical documentation late at night or on weekends. The arrival of the EHR in American hospitals coincided with increasing administrative burdens, paperwork, shorter patient visits, and increased clinical productivity demands, all of which exacerbate provider overload and the risk of burnout.

Also of major concern is the current reimbursement system. Hospital or clinic salaries may be straightforward, but many salaried psychiatrists also see private patients and bill them directly. It has been estimated that almost half of all American psychiatrists in private outpatient practice are not on private health insurance panels (Bishop et al. 2014). The well-known reasons involve the wish to avoid laborious completion of insurance forms and the burden of contacting insurance companies for payments, all made worse by reimbursement rates that are lower than the private sector. The health system as a whole suffers from fewer psychiatrists who are available for the insured, and the cash-only fee-for-service practice is limited to only those patients who can afford such fees. This raises quality issues regarding diversity of practice by excluding those with social determinant of health problems, e.g., poverty, affordable housing, and healthcare access.

Physicians need to consider and prepare for unpredictable events, for example, becoming ill with the flu. Should the dedicated doctor continue to practice or stay home by arranging for coverage? Residents or young practitioners may feel obligated to continue to work, concerned about burdening others with coverage responsibilities, whereas the mid-career or older physician may be more likely to stay home if only to avoid infecting others. The decision to avoid work when ill is influenced by life experience and the recognition that one is not indispensable. As physicians age, illnesses become more frequent and potentially time-consuming because various conditions affect not only doctors but their families as well. Years of practice and life experiences can assist in creating the wisdom and judgment necessary to match the clinical practice with the doctor's personal needs and health demands.

Mental health issues, including anxiety and depression, are a concern for physicians just as they are for patients because doctors are just as vulnerable to such conditions (Gold et al. 2013). The time spent in medical school and specialty training may imbue clinical knowledge but does not inoculate the doctor against depression. Of course, depression with thoughts of self-harm is most concerning, and approximately 400 physicians succumb to suicide every year (Gold et al. 2013; Schernhammer and Colditz 2004), with female physicians at higher risk (Lindeman et al. 1996; Rakatansky 2016). Many of these suicides are preventable via treatment (Claassen et al. 2014), which, for various reasons, many physicians avoid. One of the reasons for such avoidance may be the perceived risk to their medical licenses (Adams et al. 2010; Center et al. 2003).

Substance use disorders are as prevalent in physicians as in the general population. About 10% of physicians will have a substance use disorder during their career (DuPont et al. 2009b; Flaherty and Richman 1993), although fewer doctors seek any assessment or treatment (Braquehais et al. 2015). Alcohol is the most prominent substance abused, followed by opioids and benzodiazepines. Stimulants and cocaine are abused less frequently (Pförringer et al. 2018; Rose et al. 2014). Marijuana abuse is problematic even as more states legalize medical marijuana, and many state licensing boards view physician use of marijuana as problematic and unprofessional (Hark 2018).

Female physicians have a higher rate of burnout, possibly related to their having more female patients. There are many possible reasons for this, including a perception that female patients have greater psychosocial complexity and possible expectations for more empathic listening compared with male patients (Linzer and Harwood 2018; Linzer et al. 2002; McMurray et al. 2000; West et al. 2018). Less is known regarding female psychiatrists, who might have more control of their practice and work-life balance, work settings, and hours. Many women also take time off or work part time to raise a family and may be better at multitasking and organizing their work schedules (Treister-Goltzman and Peleg 2016). Foreign medical graduates and international physicians are also at risk for burnout, and their particular concerns with stress need to be better identified.

Another stressor that can compromise medical practice satisfaction is the threat of a malpractice lawsuit, which can take years before a finding is determined. In addition, state licensing board investigations are very stressful and have potentially serious consequences, such as the loss of a medical license and resultant inability to practice.

Hobbies, avocations, and other interests can be integral to well-being and satisfaction with medical practice. Cultivating these outside interests and maintaining them through one's career can be critically important. Regular exercise and a healthy diet are also important components of a healthy lifestyle. In other words, the physical health of the physician needs to be maintained. Regular visits to a primary care physician are important, although physicians as a group are less likely to seek physical examinations for themselves and are more likely to delay their own medical care (Arnetz 2001).

Life Stages

The practice of medicine entails the risk of burnout because of inherent stressors that vary by career stage. This section reflects the core concerns and successes of a life in psychiatry transitioning through the career stages. Points of satisfaction and distress are illustrated in each stage. Underlying values are discussed; these include the concepts of resiliency, well-being, and maintaining joy in practice.

EARLY FORMATIVE YEARS

The early childhood years of a doctor serve as a foundation for later professional stability. Integral to that foundation is the family of origin (and whether that family provides responsive warmth and nurturing), the role of siblings, and emotional sustenance in the preschool years. The family's core values, cultural experience, and sense of ethnicity further add to the later development of a strong sense of self. Despite a less fortunate background with serious life struggles or early family dysfunction, fortitude, resilience, and a strong character can still become part of the doctor's personality structure, creating an ability to grow and endure.

Adolescence is full of tumult, excitement, confusion, and the building of one's identity and self-esteem (Erikson's stage five: identity vs. role confusion) if the phase is traversed without major dilemmas and troubles (Erikson 1950). Friendships are established and changed. Romantic relationships develop and end. School, teachers, courses, and rankings become more important. Many adolescents experiment with or use illicit drugs and alcohol for their first time. Difficult pathways can cause trouble, such as substance abuse, bullying, and emotional upheavals that include bouts of anxiety and depression. Family and parental relationships can become rife with conflict and ambivalence. College choices and decisions related to a course of study need to be made. Future career interests in medicine may or may not be apparent. Emotionally painful experiences and traumas need not indicate a bleak future because learning from these struggles can facilitate the development of resilient qualities so useful later in life.

Future medical doctors and psychiatrists must attend and do well academically in college, which can contribute to soliciting positive recommendations. The selection of a college at a young age when career direction is still unknown can be fraught with anxiety. For those who have already chosen to be future doctors, the college experience may be more directed and academically straightforward. More complex is the navigation of the extracurricular college experience, including being away from home, making new friends, contending with roommates and various temptations, and selecting one's courses, many first-time experiences. The first year can be filled with joy, expectations, fears, and concerns. Bouts of anxiety and even depressive symptoms can complicate the experience. Genetic vulnerabilities to mental illnesses can become manifest at this transitional life stage. The seeking of professional help, counseling, therapy, and medication treatment might provoke fears of compromising the medical school application process and acceptance. The later college years need to be navigated without significant turbulence in order to facilitate the medical school application process with its interviews and examinations. Many medical school applicants "take time off" between college and the application process, which affords the opportunity to broaden one's experience, work in medically related fields, or simply to travel, any of which may heighten the chances of acceptance to medical school or even acceptance at one's first-choice school.

An important aspect of the early premedical school foundation is the method by which the decision is made to be a doctor. Although there is a range of reasons, including emotional motivations to explain this career choice, a frequent central theme is to take care of patients and what that means to the future physician. The factors that may have contributed to this decision, for example, the influence of parents, the presence of a physician family member or mentor, the considerations of one's strengths and weaknesses, and any ambivalence about the field, can be related to the level of later career satisfaction.

MEDICAL SCHOOL/RESIDENCY YEARS

The first year of medical school can be stressful. A meta-analysis of 23 studies involving 16,500 medical students indicates that during the first year, 42% are emotionally exhausted, 25% experience depersonalization, and 79% fear that they have no personal accomplishments (Frajerman and Gorwood 2018). Another study surveyed medical students, residents, and early-career physicians (less than 5 years in practice) to determine if burnout symptoms differed in these three groupings and compared the burnout rate with the general population. Medical students had more anxiety and depressive symptoms relative to residents, early-career physicians, and the general population. These higher rates of problematic symptoms are thought to be due to the student's stress levels, related to the rigors of medical school, and a lower sense of personal accomplishment from roles that involve limited patient interaction (Dyrbye et al. 2014). The stresses of medical school can lead to burnout and stunting of the student's capacity for empathy, or the stresses may be handled more successfully, and both pathways can be associated with later levels of career satisfaction. Influential factors include the friendships formed in medical school, classmate relationships, the presence of role models, mentoring, and relationships with faculty members. Of course, the presence of psychiatric symptoms such as stress, anxiety, and depression are important, as are the attributes of resilience and an effective coping style. Also contributory to career satisfaction as a psychiatrist are the reasons this specialty was chosen, the expectations held for this career, and whether psychiatry was a first or second choice.

Selecting a specialty—most commonly in the fourth year of medical school—may result in a specialty choice that lasts through one's whole career. However, there are exceptions in which specialty changes are made later in the career to more closely align skills and changing interests. In fact, these evolving interests may redirect the physician more than once, as illustrated in the following example.

VIGNETTE I: RESIDENCY CHOICE

A colleague chose the psychiatry specialty as a fourth-year medical student but became disillusioned with it during the second year of residency. He thought that there was too much focus on the psychoanalytic interpretation of patients' experiences and that their illnesses were inadequately treated. He often disagreed with his teachers and supervisors. He quit the residency and entered an internal medicine program and eventually became a successful solo practitioner. Interestingly, he later became dissatisfied with that practice of medicine as well, burdened and burned out by the EHR, paperwork, and diminishing compensation. He left his solo practice, moved his family to a western state, and became a hospitalist, with a salary and defined patient responsibilities. He eventually retired, remaining dissatisfied with the trends in medicine but content with his career decisions.

This vignette illustrates the challenges of Erikson's stage five, in which the developing individual evolves a coherent identity for himself or herself by resolving the issues of "who am I" or "what can I be" as the individual tries to figure out how to fit into society. If these questions are not adequately resolved, the person can develop maladaptations, for example, repudiating the adult world or society and becoming disconnected to or cut off from others (Erikson 1950).

Internship is one's first experience as a licensed physician, and it can be rewarding and exhausting, fulfilling and confusing. Patient care can be stressful because of the newly minted intern's lack of medical knowledge, unfamiliarity with routines and algorithms, and challenges with learning a new staff, team, and EHR. Burnout can prevail, with different rotations contributing unique stressors that provoke recurrent feelings of incompetence. Additional stressors, such as feelings of inadequacy, sleep deprivation, time away from significant others and family, on-call exhaustion, and strained relations with more senior residents and physicians, can exacerbate burnout symptoms. Other internship factors can include concerns about finances and loan debt, uncertainty about a psychiatry residency as the chosen specialty, and fears of one's future in medicine. In addition, there is always an underlying concern about the health of parents, family, significant others, and siblings when the excessive time spent in the hospital leaves less time for others compared with college and medical school. One's own physical and mental health need to be prioritized, but often they are not. Although underlying chronic medical illnesses need to be regularly treated, there is usually no allotted time for a primary care provider visit, dentist visits, or other medical consultations. Those interns who have a resilient core and a well-developed sense of well-being will survive internship better than others, possibly by resourceful creation of time to address mental health issues.

The first year of psychiatry residency often brings a different type of patient care, with the focus on psychiatric disorders and the emotional demands of patients. This first year traditionally involves evaluating and treating the more seriously mentally ill. The patients are often challenging and require the resident to develop new and complex skills. Unlike with medical patients, the patient-psychiatrist relationship more frequently involves strong emotions (in both parties) and greater clinical ambiguity, which contributes to the resident's confusion about courses of treatment and even maintenance of the physician stance. In addition, the trainee is unfamiliar with aspects of psychotherapy, medications, the clinical team model, and the need for supervision from senior residents and faculty psychiatrists (Galanter et al. 2016).

As the residency progresses, familiarity with the role of a psychiatrist may improve with consequent lessening of tensions and feelings of incompetence. However, the middle and later years of psychiatry training hold their own challenges as the resident's underlying personality style, vulnerabilities, and predisposition to depression or other mental disorders can become discomforting and interfere with the resident's job expectations and clinical work. The burnout syndrome can develop, especially if the trainee chooses to hide his or her struggles from colleagues, senior residents, or attending physicians. This syndrome can be mitigated by a residency training director who is compassionate, trustworthy, and helpful (Shanafelt et al. 2015). This leader can help the trainee recognize that psychiatrists, possibly more so than other specialists, must address their own personal issues, and the earlier the better. The early recognition of stress, overwhelming anxiety, and depression can reduce the potential effect on patients and the resident himself or herself. In other words, caring for oneself first, before others, is a mantra that should be well understood by psychiatrists in training (Hadjipavlou et al. 2016).

Unfortunately, the rigors of medical school and residency training can take a toll on the participants. One-third of first-year psychiatric residents experienced burnout symptoms prior to beginning their residency, as reported in one study (Chaukos et al. 2017). These residents demonstrated diminished mindfulness and coping skills and expressed depressive symptoms of tiredness, worry, and being stressed. Participation in a mindfulness program, including learning cognitive-behavioral strategies, improved their performance and lessened their sense of burnout. In addition, on-call duties lasting 24 hours or longer contributed to burnout symptoms in residents studied in another survey (Frajerman and Gorwood 2018). Another study of psychiatry residents revealed that when second-year residents participated in individual psychotherapy, their reports of burnout increased because they felt they had a confidential opportunity to discuss their decreased empathy with their patients. These residents also demonstrated a reluctance to consult with supervisors regarding their distress and exhibited unhealthy coping strategies. Neither their age nor gender seemed to make a difference in their symptoms (Dyrbye et al. 2014). Residents often experience more burnout than medical students because residents need to take care of patients as a doctor, with all the attendant stresses, including more patient and hospital responsibilities (Ishak et al. 2009).

Prior to the conclusion of the general psychiatry residency, there is an opportunity to choose a fellowship in a subspecialty of the field; this provides an opportunity to enhance the fit with the physician's personality and the skills and interests that were developed in residency. Choosing to do a fellowship can signify career satisfaction and a sense of direction, along with optimism and contentment with psychiatry. Child and adolescent psychiatry requires a special interest in patients with often devastating illnesses and parental and family distress and a willingness to be involved with social services, courts, and other government agencies. Forensic psychiatry often involves expertise in ethical concerns, in-depth assessments that can withstand the scrutiny of attorneys, and legal proceedings. Geriatric psychiatrists deal with chronic illnesses and cognitive deficits that are best handled when the psychiatrist has resolved personal conflicts and relationships with one's own spouse, parents, and other aging relatives with similar issues. Also, end-of-life issues are often prevalent in geriatric psychiatry and can be stressful for those residents with chronically or terminally ill loved ones. Psychopharmacologists need to be comfortable with the array of medications available, time-limited visits, and the sacrifice of a deeper understanding of the patient through psychotherapy. Psychotherapeutically oriented psychiatrists often appreciate their patients' histories, relationships, and conflicts and harbor a willingness to be helpful in short-term or long-term therapy. Transference and countertransference understandings are important to the therapeutic work because these phenomena almost always influence the therapeutic relationship. The maintenance of appropriate boundaries—sexual and others—is paramount, and any boundary concerns should be identified by the therapist and resolved, often through the therapist's individual psychotherapy.

Of course, there are multiple potential sources of stress for the resident outside of clinical and academic responsibilities. It is at this time of life that female psychiatrists may consider pregnancy, wanting to start a family (Stentz et al. 2016). This fulfilling experience can be rewarding for both mother and father but can also cause stress, with family leave absences for female and male residents necessary for childcare and other responsibilities. The misuse of alcohol and other substances can become problematic, especially if continued to the point of dependence. Developing an awareness of the risks and potential consequences of this misuse is critically important, as is a ready willingness to seek assistance. Additionally, routine mental health issues (e.g., anxiety, depressive disorders) can start or worsen during the training years. If untreated, these conditions can be detrimental to the person with the symptoms and can also compromise that person's clinical work and lead to suicide (Goldman et al. 2015).

VIGNETTE 2: RESIDENCY

A postgraduate year-1 surgical resident was referred to the state PHP by the residency director for evaluation of her decreased performance. She discussed feeling out of place in the residency, a loss of interest in her patients, and feeling overly fatigued, with bouts of tearfulness. She was strongly considering leaving the residency and taking a break from medicine. This decision was complicated by the fact that her significant other was also in the same residency and was himself agitated by her emotional state and possible departure. One seemingly trivial but critical factor involved her lack of opportunity to jog with her dog, which before residency she had done daily to great personal benefit. The PHP evaluation allowed her to recognize her depressive and burnout symptoms. Importantly, she was also referred to a women physicians' support program within her hospital, which allowed her to refocus her priorities toward maintaining her well-being. After further discussion with PHP staff, she felt empowered to meet with the program director, with whom she arranged to have brief breaks in her workday to exercise with her dog. She continued in the residency and did well.

This vignette illustrates various factors related to physician trainee burnout, including the classic symptoms of exhaustion and loss of interest in the work, which became apparent to one of the trainee's supervisors (the training program director). Fortunately, that director fulfilled his role as one of the caretakers of the trainee's well-being and referred her to someone who knew how to help (Shanafelt et al. 2015). The PHP director performed a thorough evaluation and made several recommendations to which the training director was receptive. The close cooperation of all parties, including the trainee herself and a women physicians' support group, saved this young physician's career in medicine.

EARLY-CAREER YEARS

The completion of residency offers opportunities to seek, consider, and accept the first employment as a practicing psychiatrist. Issues involve include choosing the right work environment, satisfaction with employers, adequate supervision, and patient work attuned to the physician's competencies and personality. Fortunately, the field of psychiatry affords multiple work settings, for example, outpatient, inpatient, private practice, psychopharmacology, psychotherapy and research, part-time jobs, and locum tenens positions, as well as opportunities to work in organized medicine in the state psychiatric society and medical society. The following vignette suggests the complexities involved in early-career decisions.

VIGNETTE 3: EARLY-CAREER PHYSICIAN

After completing her residency, a 32-year-old single female psychiatrist accepted her first job at a well-regarded outpatient mental health clinic where she knew other physicians as well as the medical director. She thought it was a good fit. After a few months, however, she felt anxious and doubtful of her competence, experiencing difficulty with the many 15-minute appointments and the voluminous resultant EHR documentation. She had previously enjoyed doing psychotherapy and observing its benefits to her patients, but now she had to focus exclusively on symptoms and psychopharmacology. She became increasingly discouraged and disengaged, with little interest in patient care (i.e., symptoms of burnout). She started to drink a glass of wine in the evening to help her relax and sleep, and as her work problems continued, she gradually increased her nightly alcohol intake to almost a full bottle.

Over time, she also slowly withdrew from others, including her family, who voiced concerns that she ignored. Her work performance declined as she felt ever-decreasing satisfaction and enjoyment from her patients and colleagues. At a weekend social function, her friends noticed that she drank too much, and they confronted her. She reluctantly agreed to an evaluation by the director of the state PHP, to whom she gave permission to hear the concerns of her medical director, a caring and supportive leader. She agreed to enter a short-term intensive treatment program, where she was treated for her burnout, alcohol abuse, and depression. Upon discharge, she followed up with the PHP and returned to work, initially part-time. She also started individual therapy, a 12-step support group, and random urine screening for substances. With this support, she was able to successfully regain pleasure in her life and work, which included a greater focus on self-care and wellness along with re-involvement with her family, colleagues, and the medical community.

This vignette describes the importance of Erikson's stage six: intimacy versus isolation (Erikson 1950). After developing a sense of self and engaging in treatment, the physician, through support and therapy, realized the importance of connection with others and regained her role as a valued, employed psychiatrist in the clinic workforce.

There are many avenues to prevent burnout in the early-career stage. Involvement in organized medicine at the local, state, and national levels can be very rewarding, including the state and national chapters of the American Psychiatric Association and the American Medical Association. Social media involvement can be useful to minimize stress and enhance collegial relationships. Work-life balance issues can be addressed with workable schedules that include time for exercise and healthy eating in the daily routine. In addition, it is essential to avoid isolation by prioritizing collaboration, communication, consultation, and coordination with colleagues, friends, and family.

MID-CAREER YEARS

Mid-career psychiatrists are busy maintaining their practices, which can be at a single site or of various types at multiple sites. In addition to focusing on work, mid-career psychiatrists are also often involved with their families, choosing to spend precious time with a spouse, significant other, and children. Community and spiritual pursuits may also be important. Caring for one's physical health via collaboration with a primary care physician, regular checkups, dental care, obstetric/gynecologic care, and prescribed medications are essential to the overall health and well-being of the mid-career physician. Contending with compromised health or a chronic or terminal illness is certainly stressful and can contribute to work dissatisfaction. Other work-related factors, including long work hours with high clinical intensity, understaffing, on-call responsibilities, and major systemic changes can lead to burnout or discouragement with one's job (Gengoux and Roberts 2018).

VIGNETTE 4: MID-CAREER PHYSICIAN

A 55-year-old psychiatrist had the tendency to change jobs every 5 years to take advantage of new opportunities as they arose. One such opportunity was a high-level administrative position at an academic hospital where years before he had trained as a resident. Although the first few years were professionally gratifying for the psychiatrist, hospital leadership soon decided to drastically reorganize the hospital's mental health program for financial reasons. This resulted in the physician's job becoming one that included much more responsibility with little to no authority. He felt increasingly overworked, ineffective, and unhappy. This was compounded by strains in his marriage because he often brought the stresses home. The final blow came when the hospital advertised for a replacement for his position without informing him; he reacted by disengaging altogether from the job, and he seriously considered retiring early. However, he accepted a position at another hospital, believing that the new job would be largely administrative. Unfortunately, he quickly learned that the demands of the new job had been misrepresented and that it was actually heavily patient oriented, with a strong focus on clinical productivity. He worked on an inpatient unit that treated very ill, complex patients very briefly, which the physician found baffling and exhausting. The physician quickly felt demoralized and burned out again, and he resigned. Within a year, he was able to find a suitable administrative position at a well-functioning organization that also allowed him to continue his rewarding private practice. He regained his joy as a practicing psychiatrist and successfully continued his career.

This vignette illustrates the seventh Eriksonian stage of development, generativity versus stagnation (Erikson 1950), wherein the psychiatrist, because of changing unfavorable circumstances, almost unhappily retired, succumbing to stagnation. Instead, fortunately, he found employment that allowed him to continue to use his skills and talents for organizational leadership, mentorship, and caring for colleagues in distress, much of which he described in published articles. He found a way to be generative as a psychiatrist in areas that he valued.

As an alternative to clinical responsibilities, mid-career psychiatrists can become involved in hospital leadership and play a role in designing hospital policies and procedures that advance the well-being of residents and staff physicians. Positions in organized psychiatry and medicine can likewise provide opportunities to collaborate with colleagues to effect policy changes that endorse wellness and reduce the prevalence of burnout (Barbe 2018). In the spring of 2018, the Collaborative for Healing and Renewal in Medicine developed the "Charter on Physician Well-being," which provides guidelines for medical organizations in promoting physician wellness, another initiative in the campaign to prevent burnout (Thomas et al. 2018). Physicians can take advantage of the varieties of work settings available in psychiatry by periodically changing jobs and the types of work therein.

SENIOR PHASE

The senior physician category is usually defined as age 65 and older, and for some it is the winding-down phase of their medical careers. Psychiatrists often have an advantage over other specialties in their ability to maintain a practice that needs minimal office equipment and staff, if any. Because of this, psychiatrists can more easily extend their practice years.

Part-time practice might be a consideration, with a reduction of the patient load or a less stressful practice, to begin a pathway to eventual retirement. Personal and family health issues can be significant; caring for elderly parents and family with health concerns is common at this life stage.

Mentoring and coaching of younger physicians and psychiatrists afford an opportunity to stay involved with the larger psychiatric community while sharing one's experience and expertise. Continued teaching in an academic institution can also provide ongoing satisfaction to the senior physician.

This phase also offers an opportunity for reflection, reconciling the ambition and goals set as a younger doctor with the inevitable career disappointments. The "almost-retired" psychiatrist must also reconcile his identity as a doctor with his nonclinical interests, concerns, and lifestyle.

The senior phase of the medical career is the time for retirement planning and taking steps toward this goal. Retirement can be a complex endeavor that needs to be thoughtfully planned, and sharing those plans with the spouse, family, and colleagues can be fruitful. Considerations need to be more than financial, although wills, trusts, investments, and other aspects need to be addressed to maintain one's desired lifestyle without the income from work. The retirement checklist can include categories of professional, personal, and medical, as well as volunteering, exercise, hobby, educational, friendship, travel, community, and spiritual considerations.

VIGNETTE 5: SENIOR PHYSICIAN

A 65-year-old psychiatrist retired following a successful career as a private-practice psychodynamic psychotherapist. Six months into his retirement he became bored, was more irritable with his wife, and missed caring for patients. He then accepted a part-time job at a local outpatient mental health clinic and was very unpleasantly surprised that the work consisted exclusively of 15- to 20-minute psychopharmacology visits and documentation in a confusing EHR. In addition, he was also completely unfamiliar with the new psychotropic medications and felt devalued and unappreciated by the clinic staff. He felt increasingly demoralized, despondent, and rudderless. He recognized that he was burned out.

The psychiatrist self-referred to the state's PHP. With the PHP director's help, he met with a coach with whom he explored his identity as a physician and psychiatrist. His coach and a psychiatrist colleague/mentor helped him to view his new work as an educational opportunity and encouraged him to learn much more about the EHR and psychopharmacology via various courses. The psychiatrist also reached out to the clinic staff to consult on psychodynamic issues, and he became active in the local medical society. He and his wife benefited from short-term counseling focused on improved communication and shared interests, such as travel and socializing with friends. His return to practice was successful, and he reevaluated his future retirement plans.

This vignette illustrates the eighth Eriksonian stage of development, integrity versus despair (Erikson 1950), with the 65-year-old psychiatrist experiencing a variant of the latter condition, ultimately checked by his choosing to contribute to various communities and relationships, thereby cultivating a sense of pride and purpose for his life and career.

Some physicians will consider early retirement because of stress, burnout, health issues, and dissatisfaction with medical practice. As mentioned in the section "Physician Satisfaction," stresses related to the EHR, billing, reimbursement, documentation, and prior approvals can cause considerable distress and often complicate patient care. Of course, a paramount concern for all physicians in this phase is continued competency to practice. The aging process can include a degree of loss of cognitive function (LoboPrabhu et al. 2009). All aging physicians need to be attuned to their cognitive status and the ability to practice safely and competently.

Physician colleagues also have a responsibility to recognize competency difficulties in colleagues and to take steps to address these concerns when they arise. The physician community needs to do better in this regard to more effectively address concerns about a colleague's competency or take action with the relevant department chairs, administrators, or if need be, the state licensing board.

VIGNETTE 6: PSYCHIATRIST SATISFACTION AND A SUCCESSFUL CAREER

A young psychiatrist after leaving military service accepted a job as a residency training director at a large urban academic medical center that prioritized the delivery of care to the poor and indigent. He became proficient in the intricacies of community mental health care and in establishing authority in a large institution. He published widely and was academically well respected. After 20 years, he accepted the role of chief of psychiatry at a rival academic center across town, where his division was in the department of medicine. He expanded the division by hiring young, capable clinicians and researchers. He felt his real talent was bringing together people with potential and nurturing them in their professional development. His division of psychiatry eventually became an independent department, with him as chair. The affiliated medical school created an annual mentorship award in his honor. He later stepped down as the chair and accepted an executive administrative hospital role. Years later, he fully retired, recognized his success in many areas, managed losses as he could, and ultimately earned the respect of trainees, clinical colleagues, and administrative leaders. He viewed his career as successful with much personal satisfaction.

This vignette reflects a psychiatrist's career of well-being and satisfaction, demonstrating Erikson's highest degree of integrity and psychosocial development in the eighth stage (Erikson 1950).

Conclusion

Each phase of a physician's career, from medical student through senior physician, provides opportunities for both professional satisfaction and personal exhaustion and burnout. A significant percentage of participants will experience either or both, and successful navigation through these stages often hinges on the recognition of and remedial efforts to address burnout. Medical students and psychiatry residents need to be assured that the early stages of a medical career are stressful but ultimately rewarding. Early-career psychiatrists face the stresses of entering new employment or a psychiatric practice and will benefit from mentoring, supervision, and collegial support, allowing the early-career psychiatrist to adjust to patient and administrative demands without becoming overwhelmed. Mid-career psychiatrists can use their experience and leadership skills to shape their academic, hospital-based, or private practice to meet their expectations and work-life balance needs. Senior psychiatrists can use their wisdom and experience to assist younger psychiatrists to pursue their careers positively while restructuring their own work as they wind down and plan retirement.

KEY POINTS

- The practice of medicine entails the risk of burnout because of the inherent contribution of stressors that can vary by career stages.

- Early-career stressors are worsened by the false belief that the early-career physician should be able to handle multiple stressors without support, such as sleep deprivation, separation from loved ones, personal illness, and a steep learning curve.

- Mid-career stressors often include systemic changes, such as introduction of an EHR, a new chair or director, or new areas of responsibility, which often require the integration of new learning by the physician.

- Late-career stressors can include boredom, feeling underappreciated, and personal and/or family health concerns.

- A healthy response to stress includes candidly acknowledging the situation and discomfort, discussing it with others, and collectively deciding on a mitigating path that includes self-care.

———————■———————

References

Adams EF, Lee AJ, Pritchard CW, et al: What stops us from healing the healers: a survey of help-seeking behaviour, stigmatisation and depression within the medical profession. Int J Soc Psychiatry 56(4):359–370, 2010 19617278

American Medical Association: AMA Principles of Medical Ethics. Chicago, IL, American Medical Association, 2016. Available at https://www.ama-assn.org/delivering-care/ama-principles-medical-ethics. Accessed November 26, 2018.

Arnetz BB: Psychosocial challenges facing physicians of today. Soc Sci Med 52(2):203–213, 2001 11144776

Barbe D: Dousing the physician burnout epidemic: an AMA perspective. Pract Pain Manag 18(3):34–35, 2018

Bishop TF, Press MJ, Keyhani S, et al: Acceptance of insurance by psychiatrists and the implications for access to mental health care. JAMA Psychiatry 71(2):176–181, 2014 24337499

Braquehais MD, Tresidder A, DuPont RL: Service provision to physicians with mental health and addiction problems. Curr Opin Psychiatry 28(4):324–329, 2015 26001924

Center C, Davis M, Detre T, et al: Confronting depression and suicide in physicians: a consensus statement. JAMA 289(23):3161–3166, 2003 12813122

Chaukos D, Chad-Friedman E, Mehta DH, et al: Risk and resilience factors associated with resident burnout. Acad Psychiatry 41(2):189–194, 2017 28028738

Claassen CA, Pearson JL, Khodyakov D, et al: Reducing the burden of suicide in the U.S.: the aspirational research goals of the National Action Alliance for Suicide Prevention Research Prioritization Task Force. Am J Prev Med 47(3):309–314, 2014 24750971

DuPont RL, McLellan AT, Carr G, et al: How are addicted physicians treated? A national survey of Physician Health Programs. J Subst Abuse Treat 37(1):1–7, 2009a 19482236

DuPont RL, McLellan AT, White WL, et al: Setting the standard for recovery: Physicians' Health Programs. J Subst Abuse Treat 36(2):159–171, 2009b 19161896

Dyrbye LN, West CP, Satele D, et al: Burnout among U.S. medical students, residents, and early career physicians relative to the general U.S. population. Acad Med 89(3):443–451, 2014 24448053

Erikson E: Childhood and Society. New York, WW Norton, 1950

Flaherty JA, Richman JA: Substance use and addiction among medical students, residents, and physicians. Psychiatr Clin North Am 16(1):189–197, 1993 8456044

Frajerman A, Gorwood P: Burnout in medical students before residency: systematic review and meta-analysis. Abstract presented at the 26th European Congress of Psychiatry, Nice, France, March 2018

Galanter CA, Nikolov R, Green N, et al: Direct supervision in outpatient psychiatric graduate medical education. Acad Psychiatry 40(1):157–163, 2016 25424638

Gengoux GW, Roberts LW: Enhancing wellness and engagement among healthcare professionals. Acad Psychiatry 42(1):1–4, 2018 29297148

Gold KJ, Sen A, Schwenk TL: Details on suicide among US physicians: data from the National Violent Death Reporting System. Gen Hosp Psychiatry 35(1):45–49, 2013 23123101

Goldman ML, Shah RN, Bernstein CA: Depression and suicide among physician trainees: recommendations for a national response. JAMA Psychiatry 72(5):411–412, 2015 25738529

Hadjipavlou G, Halli P, Hernandez CA, et al: Personal therapy in psychiatry residency training: a national survey of Canadian psychiatry residents. Acad Psychiatry 40(1):30–37, 2016 26289116

Hark R: Medical marijuana and the licensed professional—just say no. The Legal Intelligencer, July 5, 2018

Ishak WW, Lederer S, Mandili C, et al: Burnout during residency training: a literature review. J Grad Med Educ 1(2):236–242, 2009 21975985

Kohlberg L: Essays on Moral Development, Vol. I: The Philosophy of Moral Development. San Francisco, CA: Harper and Row, 1981

Krall EJ, Niazi SK, Miller MM: The status of physician health programs in Wisconsin and north central states: a look at statewide and health systems programs. WMJ 111(5):220–227, 2012 23189455

Lindeman S, Läärä E, Hakko H, et al: A systematic review on gender-specific suicide mortality in medical doctors. Br J Psychiatry 168(3):274–279, 1996 8833679

Linzer M, Harwood E: Gendered expectations: do they contribute to high burnout among female physicians? J Gen Intern Med 33(6):963–965, 2018 29435727

Linzer M, McMurray JE, Visser MR, et al: Sex differences in physician burnout in the United States and The Netherlands. J Am Med Womens Assoc (1972) 57(4):191–193, 2002 12405233

LoboPrabhu SM, Molinari VA, Hamilton JD, et al: The aging physician with cognitive impairment: approaches to oversight, prevention, and remediation. Am J Geriatr Psychiatry 17(6):445–454, 2009 19461256

Massachusetts Board of Registration in Medicine: Physician Regulations, Policies, and Guidelines: Mandated Reporting, 2018. Available at: https://www.mass.gov/service-details/mandated-reporting. Accessed September 1, 2018

McMurray JE, Linzer M, Konrad TR, et al: The work lives of women physicians: results from the physician work life study. J Gen Intern Med 15(6):372–380, 2000 10886471

Pförringer D, Mayer R, Meisinger C, et al: Health, risk behaviour and consumption of addictive substances among physicians—results of an online survey. J Occup Med Toxicol 13:27, 2018 30158999

Rakatansky H: Physicians at high risk for suicide in US; incidence higher in women doctors Physician Health Programs (PHP) offer confidential treatment. R I Med J (2013) 99(11):11–12, 2016 27801912

Rose JS, Campbell M, Skipper G: Prognosis for emergency physician with substance abuse recovery: 5-year outcome study. West J Emerg Med 15(1):20–25, 2014 24696748

Schernhammer ES, Colditz GA: Suicide rates among physicians: a quantitative and gender assessment (meta-analysis). Am J Psychiatry 161(12):2295–2302, 2004 15569903

Shanafelt TD, Gorringe G, Menaker R, et al: Impact of organizational leadership on physician burnout and satisfaction. Mayo Clin Proc 90(4):432–440, 2015 25796117

Stentz NC, Griffith KA, Perkins E, et al: Fertility and childbearing among American female physicians. J Womens Health (Larchmt) 25(10):1059–1065, 2016 27347614

Thomas LR, Ripp JA, West CP: Charter on physician well-being. JAMA 319(15):1541–1542, 2018 29596592

Treister-Goltzman Y, Peleg R: Female physicians and the work-family conflict. Isr Med Assoc J 18(5):261–266, 2016 27430080

West CP, Dyrbye LN, Shanafelt TD: Physician burnout: contributors, consequences and solutions. J Intern Med 283(6):516–529, 2018 29505159

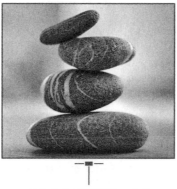

CHAPTER 10

BURNOUT AMONG MEDICAL STUDENTS AND RESIDENTS

Lisa Boyars, M.D.

Constance Guille, M.D., MSCR

Physician burnout is a topic of national discussion because of its prevalence and negative impact on physicians, their families, and patients. Symptoms of burnout can occur very early on in graduate medical education and persist throughout medical training. The purpose of this chapter is to review the literature related to medical student and resident burnout and highlight the significant cost associated with burnout, as well as factors shown to be associated with it, in order to inform the development of system- and individual-level interventions to reduce the significant burden of burnout. Furthermore, we review the gaps in research, which may help to direct future interventions. To date, many interventions have not proven effective at reducing burnout in medical students and residents.

Prevalence of Burnout in Medical Students

It is estimated that 35%–45% of medical students experience symptoms suggestive of burnout (Boni et al. 2018; Dyrbye and Shanafelt 2016; Paro et al. 2014). It is clear that burnout increases over the course of medical training and that the increase in burnout is greater in medical students compared with nonmedical graduate students. Prior to the start of medical school, levels of burnout in matriculating students are lower in comparison with students entering graduate school; however, upon completion of medical school, levels of burnout in medical students are higher compared with their nonmedical graduate school peers (Dyrbye and Shanafelt 2016). The onset of burnout in medical students is present prior to clinical rotations, before medical students engage in their first patient experiences (Boni et al. 2018; Dyrbye and Shanafelt 2016). Extant research suggests that burnout increases as medical education continues into clinical rotations, internships, and residency (Dyrbye and Shanafelt 2016; Paro et al. 2014).

Factors Associated With Medical Student Burnout

The consequences of medical student burnout are significant for individuals and for their patients. Students with high levels of burnout are more likely to experience suicidal ideation, use or abuse substances, engage in unprofessional behaviors, have poor academic performance, lack empathy, and consider withdrawal from the medical profession (Dahlin et al. 2007; Dyrbye and Shanafelt 2016; Dyrbye et al. 2010a, 2010b; Frank et al. 2008; Hojat et al. 2004; Jackson et al. 2016; Thomas et al. 2007).

The estimated prevalence of depression and suicidal ideation in medical students is 27.2% and 11.1%, respectively (Rotenstein et al. 2016), and these rates are nearly twice the rate of depression and suicidal ideation found among university students of similar age (Eisenberg et al. 2007). Burnout is associated with an increased likelihood of suicidal ideation, and recovery from burnout is associated with less suicidal ideation (Dyrbye and Shanafelt 2016). In a longitudinal cohort study of medical students, only 26.8% of students recovered from burnout (Dyrbye and Shanafelt 2016). Fortunately, among those who recovered the rate of suicidal ideation was similar to those who never experienced burnout. However, more than 70% of students in this study did not recover from burnout.

Alcohol use, and in particular binge drinking, is common among medical students and may be associated with burnout. In a multi-institutional review of 16 U.S. medical schools, nearly one-third of medical students at various levels of education reported excessive alcohol consumption within the past month, with men having a greater prevalence of excessive alcohol use compared with women, 43% versus 24%, respectively (Frank et al. 2008).

Of those who met criteria for excessive drinking, nearly all reported binge drinking (consuming five or more drinks in one sitting) in the past month. Similarly, alcohol abuse or dependence was found in one-third (32.4%) of medical students, which was greater than the 15.6% found in their nonmedical college-educated peers (Jackson et al. 2016). Although there are few studies examining the relationship between burnout in medical students and alcohol abuse or dependence, study findings suggest they are highly correlated. Medical students with alcohol abuse or dependence are also more likely to be experiencing burnout, depression, and poor mental and emotional quality of life (Jackson et al. 2016).

Medical students with high levels of burnout are significantly more likely to have engaged in dishonest clinical behavior, and altruistic professional values showed an inverse relationship to burnout (Dyrbye et al. 2010a). Examples of dishonest clinic behavior include reporting a physical examination finding as normal when it had been omitted or reporting a laboratory test as pending when it is unclear that one has been collected. Examples of altruistic professional values include concern about the problems facing the medically underserved or wanting to provide care to this population. Although both burnout and depression have substantial consequences for medical students, students with depression or poor mental or physical quality of life were not more likely to engage in dishonest clinical behavior or have less altruistic professional values (Dyrbye et al. 2010a).

Declining empathy is inversely associated with medical student burnout (Thomas et al. 2007). Cultivation of empathy and its perseverance through medical training has important implications for patient care, yet empathy seems to decline during medical school (Hojat et al. 2004). Interestingly, the capacity for empathy and maintenance of a positive attitude among female students is less subject to fluctuations over the course of medical school compared with that of male medical student peers (Woloschuk et al. 2004), yet female medical school graduates are more likely to experience symptoms of burnout (Dahlin et al. 2007; Dyrbye and Shanafelt 2016), suggesting that empathy is only in part impacted by burnout.

Attrition from the medical profession appears to be associated with burnout. Approximately 11% of students have serious thoughts of "dropping out" of medical school each year, and although a causal relationship cannot yet be established, burnout precedes serious thoughts of dropping out. Elevated symptoms of burnout are associated with a threefold increased risk of having serious thoughts of leaving medical school (Dyrbye et al. 2010b). Among students whose symptoms of burnout decreased over time, there was also a reduction in thoughts about leaving medical school. Serious thoughts of dropping out also appear to be associated with significant life events (i.e., divorce, major personal illness, major illness or death of a close family member), which are also associated with burnout (Dyrbye et al. 2010b). Unfortunately, because negative life events are unpredictable, it is difficult to know if negative life events precede symptoms of burnout and thoughts of attrition from medical training, but there appears to be an association between all three factors. Furthermore, a low frequency of time spent with family, lack of leisure time, and low physical activity are associated with burnout among medical students in Brazil (Boni et al. 2018).

Factors related to the educational training process are associated with burnout in medical students (Dyrbye and Shanafelt 2016). A number of curricular elements have been evaluated, such as total number of lecture hours, number of tests, amount of time spent taking exams during the academic year, and hours spent on learning experiences. In one study, the type of grading scale used was most strongly associated with medical student well-being (Reed et al. 2011). Students graded on scales of three or more categories (e.g., honors/pass/fail or A through F letter grade as opposed to pass/fail) had higher levels of burnout as well as high levels of perceived stress and poorer mental quality of life (Reed et al. 2011).

The learning environment changes between the preclinical (years 1 and 2) and clinical (years 3 and 4) years of medical school. Some learning environment factors negatively impact burnout throughout all 4 years, with some additional factors negatively impacting burnout during the clinical years. In a cross-sectional study, burnout in year-1 and year-2 students was associated with dissatisfaction with the learning environment and perceived level of support by faculty (Dyrbye and Shanafelt 2016). Among year-3 and year-4 medical students, burnout was associated with dissatisfaction with the overall learning environment, clerkship organization, and working with a cynical resident (Dyrbye and Shanafelt 2016). Students on hospital ward rotations were more likely to experience burnout compared with peers on outpatient, intensive care unit, research, or consult services (Dyrbye and Shanafelt 2016). Students on rotations requiring overnight call also experienced higher levels of burnout, compared with those not on rotations requiring overnight call (Dyrbye and Shanafelt 2016). In students on rotations requiring being on call, there was no difference in burnout based on frequency of call shifts per rotation, and furthermore, the number of patients seen per day in any setting was not independently associated with burnout (Dyrbye and Shanafelt 2016).

Interventions to Reduce Medical Student Burnout

Prior to the twenty-first century, there were few empirical studies that employed rigorous scientific methods to evaluate the benefit of interventions to reduce burnout and improve wellness in medical students (Shapiro et al. 2000). More recently, however, there are a number of studies evaluating the benefits of mindfulness techniques or mindfulness-based stress reduction (MBSR) to reduce burnout and improve overall medical student wellness (Dyrbye et al. 2017; Erogul et al. 2014; Finkelstein et al. 2007; Shapiro et al. 1998). All first-year medical students at the Mayo Clinic School of Medicine in 2014 and 2015 participated in a longitudinal MBSR course as part of their formal curriculum (Dyrbye et al. 2017), but unfortunately, this did not lead to measurable improvements in student burnout. Similarly, other studies examining mindfulness interventions have not yielded overwhelming positive results. In a 2018 systematic review of 12 articles that employed MBSR or mindfulness exercises for the reduction of stress, depression, fatigue, and burnout within a medical student population, three studies included a measure of burnout (Daya and Hearn 2018). Of these, two reported no significant reductions in burnout, and the third showed significant improvement in the emotional exhaustion subscale of the Maslach Burnout Inventory but not the other related subscales, including personal accomplishment and depersonalization (Barbosa et al. 2013; Daya and Hearn 2018; de Vibe et al. 2013; Garneau et al. 2013).

Mindfulness and MBSR interventions, however, have demonstrated significant benefit in reducing anxiety and depressive symptoms as well as perceived stress. In a randomized, controlled trial, medical and premedical students assigned to an 8-week course of MBSR indicated fewer self-reported depressive and anxiety symptoms and increased empathy and spirituality, compared with the wait-list control group (Shapiro et al. 1998). In addition, two nonrandomized, controlled trials also support the benefit of mindfulness techniques in reducing anxiety and depressive symptoms (Finkelstein et al. 2007). Importantly, anxiety levels remained low in students 3 months after taking part in the mind-body elective and during final examinations.

Mindfulness techniques have also helped to improve perceived stress and well-being in medical students. In a randomized, controlled trial of MBSR in 59 first-year medical students, students assigned to the MBSR intervention demonstrated significant improvements in self-compassion and perceived stress following completion of the MBSR program compared with the control group (Erogul et al. 2014). To summarize, studies evaluating the benefit of mindfulness techniques and MBSR suggest that this intervention may be more beneficial for reducing stress and improving mood and anxiety symptoms as opposed to reducing rates of burnout in medical students.

Interestingly, medical student engagement in the humanities such as singing, playing a musical instrument, reading for pleasure, listening to music, or going to a museum has been associated with a reduction in symptoms of burnout. A recent study showed that as exposure to either active or passive involvement with the humanities increased, some measures of burnout (physical fatigue, emotional exhaustion, and cognitive weariness) decreased in medical students (Mangione et al. 2018). These findings suggest that students' well-being may benefit from engagement in nonmedical activities.

Burnout in Residents

Unfortunately, many residents are beginning their residency training with elevated symptoms of burnout, and the rates of burnout during residency training increase over time. Close to half of all graduating medical students report elevated symptoms of burnout, and its prevalence increases throughout residency training (Dyrbye and Shanafelt 2016). A prospective study of internal medicine interns at five different U.S. institutions revealed the prevalence of burnout was 14%–36% just prior to the start of internship year and 50%–81% at the end of internship year (Ripp et al. 2011). The incidence of burnout among residents ranges from 50% to 75%. The range of estimates is accounted for by the variability in the definition of burnout, with stricter definitions of burnout demonstrating lower estimates. Rates of burnout among medical students entering different specialties do not differ; however, the types of symptoms experienced by students vary by specialty. Pooled data collected during the 2006, 2007, and 2009 academic years revealed no difference in the prevalence of burnout among students entering different residency specialty areas (primary care, surgical field, nonprimary care/nonsurgical fields); however, there were subtle differences in the manifestation of burnout (Dyrbye and Shanafelt 2016). Students entering surgical fields had significantly lower emotional exhaustion scores compared with all other students. Students entering primary care fields had significantly lower depersonalization scores, and students entering nonprimary care/nonsurgical fields reported the lowest score for personal accomplishment compared with those entering other fields. During residency, however, the manifestation of burnout does not appear to vary by specialty (Ishak et al. 2009; Martini et al. 2006). Although not statistically significant, rates of burnout appear to be highest in obstetrics-gynecology residents (75%), and family medicine residents report the least amount of burnout (27%) (Martini et al. 2006).

Factors Associated With Resident Burnout

Resident burnout is highly associated with depression (Lebares et al. 2018; Shanafelt et al. 2002). Studies in this area are cross-sectional; therefore, a temporal relationship between onset of burnout and onset of depression cannot be established. Rates of depression and suicidal ideation are quite elevated in residents. In a systematic review and meta-analysis of 17,560 residents, rates of depression were, on average, 28.8% (Mata et al. 2015). Perhaps one of the most significant consequences of depression is suicide. From 2000 through 2014, the second leading cause of death among residents was suicide (Yaghmour et al. 2017). Among male residents, suicide was the most common cause of death, with the majority of suicides taking place early in training.

Both burnout and depression highly correlate with poor patient care. Residents with burnout report less ability to respond empathetically to patients (Kealy et al. 2016) and are more likely to report suboptimal patient care and medical errors (de Oliveira et al. 2013; Fahrenkopf et al. 2008; Shanafelt et al. 2002; West et al. 2006). Interestingly, although residents with higher levels of burnout report making a greater number of medical errors, rates of medical errors measured by objective means are similar between residents with high and low levels of burnout (Fahrenkopf et al. 2008). This may suggest that, similar to episodes of major depressive disorder, individuals with burnout may have a more negative view of events. This underscores the significant need for interventions to reduce depression and burnout because this negative line of thinking or belief that one has committed a medical error may perpetuate burnout or increase the risk of anxiety, concentration issues, and sleep disturbance (Gallagher et al. 2003).

Resident burnout is potentially associated with excessive alcohol use or abuse. A survey of 556 U.S. surgical residents revealed that one-third (33%) of surgical residents endorsed criteria for alcohol abuse or dependence (Lebares et al. 2018). Although the association between burnout and alcohol abuse trended toward significance in this study, a statistically significant association was not established. Another cross-sectional survey of anesthesiology residents revealed that having more than five alcoholic drinks per week was associated with higher burnout scores (de Oliveira et al. 2013). Interestingly, some residents may see alcohol as a way to cope with burnout, even though alcohol use significantly correlates with increased emotional exhaustion and depersonalization (Eckleberry-Hunt et al. 2009; Kealy et al. 2016).

Individual and demographic characteristics of medical residents have been examined in relation to burnout. Some individual characteristics noted to be associated with resident burnout include self-described trait of indecisiveness (Ramey et al. 2017), disorganized personality style (Ripp et al. 2011), and intolerance of uncertainty (Kimo Takayesu et al. 2014). The relationship between burnout and these characteristics is not surprising given the nature and demands of internship and the practice of medicine.

Demographic variables such as gender and having children have both been evaluated in relation to symptoms of burnout with mixed results. Some studies identify an association between female gender or having children with burnout (de Oliveira et al. 2013; Gunasingam et al. 2015; Kimo Takayesu et al. 2014; Martini et al. 2006), whereas others do not (Fahrenkopf et al. 2008; Ramey et al. 2017; Ripp et al. 2011; Shanafelt et al. 2002; Woodside et al. 2008). It is more than likely that stressors associated with these demographic characteristics may increase the risk for burnout but are not captured solely based on these general demographic categories.

Multiple studies suggest that international medical school graduates are less likely to report high levels of emotional exhaustion and depersonalization (Eckleberry-Hunt et al. 2009; West et al. 2011; Woodside et al. 2008) and depression (Sen et al. 2010) in comparison with U.S. medical school graduates. The reason for this is unknown, but it has been speculated that international medical school graduates have already overcome significant hurdles to establish a U.S. residency position and are therefore highly resilient individuals. It has also been suggested that cultural differences or concerns about ramifications of disclosure may deter international medical school graduates from endorsing symptoms of burnout or depression.

In both 2003 and 2011, the Accreditation Council for Graduate Medical Education mandated restrictions of total weekly resident work hours and consecutive work hours (Accreditation Council of Graduate Medical Education 2011). Despite measures to limit work hours, burnout has not been reduced (Martini et al. 2006; Ripp et al. 2015), nor have depressive symptoms improved (Sen et al. 2013). These findings are not surprising given that many studies have shown that the amount of work hours, the number of on-call shifts, and sleep have no association with burnout (Chaput et al. 2015; Fahrenkopf et al. 2008; Ramey et al. 2017; Ripp et al. 2011). In order for residency programs to institute these mandated work-hour changes, many residency programs have started to rely on night float rotations in which residents work nights only in order to comply with duty-hour restrictions. Unfortunately, it appears that the night float system has not improved resident well-being and may increase rates of burnout. Internal medicine residents on night float rotations, in comparison with internal medicine residents on non–night float rotations, experienced the most symptoms of burnout despite generally working fewer hours overall compared with their colleagues (Elmariah et al. 2017).

With the establishment of the electronic health record (EHR) and increased time spent on clinical documentation, investigators have examined the impact of EHR on healthcare worker satisfaction and well-being. Among practicing physicians, there appears to be an increased risk for burnout in physicians who frequently use EHRs for their professional work (Babbott et al. 2014; Shanafelt et al. 2016). Although the relationship between burnout and EHRs has not been specifically studied in residents, there is some evidence to suggest that EHRs are having a negative impact on residents because of increased documentation in lieu of patient care (Christino et al. 2013; Oxentenko et al. 2010). It is likely that the EHR interference with patient care is impacting resident burnout, but systematic studies are needed to address this topic.

Interventions to Reduce Resident Burnout

A systematic review and meta-analysis of studies of interventions to prevent and reduce physician burnout was conducted by West et al. (2016) and demonstrated that interventions aimed at reducing burnout are effective, but the effect is small. Notably, interventions among practicing physicians were more effective than those among residents. Similarly, Panagioti et al. (2017) conducted a systematic review and meta-analysis to evaluate the effectiveness of interventions in reducing physician burnout and found a small but significant reduction in burnout. Organization-directed interventions (i.e., reduced workload, improved practice efficiency) were associated with greater treatment effects compared with physician-directed interventions (i.e., stress management, self-care training, MBSR). Although some studies have attempted to identify interventions aimed at modifying call shifts (e.g., in-house vs. home call, protected sleep on call) to reduce resident burnout, collectively, there is not a consensus on work hours or call shift type or length that produce significant improvements in resident burnout (Parshuram et al. 2015; Ripp et al. 2015; Shea et al. 2014). Practice delivery changes that reduce workload and improve efficiency may potentially be beneficial in reducing burnout among residents, as demonstrated in practicing physicians, and is an important area for future investigation.

Several interventions have focused on resident self-care and wellness, yet few have led to a meaningful reduction in burnout. In a prospective randomized, controlled study, residents were randomly assigned to a group that received four debriefing sessions ($n = 13$) or to a control group that received none ($n = 18$) (Gunasingam et al. 2015). Debriefing sessions covered topics such as work-related stressors, coping mechanisms, and ways to improve resident well-being. The intervention did not improve resident burnout scores, perhaps because of the study's small sample size; however, the intervention was well received, and most residents stated they would recommend the sessions to future residents. In a larger study, residents were randomly assigned to participate in an experimental group ($n = 37$) that received two 2.5-hour self-care workshops or a control group ($n = 37$) that did not receive any intervention (Martins et al. 2011). Although depersonalization scores improved, overall burnout did not. Another randomized, controlled trial of first-year internal medicine residents failed to show improvement in burnout after the intervention group received 18 facilitated group discussions related to stress, balance, and job satisfaction over the duration of their intern year (Ripp et al. 2016). This negative study may, in part, be explained by the fact that interns were not freed of their clinical responsibilities while attending the 1-hour discussions, so this intervention may have added additional burden to their already full schedules. In 2011, the Mayo Clinic in Rochester, Minnesota, invited all residents and fellows to participate in a 12-week, incentivized exercise program (Weight et al. 2013). After study completion, burnout was lower in those who participated in the program in comparison with those that did not take part, although the reduction in burnout was not statistically significant. There were, however, statistically significant improvements in personal accomplishment and improved quality of life. Overall, these studies suggest that prior interventions do not appear to improve burnout, but it appears that residents are willing to take part in activities related to reducing burnout, and, overall, the interventions are well received and can potentially result in improved higher quality of life.

Residents are often tasked with delivering bad news or communicating complicated information to patients and families, and a longitudinal trial sought to determine if burnout could be improved by enhancing residents' communication skills. Medical residents were randomly assigned to receive communication and stress management skills training in small groups or to a usual-care group in which residents did not receive any additional training (Bragard et al. 2010). Although residents reported feeling less stress and had a greater sense of self-efficacy in communicating with patients, there was no appreciable improvement in burnout among residents who received this intervention. Regardless of the impact of this intervention on burnout, residents and their patients would likely benefit from having this type of intervention prior to the start of their internship year.

Mindfulness-based interventions have been shown to reduce burnout in practicing physicians in at least some studies (Panagioti et al. 2017; West et al. 2016). Interestingly, prior to starting residency, residents with burnout have significantly lower levels of mindfulness and coping skills (Chaukos et al. 2017), and some studies have shown that mindfulness is an individual skill that may protect residents from burnout (Lebares et al. 2018; Olson et al. 2015). Therefore, interventions that target mindfulness may be of benefit to residents. Ophthalmology residents who participated in one 3-hour mindfulness-based session showed improvement in burnout scores (Rosdahl and Kingsolver 2014); thus, a larger study was conducted that included more resident specialties. This larger prospective study utilized residents that elected to participate in two or three 1-hour sessions of mindfulness-based resilience activities (Goldhagen et al. 2015). After completion of these sessions, residents did not demonstrate a reduction in burnout scores; however, 30 days after the intervention there was a trend toward lower burnout scores. Residents in the Netherlands were randomly selected to receive MBSR or no intervention (Verweij et al. 2018). Although residents receiving MBSR reported improved personal accomplishment, no significant difference was found in emotional exhaustion between groups. Notably, residents with high baseline levels of emotional exhaustion seemed to benefit more from MBSR training. Some studies have started to look at the feasibility and impact of mindfulness interventions using a smartphone application (Wen et al. 2017). To summarize, more studies are needed to clarify the most effective intervention for resident burnout as well as the most efficient way to deliver these interventions.

What Can Be Done Now

Only one-third of medical students with burnout seek help (Dyrbye and Shanafelt 2016). Students with burnout are reluctant to seek treatment for many reasons, including perceived stigma and fear of discrimination. Medical schools need to not only ensure rapid and easy access to professional help but also work to destigmatize help-seeking behavior.

Positive role models and mentors are important relationships that help residents develop into competent and confident physicians and may potentially help to mitigate the risk of burnout. Residents who perceive that their residency program values their education and report positive interactions with faculty and staff have a decreased risk of burnout (Ramey et al. 2017). Likewise, there is an association between resident burnout and decreased perceived support from faculty (Martini et al. 2006; Ramey et al. 2017). Doing rounds with an attending physician and regular staff meetings limit depersonalization and improve personal accomplishment, thereby protecting against burnout (Chaput et al. 2015). Organizational interventions that support faculty as positive role models and facilitate the time necessary to teach are not only critical to medical education and training but also may decrease the risk for resident burnout.

Several newly formed organizations as well as established national organizations have developed guidelines and concrete steps that can be taken to support physicians and residents confronting burnout. The American College of Emergency Physicians (www.acep.org) provides a wellness guide book, *Being Well in Emergency Medicine: ACEP's Guide to Investing in Yourself* (Manfredi and Huber 2017), part of which is dedicated to educating readers on the identification of resident burnout and discusses ways that residents and residency programs can foster wellness and prevent and reduce resident burnout. Moreover, residents are taking a more active role in preventing burnout. In March 2017, residents from 100 different programs convened at the Emergency Medicine Resident Wellness Consensus Summit and presented comprehensive lesson plans on practical skills for residents that could be used by residency programs (Battaglioli et al. 2018). Another recent initiative was the pilot study of curriculum that highlighted the feasibility of a resident-led resiliency curriculum (Chaukos et al. 2018). Stress Management and Resiliency Training Program for Residents is a group-based curriculum that teaches meditation, behavioral skills, and positive perspective-taking strategies. Resident-led initiatives have the ability to empower residents as the agents of change themselves.

Conclusion

Burnout is a syndrome that starts early in medical education and persists through medical school and into residency. In medical students, burnout is associated with dishonest clinical behavior (Dyrbye et al. 2010a), while in residents it is associated with perception of medical errors and suboptimal patient care (de Oliveira et al. 2013; Fahrenkopf et al. 2008; Shanafelt et al. 2002). From 2000 through 2014, the second leading cause of death among residents was suicide, and it was the most common cause of death among male residents (Yaghmour et al. 2017). The depth of the consequences of burnout on the individual cannot yet be truly appreciated because large, multi-institutional studies are lacking in student and resident populations.

To date, most studies examining burnout in medical student and resident populations investigate individual interventions, such as skills-based training in mindfulness, communication, or self-care. Although mindfulness and MBSR interventions often show a small or insignificant benefit on burnout reduction in medical students, symptoms such as anxiety, depressive symptoms, and perceived stress have been shown to improve as a result of these techniques (Erogul et al. 2014; Finkelstein et al. 2007; Shapiro et al.

1998). The few institutional/organizational studies on burnout in medical student and resident populations that exist have not proven to be of great benefit. Interventions aimed at reducing burnout in practicing physicians appear more effective than those targeting residents; therefore more research is needed to clarify how best to reach these populations.

It will be critical for continuing research on burnout in medical student and resident populations to consider how to effectively inform university healthcare organizations and trainees on burnout in order to promote wellness. Organizations like the American College of Emergency Physicians have recently produced books dedicated to promoting wellness and decreasing resident burnout. Additionally, residents and medical students are now taking a more active role than they had been afforded in the past.

KEY POINTS

- Burnout appears to occur very early on in medical education and increases throughout residency training.

- Burnout in medical students and residents is costly and is associated with increased risk of alcohol and other substance use/abuse, depression, suicidal ideation, career attrition, and poor patient care.

- Between 2000 and 2014, suicide was the second leading cause of death among residents and was the most common cause of death among male residents.

- Interventions aimed at reducing burnout among medical students and residents include individual-based interventions (mindfulness, self-care, exercise) and organizational interventions (duty-hour requirement changes, rotation and call schedules). Overall, these types of interventions have shown very little benefit in reducing symptoms of burnout but may have some mental health or quality of life benefits.

- Continued research is needed to identify factors that both predict and are associated with medical student and resident burnout to inform the development of effective preventive and selective interventions to reduce the burden associated with this syndrome.

- University healthcare organizations can promote wellness and reduce burnout by investing in the health and well-being of their faculty, residents, and students.

- Medical students and residents can take part in local and national organizations that promote wellness and reduce burnout in the medical profession.

References

Accreditation Council of Graduate Medical Education: Common Program Requirements. Chicago, IL, Accreditation Council for Graduate Medical Education, 2011

Babbott S, Manwell LB, Brown R, et al: Electronic medical records and physician stress in primary care: results from the MEMO Study. J Am Med Inform Assoc 21(e1 E2):e100–e106, 2014 24005796

Barbosa P, Raymond G, Zlotnick C, et al: Mindfulness-based stress reduction training is associated with greater empathy and reduced anxiety for graduate healthcare students. Educ Health (Abingdon) 26(1):9–14, 2013 23823667

Battaglioli N, Ankel F, Doty CI, et al: Executive summary from the 2017 emergency medicine resident wellness consensus summit. West J Emerg Med 19(2):332–336, 2018 29560062

Boni RADS, Paiva CE, de Oliveira MA, et al: Burnout among medical students during the first years of undergraduate school: prevalence and associated factors. PLoS One 13(3):e0191746, 2018 29513668

Bragard I, Etienne AM, Merckaert I, et al: Efficacy of a communication and stress management training on medical residents' self-efficacy, stress to communicate and burnout: a randomized controlled study. J Health Psychol 15(7):1075–1081, 2010 20453053

Chaput B, Bertheuil N, Jacques J, et al: Professional burnout among plastic surgery residents: can it be prevented? Outcomes of a national survey. Ann Plast Surg 75(1):2–8, 2015 25954838

Chaukos D, Chad-Friedman E, Mehta DH, et al: Risk and resilience factors associated with resident burnout. Acad Psychiatry 41(2):189–194, 2017 28028738

Chaukos D, Chad-Friedman E, Mehta DH, et al: SMART-R: a prospective cohort study of a resilience curriculum for residents by residents. Acad Psychiatry 42(1):78–83, 2018 29098597

Christino MA, Matson AP, Fischer SA, et al: Paperwork versus patient care: a nationwide survey of residents' perceptions of clinical documentation requirements and patient care. J Grad Med Educ 5(4):600–604, 2013 24455008

Dahlin M, Joneborg N, Runeson B: Performance-based self-esteem and burnout in a cross-sectional study of medical students. Med Teach 29(1):43–48, 2007 17538833

Daya Z, Hearn JH: Mindfulness interventions in medical education: a systematic review of their impact on medical student stress, depression, fatigue and burnout. Med Teach 40(2):146–153, 2018 29113526

de Oliveira GS Jr, Chang R, Fitzgerald PC, et al: The prevalence of burnout and depression and their association with adherence to safety and practice standards: a survey of United States anesthesiology trainees. Anesth Analg 117(1):182–193, 2013 23687232

de Vibe M, Solhaug I, Tyssen R, et al: Mindfulness training for stress management: a randomised controlled study of medical and psychology students. BMC Med Educ 13(1):107, 2013 23941053

Dyrbye L, Shanafelt T: A narrative review on burnout experienced by medical students and residents. Med Educ 50(1):132–149, 2016 26695473

Dyrbye LN, Massie FS, Eacker A, et al: Relationship between burnout and professional conduct and attitudes among US medical students. JAMA 304(11):1173–1180, 2010a 20841530

Dyrbye LN, Thomas MR, Power DV, et al: Burnout and serious thoughts of dropping out of medical school: a multi-institutional study. Acad Med 85(1):94–102, 2010b 20042833

Dyrbye LN, Shanafelt TD, Werner L, et al: The impact of a required longitudinal stress management and resilience training course for first-year medical students. J Gen Intern Med 32(12):1309–1314, 2017 28861707

Eckleberry-Hunt J, Lick D, Boura J, et al: An exploratory study of resident burnout and wellness. Acad Med 84(2):269–277, 2009 19174684

Eisenberg D, Gollust SE, Golberstein E, et al: Prevalence and correlates of depression, anxiety, and suicidality among university students. Am J Orthopsychiatry 77(4):534–542, 2007 18194033

Elmariah H, Thomas S, Boggan JC, et al: The burden of burnout. Am J Med Qual 32(2):156–162, 2017 26917807

Erogul M, Singer G, McIntyre T, et al: Abridged mindfulness intervention to support wellness in first-year medical students. Teach Learn Med 26(4):350–356, 2014 25318029

Fahrenkopf AM, Sectish TC, Barger LK, et al: Rates of medication errors among depressed and burnt out residents: prospective cohort study. BMJ 336(7642):488–491, 2008 18258931

Finkelstein C, Brownstein A, Scott C, et al: Anxiety and stress reduction in medical education: an intervention. Med Educ 41(3):258–264, 2007 17316210

Frank E, Elon L, Naimi T, Brewer R: Alcohol consumption and alcohol counselling behaviour among US medical students: cohort study. BMJ 337(7679):a2155, 2008 18996938

Gallagher TH, Waterman AD, Ebers AG, et al: Patients' and physicians' attitudes regarding the disclosure of medical errors. JAMA 289(8):1001–1007, 2003 12597752

Garneau K, Hutchinson T, Zhao Q, et al: Cultivating person-centered medicine in future physicians. Eur J Pers Cent Healthc 1(2):468–477, 2013

Goldhagen BE, Kingsolver K, Stinnett SS, et al: Stress and burnout in residents: impact of mindfulness-based resilience training. Adv Med Educ Pract 6:525–532, 2015 26347361

Gunasingam N, Burns K, Edwards J, et al: Reducing stress and burnout in junior doctors: the impact of debriefing sessions. Postgrad Med J 91(1074):182–187, 2015 25755266

Hojat M, Mangione S, Nasca TJ, et al: An empirical study of decline in empathy in medical school. Med Educ 38(9):934–941, 2004 15327674

Ishak WW, Lederer S, Mandili C, et al: Burnout during residency training: a literature review. J Grad Med Educ 1(2):236–242, 2009 21975985

Jackson ER, Shanafelt TD, Hasan O, et al: Burnout and alcohol abuse/dependence among U.S. medical students. Acad Med 91(9):1251–1256, 2016 26934693

Kealy D, Halli P, Ogrodniczuk JS, et al: Burnout among Canadian psychiatry residents: a national survey. Can J Psychiatry 61(11):732–736, 2016 27310237

Kimo Takayesu J, Ramoska EA, Clark TR, et al: Factors associated with burnout during emergency medicine residency. Acad Emerg Med 21(9):1031–1035, 2014 25269584

Lebares CC, Guvva EV, Ascher NL, et al: Burnout and stress among US surgery residents: psychological distress and resilience. J Am Coll Surg 226(1):80–90, 2018 29107117

Manfredi RA, Huber JM (eds): Being Well in Emergency Medicine: ACEP's Guide to Investing in Yourself. Washington, DC, American College of Emergency Physicians, 2017

Mangione S, Chakraborti C, Staltari G, et al: Medical students' exposure to the humanities correlates with positive personal qualities and reduced burnout: a multi-institutional U.S. survey. J Gen Intern Med 33(5):628–634, 2018 29380213

Martini S, Arfken CL, Balon R: Comparison of burnout among medical residents before and after the implementation of work hours limits. Acad Psychiatry 30(4):352–355, 2006 16908615

Martins AE, Davenport MC, Del Valle MP, et al: Impact of a brief intervention on the burnout levels of pediatric residents. J Pediatr (Rio J) 87(6):493–498, 2011 22170452

Mata DA, Ramos MA, Bansal N, et al: Prevalence of depression and depressive symptoms among resident physicians: a systematic review and meta-analysis. JAMA 314(22):2373–2383, 2015 26647259

Olson K, Kemper KJ, Mahan JD: What factors promote resilience and protect against burnout in first-year pediatric and medicine-pediatric residents? J Evid Based Complementary Altern Med 20(3):192–198, 2015 25694128

Oxentenko AS, West CP, Popkave C, et al: Time spent on clinical documentation: a survey of internal medicine residents and program directors. Arch Intern Med 170(4):377–380, 2010 20177042

Panagioti M, Panagopoulou E, Bower P, et al: Controlled interventions to reduce burnout in physicians: a systematic review and meta-analysis. JAMA Intern Med 177(2):195–205, 2017 27918798

Paro HB, Silveira PS, Perotta B, et al: Empathy among medical students: is there a relation with quality of life and burnout? PLoS One 9(4):e94133, 2014 24705887

Parshuram CS, Amaral AC, Ferguson ND, et al: Patient safety, resident well-being and continuity of care with different resident duty schedules in the intensive care unit: a randomized trial. CMAJ 187(5):321–329, 2015 25667258

Ramey SJ, Ahmed AA, Takita C, et al: Burnout evaluation of radiation residents nationwide: results of a survey of United States residents. Int J Radiat Oncol Biol Phys 99(3):530–538, 2017 29280446

Reed DA, Shanafelt TD, Satele DW, et al: Relationship of pass/fail grading and curriculum structure with well-being among preclinical medical students: a multi-institutional study. Acad Med 86(11):1367–1373, 2011 21952063

Ripp J, Babyatsky M, Fallar R, et al: The incidence and predictors of job burnout in first-year internal medicine residents: a five-institution study. Acad Med 86(10):1304–1310, 2011 21869661

Ripp JA, Bellini L, Fallar R, et al: The impact of duty hours restrictions on job burnout in internal medicine residents: a three-institution comparison study. Acad Med 90(4):494–499, 2015 25607940

Ripp JA, Fallar R, Korenstein D: A randomized controlled trial to decrease job burnout in first-year internal medicine residents using a facilitated discussion group intervention. J Grad Med Educ 8(2):256–259, 2016 27168899

Rosdahl JA, Kingsolver K: Mindfulness training to increase resilience and decrease stress and burnout in ophthalmology residents: a pilot study. Invest Ophthalmol Vis Sci 55(13):5579, 2014

Rotenstein LS, Ramos MA, Torre M, et al: Prevalence of depression, depressive symptoms, and suicidal ideation among medical students: a systematic review and meta-analysis. JAMA 316(21):2214–2236, 2016 27923088

Sen S, Kranzler HR, Krystal JH, et al: A prospective cohort study investigating factors associated with depression during medical internship. Arch Gen Psychiatry 67(6):557–565, 2010 20368500

Sen S, Kranzler HR, Didwania AK, et al: Effects of the 2011 duty hour reforms on interns and their patients: a prospective longitudinal cohort study. JAMA Intern Med 173(8):657–662, discussion 663, 2013 23529201

Shanafelt TD, Bradley KA, Wipf JE, et al: Burnout and self-reported patient care in an internal medicine residency program. Ann Intern Med 136(5):358–367, 2002 11874308

Shanafelt TD, Dyrbye LN, Sinsky C, et al: Relationship between clerical burden and characteristics of the electronic environment with physician burnout and professional satisfaction. Mayo Clin Proc 91(7):836–848, 2016 27313121

Shapiro SL, Schwartz GE, Bonner G: Effects of mindfulness-based stress reduction on medical and premedical students. J Behav Med 21(6):581–599, 1998 9891256

Shapiro SL, Shapiro DE, Schwartz GER: Stress management in medical education: a review of the literature. Acad Med 75(7):748–759, 2000 10926029

Shea JA, Bellini LM, Dinges DF, et al: Impact of protected sleep period for internal medicine interns on overnight call on depression, burnout, and empathy. J Grad Med Educ 6(2):256–263, 2014 24949128

Thomas MR, Dyrbye LN, Huntington JL, et al: How do distress and well-being relate to medical student empathy? A multicenter study. J Gen Intern Med 22(2):177–183, 2007 17356983

Verweij H, van Ravesteijn H, van Hooff MLM, et al: Mindfulness-based stress reduction for residents: a randomized controlled trial. J Gen Intern Med 33(4):429–436, 2018 29256091

Weight CJ, Sellon JL, Lessard-Anderson CR, et al: Physical activity, quality of life, and burnout among physician trainees: the effect of a team-based, incentivized exercise program. Mayo Clin Proc 88(12):1435–1442, 2013 24290117

Wen L, Sweeney TE, Welton L, et al: Encouraging mindfulness in medical house staff via smartphone app: a pilot study. Acad Psychiatry 41(5):646–650, 2017 28795335

West CP, Huschka MM, Novotny PJ, et al: Association of perceived medical errors with resident distress and empathy: a prospective longitudinal study. JAMA 296(9):1071–1078, 2006 16954486

West CP, Shanafelt TD, Kolars JC: Quality of life, burnout, educational debt, and medical knowledge among internal medicine residents. JAMA 306(9):952–960, 2011 21900135

West CP, Dyrbye LN, Erwin PJ, et al: Interventions to prevent and reduce physician burnout: a systematic review and meta-analysis. Lancet 388(10057):2272–2281, 2016 27692469

Woloschuk W, Harasym PH, Temple W: Attitude change during medical school: a cohort study. Med Educ 38(5):522–534, 2004 15107086

Woodside JR, Miller MN, Floyd MR, et al: Observations on burnout in family medicine and psychiatry residents. Acad Psychiatry 32(1):13–19, 2008 18270276

Yaghmour NA, Brigham TP, Richter T, et al: Causes of death of residents in ACGME-accredited programs 2000 through 2014: implications for the learning environment. Acad Med 92(7):976–983, 2017 28514230

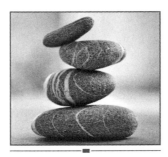

PART IV

ADDRESSING AND PREVENTING PHYSICIAN BURNOUT

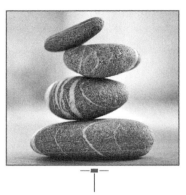

CHAPTER 11

A MODEL FOR MAINTAINING WELL-BEING AND PREVENTING BURNOUT FOR PSYCHIATRISTS

Linda L. M. Worley, M.D.

Cynthia M. Stonnington, M.D.

"People change for two reasons: (1) pain, and
(2) great pain."

William H. Swiggart, M.S.
Co-Director of the Vanderbilt Center for Professional Health

Disclaimer: The stories in this chapter capture common contributors to burnout in the lives of psychiatrists. If a story feels familiar, this is merely a coincidence reinforcing that you are not alone.

One might presume that psychiatrists, whose expertise it is to help others achieve happiness and health, would be spared the epidemic of physician burnout. Sadly, this is not the case. It is time to proactively recapture our well-being and our enthusiasm for life and for the powerful work we do as psychiatrists.

In this chapter, we provide a framework for preventing burnout by using the "Smooth Sailing Life Nautical Metaphor."[1] Important contributors to burnout are illustrated within five stories of psychiatrists' lives, followed by the application of the metaphor identifying specific problems and solutions. The chapter concludes with take-home tips to thrive.

Crystallization of the Smooth Sailing Life Nautical Metaphor

VIGNETTE 1: "I'M CAPSIZING!"

I was 32, in my second year of an academic faculty position as an assistant professor of psychiatry. My personal life as the wife of a resident and mother of a 4-year-old daughter and an 8-year-old son was demanding. Our family relied on my faculty salary to make ends meet.

I was responsible for running three busy clinical services: the hospital consultation-liaison psychiatry service, the College of Medicine Student Mental Health Service, and my outpatient psychiatric clinic, in addition to covering a grueling 24/7 call for a week at a time.

It was through this on-call duty that I discovered how severely broken our state mental health system was. Increasing numbers of seriously mentally ill patients were seeking help in our university hospital emergency department. We did not have an inpatient unit, and most gravely ill patients did not have any ability to pay for treatment. We would conduct thorough evaluations of patients and whenever possible come up with a viable alternative to inpatient hospitalization. When a patient was too ill for this approach, we would contact the state mental health screener (a social worker), who would arrive at the emergency department hours later to conduct their own evaluation and determination of necessary disposition. Increasingly, the screener would declare that the patient was "safe to go home" to be followed in an outpatient setting, leaving the university physician staff and residents liable if the patient had a bad outcome. We had no good options for placement, and the state funds designated for uninsured mentally ill patients were not being authorized to be used. Eager to fix the problem, I scheduled a sit-down meeting with my service chief and carefully outlined the situation and how serious it was becoming.

I was stunned by his response.

"Don't be a lightning rod." His back stiffened. He leaned forward, "You're on the tenure track. If you want to keep your job 6 years from now, you'd best pick up the pace and get moving on your research and publications."

I felt a pressure rising in my chest, my heart pounded, and I bit the inside of my cheek holding back my fury, disappointment, and disbelief and made a composed, hasty departure. It seemed like an eternity until I was safely in the sanctuary of home, where my exhaustion and tears could erupt. Completely unaccustomed to seeing me in this state, my alarmed husband rushed in. "What's happened? What's wrong?"

I looked up at him. "I just can't do this.... I'm capsizing!"

He gently wrapped his strong arm around my shoulders and held me closely, tenderly kissing my head, and whispered, "Reef[2] in your sails my love. Just reef in your sails."

The early crystals of the nautical metaphor that formed that day have continued to grow into the Smooth Sailing Life Nautical Metaphor, an easy to remember biopsychosocial-spiritual model that provides an accessible framework for understanding and solving burnout. May it light your way!

SMOOTH SAILING LIFE NAUTICAL METAPHOR DEFINED

Each of us is born into a single sailboat for our entire lifetime. The metaphor being used here for a physician's professional and personal life is that of a sailboat/yacht.[3] The yacht, including the crew, are all the parts of a single physician. Other yachts represent other people in the physician's life, including patients, coworkers, significant others, supervisors and administrators, and so on. Yacht components are shown in Figure 11–1. Definitions are as follows:

- The *hull* is the body of the sailboat that keeps you afloat. In the metaphor, the hull represents your entire physical self, including all your organs, especially your brain.
- The *mast* is the sturdy pole anchored at its base within the body of the boat. It serves as the secure frame for the sails. It represents your knowledge.
- The *sails* come in many sizes, shapes, and colors. They represent your skills. Over time, they wear out and require updating as new technologies and advances in the field emerge.
- The *wind gusts* that fill the sails are your tasks and responsibilities.
- The *keel* is a dense structure on the belly of the yacht that provides a stabilizing counterbalance against the force of the wind. It represents being connected to love and to one's deepest, most meaningful values and spiritual beliefs. The keel protects the yacht from capsizing. It also provides a

---

[2]"Reefing in one's sails" means to pull in some of the exposed sail so that it catches less wind. This prevents the high winds from capsizing the boat.
[3]The terms sailboat and yacht are used interchangeably throughout this chapter.

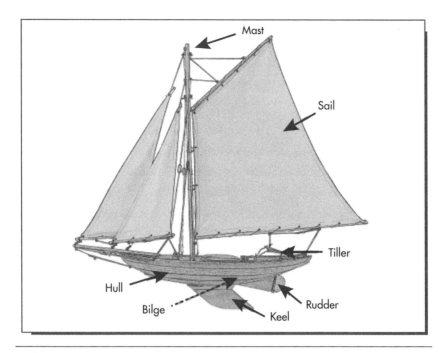

FIGURE 11–1. Anatomy of a sailboat.
Source.   Smooth Sailing Life Nautical Metaphor.® Image © Linda L. M. Worley, M.D. All rights reserved. Reproduced here with permission.

force beneath the water enabling the yacht to sail a straight course rather than being helplessly pushed sideways across the surface of the water.

- The *rudder,* at the back of the boat beneath the water, is turned side to side by the tiller (a handle on smaller boats) or by the captain's steering wheel (on large yachts). This controls the direction the yacht will travel. It represents your mind and your ability to choose.
- The *bilge* is a compartment within the hull where excess water collects so it can be emptied back into the ocean where it belongs. This contained water represents uncomfortable or painful emotions (e.g., sadness, disappointment, grief, anxiety, nervousness, fear, frustration, irritation, anger). The ability to recognize and name emotions, to understand their triggers, and then to choose optimal responses is emotional intelligence. Most times, uncomfortable emotions are a normal, adaptive response to life's challenges, but when they persist, it is essential to search deeper for an underlying treatable physical illness, such as hypothyroidism, mania, and so on.
- The *journey* represents your lifetime accomplishments and the legacy that you will leave.

Important messages can be derived from negative emotions:

- *Sadness/disappointment/grief* is experienced when a person has a significant loss. It is important to be self-aware (check the bilge), identify the etiology of the sadness, and then name it and express it, honoring its importance in your life and allowing yourself to grieve. When a person is sad, they often pull back from interacting with others, isolate, and heal. Some journal, others cry, some either listen to or play music in the minor key or watch a sad movie. Support groups after loss can be particularly helpful. When sadness does not lift despite facing it, it is important to reach out for professional help.
- *Anger/frustration/irritation* is experienced when your needs are not being met. These emotions alert you to something that needs your attention. Take the time to sort through the cause of your reaction and explore your options for resolution. When necessary, seek out consultation and mentoring as you seek solutions. For individuals raised to believe that it is unacceptable to express anger or frustration, seeking psychotherapy to gain the skills to better acknowledge, effectively express, and assertively get one's needs met can be instrumental in avoiding clinical depression.
- *Fear/anxiety/nervousness* is experienced when a person anticipates a bad outcome or harm. The accompanying increased sympathetic nervous system activity increases alertness and fuels a response-enhancing performance and in emergent situations can be lifesaving. When anxiety and fear are incapacitating, it is important to seek professional help.

When a bilge remains full of water (negative emotions), it weighs down the boat, making it more difficult to move through the water (an energy drain), reducing its efficiency and speed. An overflowing bilge also strains the structure of the hull (e.g., manifesting as suffering expressed through unexplained bodily symptoms), decreases its overall resilience, and leaves the vessel vulnerable to capsizing in high winds.

Achieving a balanced, fulfilled life, much like smooth sailing, is an ongoing challenge requiring continual readjustment, self-care, and a focus on heading toward what matters most in life.

VIGNETTE I DISCUSSION

Problems

Vignette 1 highlights the following problems:

- Attempting to stay upright in gale force winds—too many responsibilities to manage!
- The bilge is full of wastewater—uncomfortable emotions of frustration, sadness, and anxiety.
- The yacht is in need of maintenance—exhaustion.
- The keel (one's values) is hitting ground in shallow water and is being torn up—the boss's stance is violating deeply held principles of doing right by the attending physician and her mentally ill patients.

The factor most highly associated with wanting to leave a position is one's relationship with one's boss and its contribution to physician burnout. It is difficult to work for a boss who does not share the same values. Job turnover is extremely costly to the healthcare system (Shanafelt et al. 2017).

Necessary Adjustments

The adjustments to the problems that are outlined in Vignette 1 are the following:

- Reef in the sails—triage tasks, ask for help, say no to new requests whenever possible. Negotiate for realignment of duties to ensure success (Fisher and Ury 2011).
- Urgently provide tender loving care for the yacht—catch up on sleep, drink plenty of water, eat healthy foods, do a little exercise, accept and give love.
- Empty the bilge—write out what is upsetting in a journal or share with a listening trustworthy beloved friend, family member, or colleague.
- Consider possible journeys for your life—consider best fit for career aspirations and identify occupational goals, seeking out skilled mentorship both inside and outside the institution.
- Outfit the yacht for the journey seeking additional knowledge, skills, etc.—learn effective negotiation skills to pursue realignment of clinical duties with obligatory requirements for achieving promotion and tenure.
- If you are working in conditions that conflict with your values, the courageous decision may be to change course when the right opportunity presents itself (e.g., head out to sail in deeper waters capable of accommodating the depth of your keel).
- Identify and seek out a fleet leader (a new boss) who shares your values. Team well-being is strongly enhanced when mutual trust and respect is the norm and all are working together toward a unified, meaningful mission. Positive team structure and social connection at work are important factors for physician well-being (Thomas et al. 2018).
- Commit to values-based decisions both for yourself individually and, should you rise to be the leader, for your organization (Graber and Kilpatrick 2008; Mills and Spencer 2005).

VIGNETTE 2: ANTIQUATED SAILING RULES!

Outward Appearances

Dr. Steele has a great reputation. Anytime a difficult project needs to be done, we ask her. She is one of the most conscientious members of the department. Selecting her as chair last year was a great choice. Lately, she has not seemed herself. Just this morning, she had dark circles under her eyes and did not even make eye contact or smile when we passed in the hall. This is completely unlike her.

Inner World—A Glimpse Inside Dr. Steele's Journal

I just can't keep up. I'm upset with myself for NOT being more efficient. When both grants were funded last year, I saw it as a blessing. I really needed the funding to balance the departmental budget, but now, it's on me to deliver. No one else here has time to help. My entire faculty are still resentful about the newly imposed relative value unit requirements to be eligible for quarterly bonuses. I don't have the heart to ask them for more. I'm afraid they'll just walk if I do. I can't safely run our programs if I lose anyone else. My own clinic doesn't have an opening for 3 months. Just yesterday, the chair of neurosurgery called me about his mother. He was so worried about her that he literally begged me to see her for an urgent evaluation. Her condition sounds so complex and needs the kind of evaluation that I have the specialized training to do. I offered to see her early Friday if he'd bring her in before clinic hours. I don't know what I was thinking. I have so many other obligations closing in on me. I'm regularly unable to send or receive emails because I'm over the message limit. This isn't fun anymore.

VIGNETTE 2 DISCUSSION

Problems

Dr. Steele's yacht is leaning over so far that her keel is nearly out of the water, causing complete loss of steerage—she is attempting to manage an impossible number of tasks and responsibilities. She is living life (sailing) according to rules she acquired in her family of origin and in her medical training:

- Work hard and be responsible!
- Be self-sufficient, don't be weak or ask for help.
- Be conscientious and generous; be there for others.

Solutions

Take an emergency break from work to avoid capsizing. Quickly assess yacht for seaworthiness (significant leaks—symptoms of treatable medical/psychiatric conditions), get a good night of restorative sleep, eat several healthy meals, drink plenty of water, and avoid detrimental self-soothing behaviors (overeating, alcohol, or substance use). Empty the bilge (journaling for 20 minutes about what is most upsetting) and fortify the keel by connecting with sources of love and meaning.

Examine current sailing rules (rules of acceptable behavior from family of origin and from medical training) and how they contribute to present-day successes and difficulties.

- Successes: Dr. Steele has risen to be chair of the department through hard work, being there for others, and being self-sufficient.
- Difficulties: She is struggling to effectively delegate and to ask for help, and she puts others' needs first over her own to the point of making herself ineffective.

Step back and examine life to define long-term aspirations, imagining what you hope family, friends, patients, students, and colleagues will say about the impact you have had on their lives and on the world. Update outdated sailing rules to new ones that support the journey to your desired destination for this lifetime:

- Make it a priority to maximize the strength and well-being of the yacht.
- Lead the fleet (the department faculty) effectively by learning to share opportunities (wind that will be good for their career journeys).
- Set strategic limits that will enable success.

Triage obligations (current winds), choosing which ones can be reassigned or delegated and which ones to prioritize. Negotiate new due dates if necessary. Create a 4×4 table to triage the tasks (Table 11–1). Focus on completing high-value tasks.

- Focus on one task at a time; multitasking is less effective.
- Strive for excellence, doing the best job you can in the time you have.
- Tackle high-value tasks first without hesitation or procrastination. Break an onerous task down into much smaller achievable tasks.
- Intersperse a fun exercise break or a creative activity between stints of hard work to rejuvenate and energize.

Identify tasks to delegate. It helps others when you share opportunities. Your fleet (the team of colleagues you work with) will be stronger together when you relinquish some control, trusting their capabilities to manage worthwhile opportunities. Thoughtfully select the best person (another yacht) to take on the task—someone you trust and who is capable. Provide specific mentorship about the task at hand, check back, offer feedback, and express gratitude.

Seek additional skills in limit setting, working with a mentor. Practice clarifying what you can and cannot do. Understand the range of vulnerabilities leading people to say "yes" when the task would take them in the wrong direction (Lencioni 2018):

- Work equals identity: Being overcommitted reaffirms that identity.
- People pleasing: Saying "yes" feeds the need for external approval and admiration.
- Genuine wish to help others or interest in the activity: The desire to help others or to pursue an interest overshadows the true costs and benefits of saying "yes."

TABLE 11–1.   **Triage tool for obligations**

	High value	Low value
Easy (minimal time)	Prioritize	Maybe
Hard (most time)	Maybe	Discard

- Denial: The reality that there are just 24 hours in the day is dismissed.
- Escape: Emotionally difficult situations are avoided through overworking.
- Fear: Believing an important opportunity will never come again spurs taking on more than is wise.

Place a moratorium on saying "yes" to new opportunities (winds). Institute a 24-hour buffer before allowing yourself to give an answer when asked to take on something new. Consult a mentor who has your best interests at heart before you respond. Set compassionate boundaries and limits and carefully choose when to say "no," realizing that when you selectively say "no," you enhance your "yes" (Epstein and Krasner 2013; Meldrum 2010; Spiers et al. 2017; Zwack and Schweitzer 2013).

- Make strategic decisions based on your mission and what you are striving to accomplish in this lifetime. Selectively say yes to opportunities aligned with your aspirations (Creswell et al. 2005).
- With requests you cannot manage or that do not fit with your values and goals, express gratitude for the invitation and send regrets earlier rather than later. This will earn you respect because you are valuing the requester's need for time to find an alternate.
- Do not say "yes" when you mean "no"; if you say "no," refrain from being overly apologetic (Smith 1985).

Master the onslaught of emails (Song et al. 2008):

- Take control of your email in-box by taking a course that teaches the latest tips and tricks for organization.
- Silence the alerts announcing the arrival of new emails.
- Practice the golden rule of treating others as you would like to be treated. Limit your sent email messages, sending only concise messages and being judicious with "reply all."
- Use the power of shared drives for meeting agendas, minutes, daily on-call doctor information, and so on.
- Create rules for automatic filing of nonurgent messages. Periodically visit files to clean them out.

VIGNETTE 3: IGNORANCE, ROLE CONFUSION, AND HIGH-RISK CARVE OUTS

On a flight to a medical conference, the passenger next to me asked, "What's the difference between a psychologist and a psychiatrist?" It's a familiar question that I have gotten used to answering. I took a deep breath and, once again, patiently described the difference between a social worker, a psychologist, a nurse practitioner, and a psychiatrist. Shortly after returning to work, it became apparent to me that even physicians making referrals did not understand the neurobiology of psychiatric illnesses. A patient with hypoactive delirium was referred for an evaluation of "depression and poor coping." Later that day, an insurance company refused to allow a patient who had struggled with debilitating and life-threatening depression after "successful" treatment for lymphoma to be seen by the psychiatrist working in collaboration with the oncologist, because of their "carve out for mental health care." After finally convincing the insurance company to allow at least a few visits with the psychiatrist integrated with the oncology team, it turned out that a medication that the patient responded well to needed preauthorization, despite being generic and not the most expensive!

VIGNETTE 3 DISCUSSION

Problems

This widespread ignorance about the complex medical etiologies underlying psychiatric illness is frightening when it threatens the safe and effective treatment of patients with psychiatric illness. It is also demoralizing to and dismissive of our profession. The perception of being invisible and overlooked as a vital resource for providing safe and effective patient care, even if largely unintentional due to ignorance, contributes to burnout. It is both frustrating and frightening to know that patients in need of a psychiatrist's medical expertise may only be allowed to be seen by "behavioral health providers" with no medical training at all.

Solutions

On an individual level, maintain strong relationships with medical colleagues and participate in case conferences and educational opportunities. Partner with advocacy groups, (e.g., the National Alliance on Mental Illness and others) and with nonpsychiatric colleagues, using illustrative case examples to raise awareness about the medical basis for psychiatric illnesses.

Collectively join forces with the American Psychiatric Association and other professional organizations (e.g., the American Neuropsychiatric Association) to educate the public, the medical field, insurance agencies, and other stakeholders. We are stronger together, when our focus is about promoting the health and well-being of our citizens. Partner with screenwriters and producers to help create accurate portrayals of our field to educate the public on the depth, breadth, and value of the work we do so they will speak up and demand access to a psychiatrist when warranted.

Recognize that as we get better at assigning "the right work to the right person," psychiatrists' calendars will be filled with increasingly complex patients. Managing that stress may require the following:

- Team-based care, such as social workers, psychologists, nurses, psychiatrists, and nonpsychiatric providers, all working together to address the needs of the patient
- Supervision and/or regular case conferences
- Allotting sufficient time to see complex patients, despite pressures to schedule more patients to make up for declining reimbursement
- Working with advocacy groups to convince payors to reimburse for documentation time

Work diligently for reform supporting the American Psychiatric Association's combined advocacy efforts to develop viable solutions to overcome frustrating barriers being imposed on our field, ranging from documentation requirements to prior authorizations and inequities in reimbursement and in health insurance reform (American Psychiatric Association 2018; Swensen et al. 2016).

Align assigned job duties (allocating at least 1 day per week) to an area of work most meaningful to you. This is highly protective against becoming discouraged and burned out (a syndrome of emotional exhaustion, cynicism, and decreased effectiveness at work). In a study of 465 physicians, spending even 1 day per week on the aspect of work identified as most meaningful was associated with significantly lower physician burnout rates (53.8% vs. 29.9%) (Shanafelt et al. 2009).

Maximize meaning, engagement, and job satisfaction. Authentic, humanistic interactions with patients and colleagues enhance physician well-being, and physicians who are well may, in turn, provide better patient care and practice high-quality medicine. During the most challenging moments, look to the serenity prayer: "God, grant me the serenity to accept the things I cannot change, the courage to change the things I can, and the wisdom to know the difference."

VIGNETTE 4: THE DOCTOR'S OVERFLOWING BILGE

They say bad things happen in threes. I guess that is true. It has been a horrific year. One of my closest friends, Thomas, was diagnosed with pancreatic cancer. My wife announced on her birthday that, after 23 years of marriage and two kids, she "couldn't love me the way I deserved" and that she finally was strong enough to share that she is gay. Our divorce was finalized last month. Two days ago, I got the call that my medical school roommate had completed suicide. His wife said he had left a note. I am furious with him for not calling me. I could have helped him! How could I have missed the signs? I just saw him last month at the reunion.

I am exhausted, I feel as though an elephant is sitting on me. My brain is fuzzy. I'm short tempered and snapped at Jessie, our kind and gentle receptionist who would not hurt a flea. She recoiled as if I had just hit her. I felt terrible. Now all I feel is numb. I could hardly sit still through my last session today, especially when my patient began recounting how her parents had expected her to clean up the car after her younger brother shot himself in it. I haven't cried in years. I don't think I even know how to anymore. The last time I cried was when I was a kid and my dog died.

VIGNETTE 4 DISCUSSION

Problems

The bilge is filled beyond capacity (profound sadness related to catastrophic losses), and the bilge pump is broken. Thus, there is no healthy outlet for the powerful emotions that are driving feelings of exhaustion, an inability to be empathic, and displaced irritable outbursts. A functional bilge pump (which enables the identification and the effective expression of painful emotions and a sense of congruence, i.e., looking the way you feel) is vital. Without it, one's risk for burnout increases exponentially.

Solutions

High levels of distress and trauma may warrant taking one's yacht to a "maintenance bay" for immediate help emptying the bilge (seeing a trusted therapist). It is challenging for psychiatrists to seek help for themselves but invaluable in facilitating our ability to give our own patients our very best.

The following are ways to process difficult emotional experiences:

- Journaling or art expression (Keeling and Bermudez 2006)
- Engaging in psychotherapy—psychodynamically oriented, interpersonal, cognitive-behavioral, and mindfulness-based therapies—all shown beneficial for enhancing awareness of and processing strategies for difficult emotions
- Talking with peers, family, or friends (Lemaire and Wallace 2010)
- Connecting with a suicide survivor support group

Fortifying the keel can be accomplished by getting spiritually centered through cultivating mindfulness and gratitude. One approach is through regular practice of reflection and mindfulness meditation, which has been found to be an excellent strategy for skillfully responding to stress and for accepting and tolerating one's emotions without unwittingly adding more wastewater via unnecessary judgment, self-blame, and resistance (water in the bilge) (Amutio et al. 2015; Goodman and Schorling 2012; Irving et al. 2009; Siegel 1999). *Mindfulness* means paying attention to present experiences on a moment-to-moment basis with nonjudgmental awareness. It can involve focusing inward (centering), for example, awareness of the breath, body scanning, or walking meditation versus "loving kindness" meditations and "open" meditations that require a receptive attitude to whatever arises rather than focusing on one object (Kabat-Zinn 2013). Consider taking a course in mindfulness-based stress reduction (Kabat-Zinn 2013; Krasner et al. 2009), acceptance and commitment therapy (Hayes et al. 2006, 2013), and/or yoga. Begin a daily practice of noting "three good things," either at the start of the day, lunchtime, or end of the day (e.g., see phone applications at the end of this chapter).

Exercise to de-stress and rejuvenate (Lemaire and Wallace 2010; Weight et al. 2013). Strategies to turn the good intentions to exercise into a reality include the following:

- Have a regular exercise time that can work in your schedule.
- Find a partner or group to exercise with.
- Set an intention to exercise and track it.
- Remind yourself how you feel after exercising, rather than focusing on how exhausted you are feeling beforehand.

More global strategies for emptying the bilge and fortifying your keel are the following:

- Improve systems-level barriers interfering with students, trainees, and faculty seeking treatment by creating free or easily accessible mental health treatment (Ey et al. 2013; Gold et al. 2016; Worley 2008).
- Provide a platform for colleagues openly acknowledging their own journey in recovering from mental illness, removing the element of shame and secrecy (American Psychiatric Association 2018).
- Work with advocacy groups to eliminate inappropriate licensure questions about having or being treated for a mental illness (Dyrbye et al. 2015, 2017; Gold et al. 2017).

Negative emotions provide important information to inform and guide our journey; therefore, the goal is not to eliminate or avoid all negative emotions. However, difficult emotions are unpleasant, and it is common to consciously or unconsciously defend against being aware of uncomfortable emotional states. When they remain in the bilge because of suppression, repression, denial, displacement, or any number of other well-known defense mechanisms, they interfere with optimal sailing and strain the physical structure of the yacht. Emotional spillover, that is, internalizing stressful experiences, leads to depletion and exhaustion. Psychiatrists' work is often solitary and necessarily involves a one-way relationship with patients. Over time, it can become more difficult and uncomfortable to disclose information about oneself to peers, family, and friends. Importantly, when personal two-way relationships are starved, it creates vulnerability for boundary violations. For example, in this case, if the psychiatrist does not seek his own treatment or supervision, he is vulnerable to falling down a slippery slope, such as initially by hugging a patient to whom he consciously intended to show support or nurturance but unconsciously was fulfilling his need for gratification and personal support (Gabbard 1996). Left unexamined and untold, the hug could evolve to further sexual boundary violations due to the difference between conscious and unconscious intent and the "perils of secrecy" (Gabbard 1996). Good-quality clinical supervision guards against misconduct and has also been shown to be protective against burnout among mental health professionals (O'Connor et al. 2018).

This psychiatrist just experienced several traumatizing life events and was also caring for a patient with horrific trauma. Having one's own personal history of trauma increases the likelihood even further for experiencing compassion fatigue when also caring for patients with trauma. Mental health providers who experience multiple recent traumatic experiences are at higher risk for burnout (Rossi et al. 2012). A regular practice of reflection aids our ability to recognize the emotional toll of trauma as well as important countertransference responses in patient encounters. Screening tools can also be useful as a means to recognize when one is struggling (Halbesleben and Demerouti 2005; Maslach and Jackson 1981; Shanafelt et al. 2014; Trockel et al. 2018). Seeking professional help early is ideal. It is easier to repair a small leak in a yacht than a large, gaping hole that has been neglected for years.

VIGNETTE 5: SECRETS FOR THRIVING

Journal club was winding down early. The day's attending physician was Dr. Lee, so the room was packed. Her very presence was reassuring. Despite managing what appeared to be an impossible job, she remained openly accepting of others, exuding an aura of peace and kindness. Just being around her felt uplifting.

It was Dr. Byron's question, our third-year psychiatry resident with a reputation for directness, that captured our attention: "Dr. Lee, what's your secret? How do you manage so many frustrating situations and responsibilities and still have the energy you do and genuinely seem to love your job?"

Dr. Lee was caught off guard. All eyes now focused on her. Most of the residents were genuinely struggling themselves and were searching for advice and mentorship. Dr. Lee shifted her gaze out the window, deep in thought. She turned back, lowering her chin, her mouth revealing the hint of an embarrassed smile. "I think I am where I am today because of the many mistakes I've made."

She continued, "When I was a resident, I was already married like many of you. We had two little ones, and I felt guilty so much of the time. I know I didn't get enough rest. I didn't exercise, and I'd beat myself up every night about it. I just didn't have it in me to exercise. Instead, I'd collapse on the couch and mindlessly watch TV, eating a large bowl of popcorn smothered in butter and salt. It was best with a cool glass of wine. In the mornings, I could tell my clothes were getting tighter and harder to get into. They were looking old too. Out of curiosity, I stepped on our dusty bathroom scale. I literally screamed when I read the number. I'd never weighed that much in my entire life, except of course when I was pregnant. I really didn't feel good about myself at that point, and I knew I had important choices to make. I'd be lying if I said it was easy. It wasn't, and still isn't. But it's definitely been worth it."

"One of my biggest challenges was to give myself permission for down time and play time and time to take care of myself. I grew up in a family with the rule that it was unacceptable to play or rest until all the work was done. The problem is, being a physician, the work is never done. When I didn't take time for self-care, I just couldn't keep up with my previous pace. I was weary; my energy and enthusiasm for what I previously loved was fizzling. For me, this is what it meant to get burned out."

"After I began investing in self-care and just a little exercise, my energy quickly increased, my efficiency improved, and I accomplished much more than if I'd worked and worked straight through without any breaks."

"The other key secret I've discovered is the power of unconditional love and acceptance. Being spiritually centered and connected to that universal loving presence is key for me. When I extend outwardly the warmth and kindness I experience from my spiritual connection, I feel a deep satisfaction and an inner warmth. In some ways, it's a mitzvah, doing a good deed anonymously for another without any expectation of anything in return."

VIGNETTE 5 DISCUSSION

Problems From Dr. Lee's Past

Below are two problems specific to Dr. Lee's past experience:

- Obsolete sailing rules—having to complete all her work before allowing any self-care; living under the faulty premise that physicians do not need rest, food, or vacation
- Sailing aimlessly with absent keel—failing to invest time and energy in what matters most (e.g., squandering hours on mindless TV watching)

Solutions

Dr. Lee's story underscores the following solutions to avoid burnout:

- Nurture your spiritual connections (Davich 2014).
- Extend loving kindness to others, smile, look deeply, and listen with your eyes and heart.
- Persist in seeing and seeking the good in others (e.g., the diamond in the rough); reflect the brilliance you discover.

- Care for your yacht (your body) to function at your best (Weight et al. 2013).
- Advocate to advance technology to enhance our efficiency in mundane tasks to maximize the time and energy available to invest in a strong therapeutic relationship with our patients (Shanafelt et al. 2016).
- Invest in your intimate relationships, loving and being loved (Gottman and Silver 2015; Perlman et al. 2015).
- Share experiences and vulnerabilities with colleagues and be there for one another. Facilitated support groups for physician mothers have been shown to improve well-being and connectedness and were associated with an increased willingness to seek treatment (Luthar et al. 2017).
- Train clinician peers to reach out to their colleagues in response to adverse events and other stressful situations (Shapiro and Galowitz 2016).

Summary: Tips for Maintaining Well-Being and Preventing Burnout

SMOOTH SAILING LIFE NAUTICAL METAPHOR

You are a sailboat, including the entire crew that serve you for your lifetime. Each of the crew members are parts of yourself that fulfill essential roles.

CAPTAIN

Your captain is in charge of your life and stands at the helm, steering the yacht, ultimately in charge of all decisions. Have the courage to be authentic. Outline your long-term aspirations. Identify the important roles in your life. The struggles and challenges you have endured thus far are equipping you for your important purpose. Pay attention to what infuses you with love, light, and energy. Consult with your navigator/tactician to map out the short- and long-term course. Once selected, focus on staying on course. Listen to and respect your engineer's appraisal of your yacht's condition and needs. Prioritize maintenance and care of the yacht. This will ensure its longevity, strength, and ability to accomplish meaningful journeys.

Be kind to your crew. Factor in anchor-down time for vital rest and relaxation and a combination of intense upwind sailing, which requires great energy and focus, interspersed with fun, creative activities (effortless downwind sailing) that rejuvenates and refreshes.

NAVIGATOR/TACTICIAN

Your navigator/tactician is the expert who knows the globe, the currents, the sailing rules at sea, the depth of the water, and the weather conditions. In consultation with the captain, map out possible routes and strategies to reach desired destinations (life goals). Anticipate difficult barriers and hazards along the way and strategize to maneuver effectively (e.g., revising outdated sailing rules that now interfere).

ENGINEER

Your engineer is responsible for assessing and maintaining the seaworthiness of the vessel. To successfully sail long and meaningful journeys to great destinations, the yacht must be well equipped and in top form. It must be seaworthy, polished, strong, and rigged with the finest, most technologically advanced sails (knowledge and skills).

Prior to setting sail each day, the yacht must be carefully checked over, observing for any signs of leaks, weakness, or dysfunction. At the earliest signs of any difficulty, maintenance is called for (seek appropriate professional care). The earlier a difficulty is recognized, the easier it is to repair. The bilge must be checked frequently for wastewater (uncomfortable emotions) and effectively emptied.

A common weakness is a broken connection between the steerage of the yacht and the rudder (a lack of discipline), resulting in a mismatch between what the captain professes to want (e.g., to get buff and fit through regular exercise) and an ability to get there (deck hands being too weary at the end of the day to get off the couch). This inability to accomplish this goal (destination) is frustrating for the captain, and water seeps into the bilge as a result, additionally decreasing energy, resilience, and strength. This makes the journey more difficult overall. Motivational interviewing can be helpful in overcoming this dysfunction, as can strategizing with the navigator/tactician: "We are kept from our goal *not* by obstacles but by a clear path to a lesser goal" (Robert Brault, emphasis added).

DECK HANDS

Your deck hands are responsible for the hard work of handling the sails to best harness the power of the wind to efficiently propel the yacht toward desired destinations under the direction of the captain (e.g., winds represent day to day responsibilities and tasks). Maximize your efficiency in completing one task at a time to the best of your ability. Avoid veering off course, chasing after meaningless gusts of wind (e.g., electronic time wasters). Accomplish the prioritized goals each day to keep you on course, being certain self-care is included up front. By getting the hard work done efficiently, there is more time for rest, play, and rejuvenating creative activities that bolster joy and energy within the team.

KEY POINTS

- Take care of your yacht; be as physically fit as possible.

- Assess your bilge morning and night; identify emotions (e.g., sadness, anxiety, frustration). When uncomfortable, painful emotions are present; accept them and respect their underlying message—what they are asking you to pay attention to. Effectively express the emotion in a safe environment, for example, journaling or sharing verbally with a trusted colleague or friend, and thoughtfully decide the best response.

- Fortify your keel. Nurture your spiritual connections. Know what your values are and have the courage to spend time doing what matters most to you. Invest in supportive and loving relationships in your personal life.

- Face your inevitable mortality, living full out, being completely present in the moment. Live a life of no regrets, giving your very best in interactions with others.

- Avoid excessive spending and debt in order to allow you the freedom and flexibility to balance your life with play and hard work.

- Build a network of strong, supportive relationships.

- Choose to work in a setting where you have a shared *why* (mission behind all you do) with others you trust and respect. Be an inspirational leader to others.

- Work for a supportive boss (or *be* that boss) whom you respect. If life circumstances keep you working in a suboptimal position, embrace the Stockdale Paradox (Honan 2012) while gaining strength to prepare for a change in course when the right opportunity presents itself. Admiral Stockdale was the highest-ranking prisoner of war in Vietnam and survived captivity and torture. He led fellow prisoners with his Stockdale Paradox: "Hold onto the faith that you will prevail in the end, while having the discipline and courage to face the most brutal facts of your current reality, whatever they might be."

- Effectively and compassionately work through conflict and misunderstandings. Seek to understand first, then to be understood. Learn to negotiate effectively to come to win-win solutions (Miyashiro 2011).

- Focus on one task at a time. Multitasking is overrated and ineffective.

- Replace time on the computer (and focus on other electronics) with relationship time.

- Enhance joy in your life (Kondo 2014).

- Practice healthy habits. Rejuvenate through creative activities that instill energy and foster renewal. Allow and cherish down time (sailing with the wind from behind, i.e., effortless sailing).
- Remain up to date in your knowledge and skills, enabling you to give your patients the very best care you can (rigging your yacht with the latest technology in sails).
- Strive for excellence, doing the best job you can in the time you have. Remember that *perfect* is the enemy of *good*, which also applies to the mastery of smooth sailing.
- Accept help from others! Ask for it when you are struggling. Be there for others when they are struggling. (When a sailboat capsizes, we ask others to help stand with us on our keel to right the boat.)
- Leaving a position is sometimes a victory and not a failure!

What to Do When It's Not Working?

Importantly, it is not recommended to attempt to apply all of the smooth sailing tactics at once. Rather, focusing on just one aspect of the nautical metaphor framework each week will alleviate the burdens rather than creating a sense that there is "one more thing to do." To get started, do a quick, compassionate sweep of your yacht to determine which part (mast, sails, wind, keel, rudder, bilge, or journey) is in need of the greatest repair, and begin there. Addressing the parts of your yacht represents a strategy for preventing burnout and achieving professional fulfillment, and the tactic you decide to employ for repairing or bolstering a particular part is the one that fits your needs and personality. Remember that even 5 or 10 minutes of attention to that tactic will begin the journey of recapturing well-being. But you cannot do it all alone. Ultimately, the solutions for burnout need our collective community of colleagues, family, friends, our institutions, and the professional community to accomplish the following:

- Do our work well
- Be respected for it
- Be fairly compensated
- Care for ourselves
- Live fulfilling and happy lives filled with love
- Impact the world in such a way that the world is a better place because we've touched it

Phone Applications

The following apps may prove useful depending on what aspect of the smooth sailing metaphor needs attention:

Insight Timer: https://insighttimer.com
Headspace: www.headspace.com
Simply Being: https://itunes.apple.com/us/app/simply-being-guided
  -meditation-for-relaxation-presence/id347418999?mt=8
Stop, Breathe & Think: www.stopbreathethink.com
Three Good Things: A Happiness Journal: https://itunes.apple.com/us/app/
  three-good-things-a-happiness-journal/id1242079576?mt=8

References

American Psychiatric Association: Get Involved With Advocacy and APAPAC. Washington, DC, American Psychiatric Association, 2018. Available at: https://www.psychiatry.org/psychiatrists/advocacy. Accessed June 30, 2018.

Amutio A, Martínez-Taboada C, Delgado LC, et al: Acceptability and effectiveness of a long-term educational intervention to reduce physicians' stress-related conditions. J Contin Educ Health Prof 35(4):255–260, 2015 26953856

Creswell JD, Welch WT, Taylor SE, et al: Affirmation of personal values buffers neuroendocrine and psychological stress responses. Psychol Sci 16(11):846–851, 2005 16262767

Davich V: 8 Minute Meditation Expanded: Quiet Your Mind. Change Your Life. London, Penguin Group, 2014

Dyrbye LN, Eacker A, Durning SJ, et al: The impact of stigma and personal experiences on the help-seeking behaviors of medical students with burnout. Acad Med 90(7):961–969, 2015 25650824

Dyrbye LN, West CP, Sinsky CA, et al: Medical licensure questions and physician reluctance to seek care for mental health conditions. Mayo Clin Proc 92(10):1486–1493, 2017 28982484

Epstein RM, Krasner MS: Physician resilience: what it means, why it matters, and how to promote it. Acad Med 88(3):301–303, 2013 23442430

Ey S, Moffit M, Kinzie JM, et al: "If you build it, they will come": attitudes of medical residents and fellows about seeking services in a resident wellness program. J Grad Med Educ 5(3):486–492, 2013 24404315

Fisher R, Ury WL: Getting to Yes: Negotiating Agreement Without Giving In. London, Penguin Books, 2011

Gabbard GO: Lessons to be learned from the study of sexual boundary violations. Am J Psychother 50(3):311–322, 1996 8886231

Gold KJ, Andrew LB, Goldman EB, et al: "I would never want to have a mental health diagnosis on my record": A survey of female physicians on mental health diagnosis, treatment, and reporting. Gen Hosp Psychiatry 43:51–57, 2016 27796258

Gold KJ, Shih ER, Goldman EB, et al: Do US medical licensing applications treat mental and physical illness equivalently? Fam Med 49(6):464–467, 2017 28633174

Goodman MJ, Schorling JB: A mindfulness course decreases burnout and improves well-being among healthcare providers. Int J Psychiatry Med 43(2):119–128, 2012 22849035

Gottman J, Silver N: The Seven Principles for Making Marriage Work: A Practical Guide From the Country's Foremost Relationship Expert. New York, Harmony Books, 2015

Graber DR, Kilpatrick AO: Establishing values-based leadership and value systems in healthcare organizations. J Health Hum Serv Adm 31(2):179–197, 2008 18998522

Halbesleben JRB, Demerouti E: The construct validity of an alternative measure of burnout: investigating the English translation of the Oldenburg burnout inventory. Work Stress 19(3):208–220, 2005

Hayes SC, Luoma JB, Bond FW, et al: Acceptance and commitment therapy: model, processes and outcomes. Behav Res Ther 44(1):1–25, 2006 16300724

Hayes SC, Levin ME, Plumb-Vilardaga J, et al: Acceptance and commitment therapy and contextual behavioral science: examining the progress of a distinctive model of behavioral and cognitive therapy. Behav Ther 44(2):180–198, 2013 23611068

Honan D: The Stockdale Paradox: how optimism creates resilience. Big Think, Nov 9, 2012. Available at: https://bigthink.com/think-tank/the-stockdale-paradox-how-optimism-creates-resilience. Accessed July 8, 2018.

Irving JA, Dobkin PL, Park J: Cultivating mindfulness in health care professionals: a review of empirical studies of mindfulness-based stress reduction (MBSR). Complement Ther Clin Pract 15(2):61–66, 2009 19341981

Kabat-Zinn J: Full Catastrophe Living: Using the Wisdom of Your Body and Mind to Face Stress, Pain, and Illness. New York, Bantam Dell, 2013

Keeling ML, Bermudez M: Externalizing problems through art and writing: experiences of process and helpfulness. J Marital Fam Ther 32(4):405–419, 2006 17120515

Kondo M: The Life Changing Magic of Tidying Up. Berkeley, CA, Ten Speed Press, 2014

Krasner MS, Epstein RM, Beckman H, et al: Association of an educational program in mindful communication with burnout, empathy, and attitudes among primary care physicians. JAMA 302(12):1284–1293, 2009 19773563

Lemaire JB, Wallace JE: Not all coping strategies are created equal: a mixed methods study exploring physicians' self reported coping strategies. BMC Health Serv Res 10:208, 2010 20630091

Lencioni P: The 5 big causes of burn-out. The Hub, March 2018. Available at: https://www.tablegroup.com/hub/post/the-5-big-causes-of-burn-out. Accessed June 30, 2018.

Luthar SS, Curlee A, Tye SJ, et al: Fostering resilience among mothers under stress: "authentic connections groups" for medical professionals. Womens Health Issues 27(3):382–390, 2017 28410972

Maslach C, Jackson SE: The measurement of experienced burnout. Journal of Organizational Behavior 2(2):99–113, 1981

Meldrum H: Exemplary physicians' strategies for avoiding burnout. Health Care Manag (Frederick) 29(4):324–331, 2010 21045584

Mills AE, Spencer EM: Values based decision making: a tool for achieving the goals of healthcare. HEC Forum 17(1):18–32, 2005 15957266

Miyashiro MR: The Empathy Factor: Your Competitive Advantage for Personal, Team and Business Success. Encinitas, CA, Puddledancer Press, 2011

O'Connor K, Muller Neff D, Pitman S: Burnout in mental health professionals: a systematic review and meta-analysis of prevalence and determinants. Eur Psychiatry 53:74–99, 2018 29957371

Perlman RL, Ross PT, Lypson ML: Understanding the medical marriage: physicians and their partners share strategies for success. Acad Med 90(1):63–68, 2015 25099240

Rossi A, Cetrano G, Pertile R, et al: Burnout, compassion fatigue, and compassion satisfaction among staff in community-based mental health services. Psychiatry Res 200(2–3):933–938, 2012 22951335

Shanafelt TD, West CP, Sloan JA, et al: Career fit and burnout among academic faculty. Arch Intern Med 169(10):990–995, 2009 19468093

Shanafelt TD, Kaups KL, Nelson H, et al: An interactive individualized intervention to promote behavioral change to increase personal well-being in US surgeons. Ann Surg 259(1):82–88, 2014 23979287

Shanafelt TD, Dyrbye LN, Sinsky C, et al: Relationship between clerical burden and characteristics of the electronic environment with physician burnout and professional satisfaction. Mayo Clin Proc 91(7):836–848, 2016 27313121

Shanafelt T, Goh J, Sinsky C: The business case for investing in physician well-being. JAMA Intern Med 177(12):1826–1832, 2017 28973070

Shapiro J, Galowitz P: Peer support for clinicians: a programmatic approach. Acad Med 91(9):1200–1204, 2016 27355784

Siegel DJ: The Developing Mind: How Relationships and the Brain Interact to Shape Who We Are. New York, Guilford, 1999

Smith MJ: When I Say No I Feel Guilty. New York, Bantam Books, 1985

Song M, Burress T, Halsey V: The Hamster Revolution: How to Manage Your Email Before It Manages You. Oakland, CA, Berrett-Koehler, 2008

Spiers J, Buszewicz M, Chew-Graham CA, et al: Barriers, facilitators, and survival strategies for GPs seeking treatment for distress: a qualitative study. Br J Gen Pract 67(663):e700–e708, 2017 28893766

Swensen S, Kabcenell A, Shanafelt T: Physician-organization collaboration reduces physician burnout and promotes engagement: The Mayo Clinic experience. J Healthc Manag 61(2):105–127, 2016 27111930

Thomas LR, Ripp JA, West CP: Charter on physician well-being. JAMA 319(15):1541–1542, 2018 29596592

Trockel M, Bohman B, Lesure E, et al: A brief instrument to assess both burnout and professional fulfillment in physicians: reliability and validity, including correlation with self-reported medical errors, in a sample of resident and practicing physicians. Acad Psychiatry 42(1):11–24, 2018 29196982

Weight CJ, Sellon JL, Lessard-Anderson CR, et al: Physical activity, quality of life, and burnout among physician trainees: the effect of a team-based, incentivized exercise program. Mayo Clin Proc 88(12):1435–1442, 2013 24290117

Worley LL: Our fallen peers: a mandate for change. Acad Psychiatry 32(1):8–12, 2008 18270275

Zwack J, Schweitzer J: If every fifth physician is affected by burnout, what about the other four? Resilience strategies of experienced physicians. Acad Med 88(3):382–389, 2013 23348093

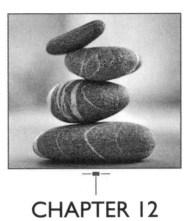

CHAPTER 12

PSYCHIATRIST BURNOUT

Prevention and Intervention

Shailesh Kumar, M.D., FRANZCP, FRCPsych,
Diploma in Psychological Medicine, MPhil

Rishi Kumar

Burnout, a term now in common usage, was first coined by Freudenberger (1974) to describe the emotional exhaustion experienced by public service workers in response to chronic stressors at work. Since then, most publications on burnout have focused on human service professions including lawyers, rehabilitation workers, relief workers, and teachers, acknowledging the unique pressures of using one's self as the "tool" in face-to-face work with needy, demanding, and often troubled populations (Carson et al. 1999). Compared with other groups, doctors experience higher rates of psychological distress, burnout, mental illness, and suicidality (Ward and Outram 2016) and indeed may be experiencing burnout in "epidemic proportions" (Rothenberger 2017; West et al. 2016).

Among doctors, psychiatrists are identified as a highly vulnerable group for experiencing burnout (Bressi et al. 2009). Studies from the United States (Vaccaro and Clark 1987), United Kingdom (Prosser et al. 1996), Australia (Rey et al. 2004), New Zealand (Kumar et al. 2006, 2011), and Italy (Ferrari et al. 2015) have reported prevalence figures of burnout in psychiatrists in excess of 50%. Burnout is seen as a major challenge in delivering sustainable mental health care (Brand et al. 2017). Low pay, excess paperwork (Clark and Vaccaro 1987), patient suicide (Chemtob et al. 1988), lack of professional support, threats of violence (Holloway et al. 2000), and health service restructuring (Kumar et al. 2006) contribute to the higher level of stress among psychiatrists.

Few studies have been conducted on intervention and prevention of burnout as a whole (Maslach 2017), and even fewer have solely investigated the issue among psychiatrists (Maslach and Leiter 2016). This chapter reviews the literature on factors associated with burnout among psychiatrists. Strategies for preventing and managing burnout in psychiatrists are identified mostly from what is reported among physicians in general.

Burnout Intervention: Principles and Strategies

Many studies on burnout assume tackling antecedents should help develop strategies to modify them. Applying this assumption in a clinical context is challenging. Knowing the association between burnout and antecedent risk factors such as younger age, female sex, single status, long working hours, and low reported job satisfaction (Amoafo et al. 2015; Montgomery 2014) has helped identify subgroups of psychiatrists at risk of experiencing burnout, but this has limited usefulness in developing preventive or treatment strategies. Other antecedents, including heavy workload, structure and length of shifts, and lack of nutrition and hydration (Hamidi et al. 2016), are modifiable through significant efforts. External factors such as weak retention rates, high turnover, heavy workloads, staffing shortages, rising societal expectations, productivity losses, and higher healthcare costs (Humphries et al. 2014; Kuster et al. 2017) are associated with burnout, but causality is difficult to prove.

Developing management strategies solely based on antecedents or associated factors may not be scientifically sound because causality has rarely been tested (Maslach 2017; Maslach and Leiter 2016, 2017). Some authors have stated that aligning personal and organizational values and enabling physicians to devote 20% of their work activities to the part of their medical practice that is especially meaningful to them is effective against burnout (Rothenberger 2017). Such opinions sound logical and are expressed by leaders in the field, but these opinions need empirical validation. Several recommendations reviewed in this chapter are not based on randomized, controlled trials and are invariably derived from studies with a single intervention group of volunteer participants with inadequate follow-up (Leiter and Maslach 2014). With these limitations in mind, three layers of intervention strategies to counter burnout in psychiatrists can be identified:

- *Primary interventions:* We know psychiatrists are at high risk of experiencing burnout. Organizational strategies to reduce or eliminate stressors by changing the nature of the job or work environment (van Wyk and Pillay-Van Wyk 2010) serve as the first port of call for preventing burnout and are hence considered primary interventions.
- *Secondary interventions:* According to van Wyk and Pillay-Van Wyk (2010, p. 3) "Secondary prevention programs aim to reduce the individual's experiences of job stress by educating the employees to manage job stress better (improved coping mechanism) and by creating supportive structures to buffer organizational stresses through improved management processes and support groups." Organization-wide screening for burnout could help deliver appropriate prevention programs to those who are at risk of developing burnout but have not yet developed it.
- *Tertiary interventions:* Highly specialized interventions against manifest burnout are considered tertiary interventions (van Wyk and Pillay-Van Wyk 2010). Burnout scores can help select an individual for tertiary interventions. More intensive intervention is offered to people with higher scores, or a specific type of intervention is delivered for a specific dimension, such as emotional exhaustion or depersonalization. Tertiary interventions are better offered by specialists with experience in the field of "treating" burnout.

The evidence to support these three layers of interventions is explored in the following sections.

PRIMARY INTERVENTIONS

The final outcome of exposure to stress is mediated by *internal* and *external* (e.g., support systems) factors (Holloway et al. 2000). Five internal factors may contribute to burnout (Maslach et al. 2001): hardiness, locus of control, coping styles, personality type, and attitude. Low hardiness is associated with lesser sense of control over events, unwillingness to accept change, and greater degree of external locus of control. Effective coping is associated with less burnout. Personality traits characterized by pessimistic outlook, the need to be in control and reluctance to delegate (Maslach and Leiter 1997), high expectations, propensity to work too hard, overinvolvement with clients (Sherman 2004), a need to please others, and prioritizing work over social life (Blom 2012) lead to exhaustion and cynicism. These factors have conceptual appeal but are difficult to measure or to achieve wide agreement on. Demographic variables such as age, gender, and ethnicity, on the other hand, are easier to measure but yield inconsistent findings with burnout (Beheshtifar and Omidvar 2013; Lloyd et al. 2002). Raising awareness about such internal risk factors may help psychiatrists deal with burnout better. This does run the risk of portraying burnout as a sign of individual weakness or fallacy and may divert attention from the environmental factors that may have contributed to the onset of burnout in the first place (Maslach 2017; Shanafelt and Noseworthy 2017).

Paying attention to external factors relating to psychiatrists' nature of work or their work environment may yield greater dividends against preventing burnout. Such external factors include the chronicity and complexity of client problems (Maslach and Jackson 1981), working with difficult patients (Schaufeli et al. 1993), high workload (Morse et al. 2012), and working with personality disordered or malingering populations (Garcia et al. 2016). Absence of job autonomy (Maslach and Leiter 1997) and lack of feedback, meaningful rewards, and job security (Demerouti et al. 2001) may also increase burnout. Sagely, Maslach et al. (2001) suggested the whole organizational context should be considered when examining burnout-favoring conditions. Despite the problems in measuring such external risk factors with precision, discussing them widely may raise awareness, facilitate discussion, and encourage early intervention against burnout.

In an attempt to bring together individual and organizational risk factors, an etiological model proposed that certain factors may predispose, precipitate, perpetuate, or protect against burnout (Kumar et al. 2005). *Predisposing factors* include personality characteristics, the mismatch between training and working environments, and increasing workload. *Precipitating factors* include violence perpetrated by patients, patient suicide, on-call duties, dealing with difficult relatives, and lack of resources, especially when personal support is limited. *Perpetuating factors* include a subjective feeling of being overworked and unsupported, dealing with patients' suffering, gender-based variation in stress appraisal, personality attributes, changes in health service delivery model, clinician-management conflicts, and time management and resource issues. *Protective factors* include being involved in academic work and having a range of interests outside of work. As is often the case in medicine, knowing the etiology of a condition is often the first step in developing intervention or prevention strategies. In the context of burnout, primary interventions or screening can be targeted for psychiatrists who may be predisposed to burnout, whereas treatment programs may be better targeted for those who are heavily exposed to precipitating and perpetuating factors. These are further explored later.

SECONDARY INTERVENTIONS

Organization-Wide Screening for Burnout

Actively screening for burnout can help raise awareness and makes help for the affected staff accessible in a timely fashion. Psychiatrists are not an easy popu-

lation to screen for burnout. They are generally hardworking and psychologically well-adjusted and fail to report changes in subjective well-being (Maslach
et al. 2001). They also continue to report high levels of job satisfaction despite feeling emotionally depleted (Kumar et al. 2007). Therefore, external or
organizational monitoring may be necessary for assessing burnout among
psychiatrists. Signals of mental or emotional exhaustion and decreased self-
efficiency are considered more useful than self-reports of burnout (Maslach et
al. 2001). Privacy issues, protection of collected data, and the potential to misuse psychiatrists' health information need to be actively considered in the
screening process. Not doing so runs the risk of undermining trust and preventing disclosure or help seeking. With these caveats, Schaufeli and Enzmann's
(1998) interpersonal signals of burnout are worth considering while screening.
Such signals are categorized into *affective* (irritability, being oversensitive, reduced empathy), *cognitive* (cynicism/dehumanized perceptions, pessimistic
outlook, derogatory labeling), *behavioral* (violent outbursts; irritability toward
clients; interpersonal, marital, and family conflicts; social isolation and withdrawal; giving mechanical responses to clients), and *motivational* (loss of interest, indifference with respect to clients). Physical signals are excluded from
screening because they can only be observed on an individual level.

Measuring Burnout

The Maslach Burnout Inventory (MBI; Maslach et al. 1996) is the most
widely used rating scale for measuring burnout. It gives scores on three subscales or dimensions that manifest in a work context: Depersonalization,
Emotional Exhaustion, and Lack of Personal Accomplishment. Elevated
scores on Depersonalization and Emotional Exhaustion and lower Personal
Accomplishment scores indicate burnout. Another tool, the Burnout Measure (BM; Pines and Aronson 1988) contains three exhaustion scales (assessing Physical, Mental, and Emotional Exhaustion). Unlike the MBI, the
items in the BM have no explicit association with work and conceptualize
burnout as a unidimensional construct (Corcoran 1995). A high correlation
between the total BM score and scores on the MBI Emotional Exhaustion
subscale scores has been reported (Pines 1988). BM scores can largely help
develop exhaustion-specific treatment programs.

Three other burnout measurement tools are available that also measure exhaustion in different forms. The Copenhagen Burnout Inventory (Kristensen
et al. 2005) measures physical and psychological exhaustion. The Oldenburg
Burnout Inventory (OLBI; Demerouti et al. 2002) measures exhaustion and
disengagement from work. In contrast to the MBI, affective, physical, and
cognitive aspects of exhaustion are covered in the OLBI, making the instrument valid for those employees who perform physical and "intellectual" work.
Furthermore, the OLBI, unlike the MBI, contains negatively and positively
worded items, rendering it more useful in measuring exhaustion, disengagement, vigor, and dedication items (Demerouti and Bakker 2008). OLBI scores
therefore can be used in improving work engagement as well as reducing burn-

out. However, MBI remains the "gold standard" to assess burnout (Shirom and Melamed 2005).

By obtaining individual scores, it is not only possible to assess the severity of burnout but also to identify target areas for intervention. These tools have enabled standardization of definition, societal acceptance, improved screening efforts, and reliable rating of burnout. Some European countries, including the Netherlands and Sweden, have accepted burnout as a medical condition, and this has enabled them to develop specialist services for treating the condition and even to grant potential access to the welfare system and compensation claims (Schaufeli et al. 2009). In North America, burnout is accepted as a nonmedical condition with minimal stigma attached (Shirom 1989). Preventive and management strategies must work in the context of the wider political environment in which psychiatrists practice and must reflect how burnout is conceptualized or measured, including perhaps the specific dimension that is affected.

Prevention Strategies Against Burnout in Psychiatrists

Preventing burnout is often a twofold exercise: enhancing the individual's strengths by either improving coping or by reducing stressors in the work environment. The multidimensional model of burnout may possibly be more useful for developing preventive strategies (Maslach and Goldberg 1998). Strategies reported to be effective against emotional exhaustion include the following: 1) changing work patterns (e.g., working less, taking more breaks, avoiding overtime work, balancing work with the rest of one's life); 2) developing coping skills (e.g., cognitive restructuring, conflict resolution, time management); 3) obtaining social support (both from colleagues and family); 4) using relaxation techniques; 5) living a healthy lifestyle; and 6) enhancing self-understanding through therapy (Maslach and Goldberg 1998). All these strategies have a common principle of replenishing the emotional reservoir in the individual. They are less effective against high levels of cynicism, which may respond to efforts to enhance collegiality, human values, and mutual respect (Leiter et al. 2011). Recognition from professional colleagues and organizational leaders could be effective against feelings of reduced personal accomplishment (Demerouti 2014; Montgomery 2014).

Although the individual-level approach has obvious advantages, it is not the entire solution. Stress from the work environment is a large contributor to the onset and perpetuation of burnout. An interactive model seeing burnout as the net result of interplay between the individual and the environment may be more effective when it comes to developing preventive strategies (Lee et al. 2013). Three levels of organizational change are recommended to reduce the risk of burnout: 1) modifying the organizational structure and work processes; 2) improving the fit between the organization and the doctor through professional development programs facilitating adaption to the work environment; and 3) individual-level actions to reduce stress through effective coping and promoting healthy behaviors (Lee et al. 2013).

These principles make sense. Like the individual strategies, they have not been evaluated for psychiatrists. Practical steps such as making psychiatrists feel valued at work through praise and other rewards and having the ability to control work volume, influence decisions that affect their work, and exercise professional autonomy can prevent burnout (Maslach and Leiter 2016, 2017). Organizations taking a supportive approach to their employees, providing child/family-friendly environments and flexible work hours, may enjoy greater employee job satisfaction (Sparks et al. 2001). Paying attention to the physical environment and providing recreational opportunities based on the Mayo Clinic's Serious Leisure Perspective (Dieser et al. 2017) may improve morale. Those individual and organizational strategies with relevance to psychiatrists are explored in more detail in the following subsections.

Building Resilience.   *Resilience*, the "ability to bounce back or recover from stress" (Tregoning et al. 2014) or "the adoption of positive coping strategies, in times of change or adversity, to enable people to carry on in their jobs and lives" (Carver 1998) is commonly identified as a preventive tool against burnout among doctors (Kumar 2016). A Canadian study (Jensen et al. 2008) found four main aspects of physician resilience: 1) developing positive attitudes and perspectives of valuing the physician role, maintaining diverse interests, and being more self-aware; 2) developing balance and prioritization (setting limits, taking effective approaches to continuing professional development, and honoring the self); 3) enhancing practice management and sound business management and employing role-specific competent staff; and 4) fostering supportive relationships with colleagues and others as well as good communication skills. These aspects of resilience building may appeal to psychiatrists and can be incorporated in the framework of regular supervision, psychotherapy, and mentoring already in existence in most countries. They can bring about attitudinal change for resilience, whereas peer support may help balance and prioritization. However, resilient psychiatrists may "soldier on" rather than seek help or may delay help seeking, thus allowing burnout to become more pronounced.

Peer Review and Support.   Receiving emotional support, feedback, and constructive criticism about one's performance from peers buffers against stress (Chang et al. 2012). Peer support, among many things, does provide informational support in the form of advice and information on proactive coping. With information from peers, psychiatrists find solutions to stressful problems, reduce the perception of the problem's significance in the bigger scheme of things, and develop a more realistic appreciation of the stressors (Cohen and Wills 1985). Fortunately, most developed countries have provisions for peer support for psychiatrists in their work environment, although their effectiveness against stress has not been investigated extensively.

Self-Care.   Taking charge of personal health and physical fitness is always a good idea for everyone and may be relatively easy. Taking care of psychological well-being, on the other hand, can be challenging. Working through one's own traumatic experiences, appreciating spirituality and human nature, taking regular breaks, achieving social recognition, and focusing on the positive aspects of life enhance psychological well-being, especially among those who work with traumatized individuals, as psychiatrists do (Maslach 2017). Regular exercise and paying attention to nutrition and hydration can help prevent burnout in other professions and could also work for psychiatrists (Hamidi et al. 2016).

Time Management.   Psychiatrists often work under considerable time pressure, which impacts their ability to find time to think and reflect. Psychiatrists, reflective by nature, may be particularly vulnerable to experiencing stress under such conditions. Most mental health services are facing cuts in resources, and psychiatrists may be forced to work under excessive time constraints. Effective time management can help enhance productivity and reduce perceived pressure (Gordon and Borkan 2014). Four strategies for time management have been identified: 1) setting short- and long-term goals, 2) setting priorities among competing responsibilities, 3) planning and organizing activities, and 4) minimizing "time wasters" (Gordon and Borkan 2014). Setting short-term (to be achieved within 1–3 years) and long-term goals (5–10 years into the future) helps physicians balance optimal professional practice and personal well-being. Prioritization of responsibilities provides structure and a sense of control. Lack of organization and poor prioritization lead to overwhelming stress and worrying. To help physicians plan and organize, Gordon and Borkan (2014) recommend Covey's Time Management Matrix Technique (Covey et al. 1996). In this matrix, responsibilities are sorted into a 2×2 table, organized according to urgent and less urgent versus important and less important. This exercise enables physicians to categorize jobs as requiring immediate attention, important, ones that can wait, and so on. Having prioritized tasks, the physician develops a plan for tackling them individually, with due attention to planning, daily lifestyle, and habits. This entire exercise requires good organizational skills, which improve with practice. Reducing inconveniences such as commute time, procrastination, logistical issues (lack of paper or ink), or physical interruptions that eat up precious time at work facilitates effective time management (Gordon and Borkan 2014). These strategies, based on a review of literature from the medical and nonmedical fields, can be easily applied to psychiatrists.

Job Crafting.   Having the ability to shape one's work to match one's interests and circumstances can be empowering. It can also be effective against burnout. Maslach and Leiter (2016) recommended that psychiatrists should accept the inherently stressful nature of their job and evaluate their workload frequently in order to reduce the risk for burnout. Developing a more versatile lifestyle, having hobbies outside work, having diverse roles (including academic, research, and administrative), and having variety in clinical work can help prevent burnout in psychiatrists (Kumar et al. 2005,

2011; Maslach 2017; Maslach and Leiter 2016). The impact of job crafting on burnout has, however, not been empirically tested.

TERTIARY INTERVENTIONS: TREATMENT AND INTERVENTION STRATEGIES FOR BURNOUT AMONG PSYCHIATRISTS

The strategies just outlined are recommended for prevention—that is, *before* burnout develops. Once burnout has manifested, treatment strategies are required. In order for treatment to be instituted, proper "diagnosis" or "caseness" using a structured validated tool is recommended. We favor the multidimensional model of burnout because it enables identifying individualized intervention strategies specific to the person's needs. General preventive strategies such as altering the characteristics of the job (making it less hindering and more motivating), separating work and nonwork domains, minimizing family-work conflicts, and actively detaching from work (Demerouti 2015) can be deployed in tandem with specific treatment strategies. Some established tertiary intervention strategies to counter burnout that can be applied to psychiatrists are reviewed in the following subsections.

Stress Management

Burnout develops because of chronic exposure to stress; hence, there is interest in stress management programs for treating burnout. A systematic review by van Wyk and Pillay-Van Wyk (2010), however, found no evidence of effectiveness of brief stress management training interventions in reducing job stress for health workers. There was low-quality evidence to support the effectiveness of stress management training of moderate intensity (defined as more than 6 hours of contact over 1 month) in the short-term reduction of job stress levels, and the beneficial effects diminished without booster sessions. The systematic review found strong levels of evidence to support the effectiveness of intensive, long-term stress management training programs in reducing job stress and risk of burnout. Intensive stress management programs with booster sessions delivered over a longer period may yield longer-lasting results against burnout.

Improving Work Environment

Stressful patient interactions are often significant contributors to the onset of burnout. Professionals experiencing burnout treat their patients with cynicism and in a depersonalized manner. A vicious cycle between negative patient interactions and burnout is often seen, with one feeding the other. This also suggests improving staff-client relationships may help manage burnout. A randomized, controlled trial of psychological interventions directed at improving staff-patient relationships (51 patients, 85 staff, across

10 psychiatric rehabilitation wards) found that staff in the intervention arm reported significantly lower level of postintervention depersonalization (Berry et al. 2016). Patients in the intervention arm also reported feeling less criticized by staff, and the overall ward atmosphere improved, but the change failed to reach statistical significance. Small size and a slow uptake would limit generalizability of this study's findings.

Simply targeting communication or interpersonal relationships as a strategy against burnout may not be effective. This view is supported by findings from a systematic review by Marine et al. (2006) that found good-quality evidence to suggest a combination of person-directed (cognitive-behavioral therapy [CBT], relaxation, music making, massage, and multicomponent programs) and work-directed (attitude change and communication, support from colleagues, participatory problem solving and decision making, and changes in work organization) strategies was effective against burnout. There was only limited evidence to support the efficacy of either person- or work-directed intervention strategies in reducing burnout in healthcare workers. The study found that the benefits of such interventions may be evident for as long as 2 years. Another recent systematic review by West et al. (2016) (2,617 articles, 15 randomized trials) pooled data from studies that evaluated structural interventions within the work environment (shortened rotation length, modifications in work processes, and shortened shifts) as well as individual-focused interventions (facilitated small group curricula, stress management, self-care training, communications skills training, "belonging intervention," and mindfulness-based approaches) and found that a combination of organization and individual strategies worked better. Overall, burnout in the studies reviewed decreased from 54% to 44% (difference 10% [95% confidence interval (CI) 5–14]; $P<0.0001$; $I^2=15\%$; 14 studies). Emotional exhaustion score decreased 23.82 points to 21.17 points (2.65 points [1.67–3.64]; $P<0.0001$; $I^2=82\%$; 40 studies) and depersonalization score decreased from 9.05 to 8.41 (0.64 points [0.15–1.14]; $P=0.01$; $I^2=58\%$; 36 studies). Studies offering mindfulness-based interventions reported greater estimated pooled reduction in emotional exhaustion (a drop of 4.68 points [2.84—6.51]; $P<0.0001$; $I^2=47\%$) and depersonalization (reduction of 2.01 [1.34–2.67]; $P<0.0001$; $I^2=0\%$). Structural and individual-focused interventions did not differ in their effectiveness in reducing emotional exhaustion or depersonalization scores. Two implications of this systematic review are worth considering: 1) more aggressive intervention should be offered to people experiencing more severe burnout, and 2) burnout measurement tools, especially multidimensional ones, should be used while deciding what intervention should be offered to which group.

Cognitive-Behavioral Therapy

As an individual intervention, CBT has been extensively examined in burnout literature. A systematic review by Ruotsalainen et al. (2015) compared CBT ($n=14$), mental and physical relaxation ($n=21$), combined CBT and relaxation ($n=6$), and organizational interventions ($n=20$). Outcomes were categorized as stress, anxiety, or general health. Low-quality evidence showed CBT, regardless of relaxation type, had the same effect on reducing stress symptoms as no intervention at 1-month follow-up in six studies. CBT by itself had no more effect than any alternative interventions. Physical relaxation (e.g., massage) led to inconsistent findings in reducing stress. Mental relaxation (e.g., meditation) led to similar stress symptom levels as no intervention at 1- to 6-months follow-up. CBT and mental/physical relaxation techniques had similar effects in reducing stress. Whether a small reduction in stress levels can translate into an improvement in corresponding burnout levels was difficult to establish from this study. A strength of the study was its focus on evaluating organizational interventions (changes in working conditions, organizing support, increasing communication skills, and changing work schedules) against burnout in comparison with individual CBT. Changing work schedules, from continuous to weekend breaks and 4-week schedules to 2-week schedules, reduced stress significantly. Some low-quality evidence emerged to suggest changing work schedules may reduce stress. Organizational interventions are likely to be more effective against burnout if they focus on reducing specific stressors.

Mindfulness Training and Meditation

Mindfulness-based stress reduction (MBSR) strategies have been widely investigated for stress management. Psychiatrists with their training in psychotherapy and familiarity with the concept of mindfulness may be adept at MBSR. Yet the effectiveness of MBSR has not been specifically evaluated for psychiatrists experiencing burnout. There are good-quality data to support the usefulness of MBSR in stress reduction in general, with improvement being maintained for up to 19 weeks of follow-up (Khoury et al. 2015). The impact of MBSR on stress was large; moderate on anxiety, depression, distress, and quality of life; and, surprisingly, only small on burnout. This suggested stress reduction should not be taken as equivalent of reduction in burnout. Another more recent systematic review found improvements in stress, anxiety, mindfulness, resiliency, and burnout symptoms with brief mindfulness interventions among hospital providers (Gilmartin et al. 2017). The effectiveness of mindfulness meditation has also been evaluated against different dimensions of burnout, with improvements in emotional exhaustion (effect size 0.37 [95% CI, 0.04–0.70]), personal accomplishment (effect size 1.18 [95% CI, 0.10–2.25]), and life satisfaction (effect size 0.48 [95% CI, 0.15–0.81]) (Dharmawardene et al. 2016). Available evidence therefore suggests that brief mindfulness interventions are effective in reducing stress and burnout and improving clinician well-being.

Computer-Based Interventions

Computer-based psychological interventions are more accessible, convenient, and cost-effective. They have also been evaluated in managing workplace stress and burnout, but results do not appear promising. A recent systematic review (Kuster et al. 2017) compared three groups of randomized controlled trials: in-person (face-to-face) or computer-based (web- and mobile-based) stress management interventions and no intervention. The study failed to establish whether one form of intervention was more effective than the other. Despite heterogeneity in data and limited follow-up, the systematic review found very low quality evidence to favor the effectiveness of computer-based stress management interventions over in-person stress management interventions. The authors had little confidence in the effect estimates and were pessimistic about whether future studies will change these conclusions.

Burnout and Impairment

Burnout is a slippery slope, potentially predisposing physicians to depression, substance abuse, and impairment, especially if help is not sought or received early. *Impairment* is defined as the inability to practice medicine with reasonable skill and safety because of personal health problems or other stressors (Gunderman and Grogan 2012). Impairment is often viewed as analogous to incompetence, which, alongside limited awareness of self-help services, can act as a barrier against help seeking. Specific interventions for impaired physicians have been developed, and some may apply to psychiatrists. Gunderman and Grogan (2012) recommend physician health programs consisting of identification, diagnosis, treatment, documentation, and monitoring of impaired physicians. Hospital-based rehabilitation programs are reported to be well received by physicians (Johnson 2009).

Many of the principles that apply to impaired physicians may also apply to psychiatrists. It is important to consider that the psychiatrist who is considered impaired is likely to feel sensitive and could be reluctant to engage, at least initially. Strategies such as two people approaching the psychiatrist together and keeping a written, confidential record of the meeting and witness accounts (Gitman 2008) are helpful. Team-based (not individual) impairment interventions with detailed preintervention data and a focus on facts, avoiding judgment and emotions (Yancey and McKinnon 2010), achieve better results. A unique approach by the Royal Australian and New Zealand College of Psychiatrists (RANZCP) is worth acknowledging. RANZCP has started embracing impaired psychiatrists on the grounds that the lived experience with mental illness or addiction contributes to planning and delivering better mental health care (McKay et al. 2015). This is a bold step in combating stigma against mental illness and addiction issues, and raises a relevant question: Without changing a profession's attitude toward its own impaired members, how can it be expected to change the attitude of society?

Organizational Changes

Making changes in work culture, volume, and accessible help can be instrumental in managing burnout. A work environment that promotes work-life balance, provides a family-friendly work environment, facilitates parental leave and flexible working hours, protects from exposure to occupational risks, and strengthens job security, is likely to enhance job satisfaction and improve employee relationships (Wiskow et al. 2010). Making the work environment positive yields great dividends against burnout. A recent systematic review (Brand et al. 2017) found evidence that whole-system healthy workplace interventions in healthcare settings improved health and well-being and promoted healthier behaviors among staff. Specifically, with regard to psychiatrists, organizations need to make attitudinal changes in acknowledging the inherently stressful aspects of psychiatry. Timely help seeking should be promoted. Many unique stressors that psychiatrists face in their work should be acknowledged. These include patients' suicides, violence or verbal abuse from patients or families, implications of homicide committed by patients, a litigious society, having to deal with psychiatric emergencies while on call, and an increasing workload while resources are being rationed. These stressors are known to affect morale and job satisfaction and contribute to burnout. Organizations that make these whole-system changes may be better equipped at tackling psychiatrist burnout.

Conclusion

Burnout among psychiatrists is a serious and increasing problem. It affects staff, their families, and the patients they care for. Individual and organizational interventions may be effective in preventing burnout. Screening for burnout improves organizational awareness and may assist in delivering early interventions. Reliable and valid tools for measuring burnout are available. Treatment strategies that combine an intensive stress management program with booster sessions delivered over a longer period may yield longer-lasting results. Both individual-focused and structural or organizational interventions are needed for significant improvement in burnout levels once it manifests. Brief stress management interventions and computer-assisted interventions do not appear promising in treating burnout.

KEY POINTS

- Limited data exist on the prevention and treatment of psychiatrist burnout. Applying research from other disciplines is necessary to develop evidence-based options.

- A multidimensional model of burnout is useful in developing prevention and treatment strategies.

- Combining an intensive stress management program with booster sessions delivered over a longer period may yield longer-lasting results.

- Individual-focused (brief stress management, computer-assisted interventions, CBT, and MBSR) and organizational interventions (attitudinal changes, improved communication, collegial support, participatory problem solving and decision making, and changes in work organization) should be combined in the management of psychiatrist burnout.

———————— ■ ————————

References

Amoafo E, Hanbali N, Patel A, et al: What are the significant factors associated with burnout in doctors? Occup Med (Lond) 65(2):117–121, 2015 25324485

Beheshtifar M, Omidvar AR: Causes to create job burnout in organizations. International Journal of Academic Research in Business and Social Sciences 3(6):107–113, 2013

Berry K, Haddock G, Kellett S, et al: Feasibility of a ward-based psychological intervention to improve staff and patient relationships in psychiatric rehabilitation settings. Br J Clin Psychol 55(3):236–252, 2016 25884235

Blom V: Contingent self-esteem, stressors and burnout in working women and men. Work 43(2):123–131, 2012 22927616

Brand SL, Thompson Coon J, Fleming LE, et al: Whole-system approaches to improving the health and wellbeing of healthcare workers: a systematic review. PLoS One 12(12):e0188418, 2017 29200422

Bressi C, Porcellana M, Gambini O, et al: Burnout among psychiatrists in Milan: a multicenter survey. Psychiatr Serv 60(7):985–988, 2009 19564233

Carson J, Maal S, Roche S, et al: Burnout in mental health nurses: much ado about nothing? Stress and Health 15(2):127–134, 1999

Carver CS: Resilience and thriving: issues, models, and linkages. J Soc Issue 54(2):245–266, 1998

Chang E, Eddins-Folensbee F, Coverdale J: Survey of the prevalence of burnout, stress, depression, and the use of supports by medical students at one school. Acad Psychiatry 36(3):177–182, 2012 22751817

Chemtob CM, Hamada RS, Bauer G, et al: Patients' suicides: frequency and impact on psychiatrists. Am J Psychiatry 145(2):224–228, 1988 3341466

Clark GH, Vaccaro JV: Burnout among CMHC psychiatrists and the struggle to survive. Hosp Community Psychiatry 38(8):843–847, 1987 3610084

Cohen S, Wills TA: Stress, social support, and the buffering hypothesis. Psychol Bull 98(2):310–357, 1985 3901065

Corcoran K: Measuring burnout: an updated reliability and convergent validity study, in Occupational Stress: A Handbook. Edited by Crandall R, Perrewe P. Washington, DC, Taylor and Francis, 1995, pp 263–272

Covey SR, Merrill AR, Merrill RR: First Things First. New York, Free Press, 1996

Demerouti E: Individual strategies to prevent burnout, in Burnout at Work: A Psychological Perspective. Edited by Leiter MP, Bakker AB, Maslach C. London, Psychology Press, 2014, pp 32–55

Demerouti E: Strategies used by individuals to prevent burnout. Eur J Clin Invest 45(10):1106–1112, 2015 26153110

Demerouti E, Bakker A: The Oldenburg Burnout Inventory: a good alternative to measure burnout and engagement, in Handbook of Stress and Burnout in Health Care. Edited by Halbesleben JR. Hauppauge, NY, Nova Science, 2008, pp 1–18

Demerouti E, Bakker AB, Nachreiner F, et al: The Job Demands-Resources Model of burnout. J Appl Psychol 86(3):499–512, 2001 11419809

Demerouti E, Bakker AB, Vardakou I, et al: The convergent validity of two burnout instruments: a multitrait-multimethod analysis. Eur J Psychol Assess 18:296–307, 2002

Dharmawardene M, Givens J, Wachholtz A, et al: A systematic review and meta-analysis of meditative interventions for informal caregivers and health professionals. BMJ Support Palliat Care 6(2):160–169, 2016 25812579

Dieser RB, Edginton CR, Ziemer R: Decreasing patient stress and physician/medical workforce burnout through health care environments: uncovering the serious leisure perspective at Mayo Clinic's campus in Rochester, Minnesota. Mayo Clin Proc 92(7):1080–1087, 2017 28624118

Ferrari S, Cuoghi G, Mattei G, et al: Young and burnt? Italian contribution to the international BurnOut Syndrome Study (BOSS) among residents in psychiatry. Med Lav 106(3):172–185, 2015 25951864

Freudenberger H: Staff burn-out. J Soc Issues 30(1):159–165, 1974

Garcia HA, McGeary CA, Finley EP, et al: The influence of trauma and patient characteristics on provider burnout in VA post-traumatic stress disorder specialty programmes. Psychol Psychother 89(1):66–81, 2016 25643839

Gilmartin H, Goyal A, Hamati MC, et al: Brief mindfulness practices for healthcare providers: a systematic literature review. Am J Med 130(10):1219.e1–1219.e17, 2017 28687263

Gitman P: Impaired physicians/physician assistants, in Administrative Policy and Procedure, in North Shore–Long Island Jewish Health System. New York, Northwell Health, 2008. Available at: https://www.northwell.edu/sites/default/files/Impaired-Physician.pdf. Accessed June 29, 2018.

Gordon CE, Borkan SC: Recapturing time: a practical approach to time management for physicians. Postgrad Med J 90(1063):267–272, 2014 24599633

Gunderman RB, Grogan K: Physician impairment and professionalism. AJR Am J Roentgenol 199(5):W543–W544, 2012 23096197

Hamidi MS, Boggild MK, Cheung AM: Running on empty: a review of nutrition and physicians' well-being. Postgrad Med J 92(1090):478–481, 2016 27215232

Holloway F, Szmukler G, Carson J: Support systems. 1. Introduction. Adv Psychiatr Treat 6(3):226–237, 2000

Humphries N, Morgan K, Conry MC, et al: Quality of care and health professional burnout: narrative literature review. Int J Health Care Qual Assur 27(4):293–307, 2014 25076604

Jensen PM, Trollope-Kumar K, Waters H, et al: Building physician resilience. Can Fam Physician 54(5):722–729, 2008 18474706

Johnson BA: Dealing with the impaired physician. Am Fam Physician 80(9):1007–1008, 2009 19873966

Khoury B, Sharma M, Rush SE, et al: Mindfulness-based stress reduction for healthy individuals: a meta-analysis. J Psychosom Res 78(6):519–528, 2015 25818837

Kristensen TS, Borritz M, Villadsen E, et al: The Copenhagen burnout inventory: a new tool for the assessment of burnout. Work Stress 19(3):192–207, 2005

Kumar S: Burnout and doctors: prevalence, prevention and intervention. Healthcare (Basel) 4(3):37, 2016 27417625

Kumar S, Hatcher S, Huggard P: Burnout in psychiatrists: an etiological model. Int J Psychiatry Med 35(4):405–416, 2005 16673840

Kumar S, Bhagat RN, Lau T, et al: Psychiatrists in New Zealand: are they burning out, satisfied at work and, in any case, who cares? Australas Psychiatry 14(1):20–23, 2006 16630192

Kumar S, Fischer J, Robinson E, et al: Burnout and job satisfaction in New Zealand psychiatrists: a national study. Int J Soc Psychiatry 53(4):306–316, 2007 17703646

Kumar S, Hatcher S, Dutu G, et al: Stresses experienced by psychiatrists and their role in burnout: a national follow-up study. Int J Soc Psychiatry 57(2):166–179, 2011 20068020

Kuster AT, Dalsbø TK, Luong Thanh BY, et al: Computer-based versus in-person interventions for preventing and reducing stress in workers. Cochrane Database Syst Rev 8(8):CD011899, 2017 28853146

Lee RT, Seo B, Hladkyl S, et al: Hum Resour Health 11:48, 2013 24074053

Leiter MP, Maslach C: Interventions to prevent and alleviate burnout, in Burnout at Work: A Psychological Perspective. Edited by Leiter MP, Bakker AB, Maslach C. London, Psychology Press, 2014, pp 145–167

Leiter MP, Laschinger HKS, Day A, et al: The impact of civility interventions on employee social behavior, distress, and attitudes. J Appl Psychol 96(6):1258–1274, 2011 21744942

Lloyd C, King R, Chenoweth L: Social work, stress and burnout: a review. J Ment Health 11(3):255–265, 2002

Marine A, Ruotsalainen J, Serra C, et al: Preventing occupational stress in health care workers. Cochrane Database Syst Rev 18(4):CD002892, 2006 17054155

Maslach C: Finding solutions to the problem of burnout. Consult Psychol J 69(2):143–152, 2017

Maslach C, Goldberg J: Prevention of burnout: new perspectives. Appl Prev Psychol 7(1):63–74, 1998

Maslach C, Jackson SE: The measurement of experienced burnout. Journal of Organizational Behavior 2(2):99–113, 1981

Maslach C, Leiter MP (eds): The Truth About Burnout. San Francisco, CA, Jossey Bass, 1997

Maslach C, Leiter MP: Understanding the burnout experience: recent research and its implications for psychiatry. World Psychiatry 15(2):103–111, 2016 27265691

Maslach C, Leiter MP: New insights into burnout and health care: strategies for improving civility and alleviating burnout. Med Teach 39(2):160–163, 2017 27841065

Maslach C, Jackson S, Leiter M: Maslach Burnout Inventory Manual, 3rd Edition. Palo Alto, CA, Consulting Psychologist Press, 1996

Maslach C, Schaufeli WB, Leiter MP: Job burnout. Annu Rev Psychol 53:397–422, 2001

McKay R, Liggins J, McMahon J, et al: Beyond impairment: using the lived experience of mental illness by psychiatrists to improve care. RANZCP Abstracts. Aust N Z J Psychiatry 49(S1):7–8, 2015

Montgomery A: The inevitability of physician burnout: implications for interventions. Burnout Research 4(1):50–56, 2014

Morse G, Salyers MP, Rollins AL, et al: Burnout in mental health services: a review of the problem and its remediation. Adm Policy Ment Health 39(5):341–352, 2012 21533847

Pines A: On burnout and buffering effects of social support, in Stress and Burnout in the Human Service Professions. Edited by Farbder B. Oxford, United Kingdom, Pergamon, 1988, pp 155–167

Pines A, Aronson E: Career Burnout: Causes and Cures. New York, Free Press, 1988

Prosser D, Johnson S, Kuipers E, et al: Mental health, "burnout" and job satisfaction among hospital and community-based mental health staff. Br J Psychiatry 169(3):334–337, 1996 8879720

Rey JM, Walter G, Giuffrida M: Australian psychiatrists today: proud of their profession but stressed and apprehensive about the future. Aust N Z J Psychiatry 38(3):105–110, 2004 14961926

Rothenberger DA: Physician burnout and well-being: a systematic review and framework for action. Dis Colon Rectum 60(6):567–576, 2017 28481850

Ruotsalainen JH, Verbeek JH, Mariné A, et al: Preventing occupational stress in healthcare workers. Cochrane Database Syst Rev 7(4):CD002892, 2015 25847433

Schaufeli WB, Enzmann D (eds): The Burnout Companion to Study and Practice. London, Taylor and Francis, 1998

Schaufeli WB, Leiter MP, Maslach C: Burnout: 35 years of research and practice. Career Development International 14(3):204–220, 2009

Schaufeli WB, Maslach C, Marek T (eds): Professional Burnout: Recent Developments in Theory and Research. Washington, DC, Taylor and Francis, 1993

Shanafelt TD, Noseworthy JH: Executive leadership and physician well-being: nine organizational strategies to promote engagement and reduce burnout. Mayo Clin Proc 92(1):129–146, 2017 27871627

Sherman DW: Nurses' stress and burnout. How to care for yourself when caring for patients and their families experiencing life-threatening illness. Am J Nurs 104(5):48–56, quiz 57, 2004 15166716

Shirom A: Burnout in work organizations, in International Review of Industrial and Organizational Psychology. Edited by Coope C, Robertson I. Oxford, United Kingdom, John Wiley and Sons, 1989, pp 26–47

Shirom A, Melamed S: Does burnout affect physical health? A review of the evidence, in Research Companion to Organizational Health Psychology. Edited by Antoniou ASG, Cooper CL. Cheltenham, United Kingdom, Edward Elgar, 2005, pp 599–622

Sparks K, Faragher B, Cooper CL: Well-being and occupational health in the 21st century workplace. J Occup Organ Psychol 74(4):489–509, 2001

Tregoning C, Remington S, Agius S: Facing change: developing resilience for staff, associate specialist, and specialty doctors. BMJ 348:g251, 2014

Vaccaro JV, Clark GH Jr: A profile of community mental health center psychiatrists: results of a national survey. Community Ment Health J 23(4):282–289, 1987 3440380

van Wyk BE, Pillay-Van Wyk V: Preventive staff-support interventions for health workers. Cochrane Database Syst Rev 3(3):CD003541, 2010 20238322

Ward S, Outram S: Medicine: in need of culture change. Intern Med J 46(1):112–116, 2016 26813903

West CP, Dyrbye LN, Erwin PJ, et al: Interventions to prevent and reduce physician burnout: a systematic review and meta-analysis. Lancet 388(10057):2272–2281, 2016 27692469

Wiskow C, Albreht T, de Pietro C (eds): How to Create an Attractive and Supportive Working Environment for Health Professionals. Geneva, Switzerland, World Health Organization, 2010

Yancey JR, McKinnon HD Jr: Reaching out to an impaired physician. Fam Pract Manag 17(1):27–31, 2010 20092233

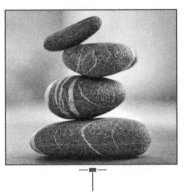

CHAPTER 13

THE ROLE OF HEALTH SYSTEM INNOVATION IN PREVENTING PSYCHIATRIST BURNOUT

Nidal Moukaddam, M.D., Ph.D.

Asim Shah, M.D.

Writers have found the life of the physician a compelling subject because they could not be indifferent to it. The physician is too intimately bound to hopes and fears of the ill in their struggle against disease and death.

McLellan (1996)

Physician engagement in the work environment and the physician-patient relationship, long viewed as cornerstones of medical treatment, have been steadily eroded. There is tension and a changing landscape in medicine with respect to the milestones that need to be measured for students, trainees, and practitioners (Boulet and Durning 2019). Assessments in medicine, whether for graduation or maintenance of certification, are knowledge based and focused. However, this may be in direct conflict with the attributes (such as values and attitudes) that contribute to physician self-image and the factors that enhance work and life satisfaction. Furthermore, these values and the attitudes of physicians are not even measured aspects of physician performance or patient satisfaction. The challenge of balancing assessments and productivity with physician satisfaction and value systems extends from the individual clinician to the very fabric of medical organizations. The balance sought here between clinical service, productivity, and advancing the academic mission, keeping in mind that healthcare organizations are among some of the most complex organizations in existence, is a precarious one. No perfect solution or model exists for this balance, and no formula for fostering a perfect equilibrium between service and scholarship is known (Pellegrini et al. 2019).

Burnout and Work Engagement Reflect the Organization

As has been discussed in other chapters in this book, burnout in medicine has reached epidemic proportions, with more than half the clinicians surveyed reporting burnout symptoms. This is inclusive of residents and medical students, even though matriculating medical students have similar or better mental health and higher quality-of-life scores than age-similar control subjects when they begin training (Brazeau et al. 2014).

Attention to organizational factors has been delayed, but the focus has gradually shifted to highlighting organizational factors as risk factors for individual burnout (West et al. 2018). This has the advantage of removing the focus from individual resilience factors, which, although important, cannot permanently and irrevocably shield an individual from burning out. In turn, burnout can alter clinicians' plans (Sinsky et al. 2017) and affect retention and job turnover. Preventing burnout becomes the shared responsibility of both the organization and the individual.

Viewing workplace environments from a systems perspective is not limited to medicine, and businesses large and small have sought to improve working environments for their staff. The ultimate goal is to promote workplace engagement, a positive view of the workplace, and a community that fosters a sense of belonging and pride in one's work and the organization they belong to. Conceptually, this exemplifies the opposite of burnout on a global level, targeting emotional and physical exhaustion, detachment and compassion fatigue, and cynicism and decreased positive outlook on the future. In a recent article, Shanafelt et al. (2017) established a suggested framework for organizational strategy to optimize physician well-being in the organizational context (Shanafelt and Noseworthy 2017). The key is transformational leadership that aims to replace inefficacy, cynicism, and exhaustion with vigor, dedication, and being healthily absorbed in work. Before we delve into the most cutting-edge solutions in the field, a look into models that provide work-related stress risk assessment is in order. These models include but are not limited to the Job Strain Model, the Cox Transactional Model, Effort-Reward Imbalance Model, and the Job Demands-Resources Model (Chirico 2016). All these models assume that job satisfaction and strain/burnout are at opposite ends of the spectrum.

1. The Job Strain Model examines the interaction between job demands (e.g., role ambiguity, role conflict, role stress, stressful events at work, workload, and work pressure) and personal or job resources (e.g., autonomy, support, feedback) (Stansfeld and Candy 2006).
2. The Effort-Reward Imbalance Model posits job satisfaction as a balance of intrinsic factors (rewards, motivations) versus extrinsic demands (workload) (Siegrist and Li 2017).
3. The Cox Transactional Model describes context factors including organizational culture and function, an individual's role in the organization, options for career development, the latitude to make decisions/control, interpersonal relationships at work, home-work interface, organizational change, and mobbing/bullying/harassment. "Content" refers to work environment and work equipment, workload/work pace/work schedule, and task design. The last element of content is how emotionally demanding the job is (Ahola et al. 2013; Santos and Cox 2000). The factors causing work stress can be viewed as context versus content factors (as specified by the Cox Transactional Model): Physical environment (content) involves the physical work setting, material conditions, commute/journey, and access. Organizational culture (content) includes schedules, structure, and interpersonal relations (e.g., how often does one get to interact with other staff, is there a community).

    Content factors interact with individual (context) conditions that reflect an individual's workload versus present resources, the balance of powerlessness versus autonomy, and rewards. Thus, at any given point, although an individual might be able to accommodate a demanding schedule, a long commute, or a schedule that is not congruent with his or her circadian rhythm, the sustainability of those parameters will depend on the individual's life circumstances and suitability to the person's temperament and preexisting factors. Organizational factors promoting temporary, though possibly long-lasting, work stress include isolation, uncertainty, and profound change and evolving standards (such as recertification and new requirements and added bureaucratic hurdles).

4. We now discuss the Job Demands-Resources Model. Looking at jobs from the point of view of maintaining a balance between demands and resources, burnout is considered to be the product of this imbalance (Demerouti et al. 2001). Any job requires a certain amount of input, which could be mental, emotional, and/or physical. These demands are balanced by rewards offered by the job, both tangible and intangible. Although the balance differs for every individual, it is important to appreciate the role of the organizational structure in promoting well-being or, conversely, undermining it.

Institutional Interventions to Decrease Burnout

An example of how an institutional intervention can be composed relates, for instance, to the algorithmic approach with difficult patients (e.g., patients with multiple comorbidities, severe illnesses/refractory cases, severe psychosocial stressors, patients on the brink of death), which includes preclinic reviews and assigning case management to patients meeting specific criteria. Clinical aspects of practice can link to worsening burnout symptoms. A high frequency of difficult cases has been shown to link to higher burnout rates, especially in family medicine (An et al. 2013). In psychiatry, working with patients with personality disorders is one of the most difficult areas and links to increased burnout, especially to desensitization (Eren 2014; Koekkoek et al. 2010). Medical encounters depend on clinician factors, patient factors, and setting-related situational factors (Cannarella Lorenzetti et al. 2013). Designing institutional interventions may thus affect 1) the setting of the encounter (e.g., office space, staff support, availability of clinic previews, availability of wraparound and other social services), 2) training clinicians to handle difficult encounters more skillfully, and 3) considering elements of flexibility or some autonomy in management of difficult patients and in a proper reward balance for challenging practice settings.

Competitive salary and generous financial compensation, also long viewed as staples of a physician's career, have dwindled in recent times, undermined by student debt, unfavorable reimbursement climate, and seismic shifts in healthcare climates. This shift has correlated with increasing burnout levels as physician allegiance to humane and proper patient care is challenged and the model shifts toward corporate profitability (Clark 2018), which no system, including academic systems, is immune to (Pellegrini et al. 2019). However, despite financial pressures, investing in physician well-being is the key to maintaining balance and safeguarding clinical and academic growth (Shanafelt et al. 2017).

Among the three elements of burnout, compassion fatigue and subsequent detachment are the least studied. The development and maintenance of compassion (which is different than empathy) has been viewed as a talent, a personality characteristic, and a component of bedside manner. A compassionate clinician may be acutely aware of another person's (e.g., the patient's or a colleague's) suffering; however, empathy carries a different level of understanding of suffering. One could feel empathy even if the feelings in question do not apply to them, by appreciating the impact those feelings have on the patient. A balance between empathy and compassion is necessary for effective practice because medicine often entails exposure to sadness, mortality, and loss. Being only compassionate (as in feeling pity or concern for another person) may decrease objectivity and render a clinician less attuned to other feelings that they do not personally relate to. Only in the past decade or less has research turned to promoting compassion among practitioners, with the hope it will trickle down to patient care and protect against dehumanization and burnout. Studies do show that compassionate medicine leads to better satisfaction in patients and practitioners (Fernando and Consedine 2014). Evidence shows that increasing the exposure that medical students have to the humanistic aspects of medicine, focusing on the ability to be vulnerable and have discussions about the humane aspects of medicine, and reinforcing the concept of being treated (and treating others) with respect and fairness contributes to decreased burnout in trainees and students (Mangione et al. 2018; Rider et al. 2018). The International Charter for Human Values in Healthcare outlines five dimensions of human values for humane, fair healthcare interactions—compassion, respect for persons, commitment to integrity and ethical practice, commitment to excellence, and justice in healthcare (Rider et al. 2014). These values can be used as a template to shape organizational cultures positively and humanistically (American Board of Internal Medicine et al. 2002; Rider et al. 2018). In a survey of physicians at eight institutions, these values were clearly shown to be important as mitigating factors for burnout, whereas organizational obstacles were listed as unsupportive leadership, inadequate time with patients, bureaucratic pressures, and nonfacilitative practice structures (Rider et al. 2018). Therefore, designing institutional policies to promote a more humane practice environment can target these obstacles.

In the model promoted by Shanafelt and Noseworthy (2017), building a wellness-rich environment is the result of individual, work unit, organizational, and even national factors as well as a challenge to healthcare leadership. The first two strategies revolve around acknowledging not only the existence, high prevalence, and cost of burnout and responsibility but also the power of leadership to significantly modify organizational conditions. Steps 3 and 4 revolve around customizing interventions while building a community spirit that enhances employees' sense of belonging. The next three steps combine using incentives and rewards in ways that align with institutional cultures, strengthen community bonds, and, lastly, integrate work-life balance rather than viewing work-related well-being as an isolated entity. A crucial step emphasized by Shanafelt and Noseworthy is the duty of the organization to facilitate self-care and invest in scientific advances to sustain physician engagement.

Innovative Systemic Approaches to Burnout

Fine institutions, academic and private, have made promoting well-being and improving their organizational culture a priority. In this section, we describe some institutional efforts across the United States serving this purpose.

Starting with improved detection and facilitating the ability to self-diagnose one's level of burnout, the Well-Being Index (www.mededwebs.com/well-being-index) is an excellent resource devised at the Mayo Clinic that allows an individual to assess his or her own well-being/burnout status, get personalized recommendations, and, more importantly, compare one's score with national averages.

At the Mayo Clinic, the experience of decreasing burnout levels to below national standards occurred via the development of the Listen-Act-Develop model (Swensen et al. 2016), which includes personalized wellness assessments as well as physician engagement groups, among other components. The model facilitates social connectedness and emphasizes the connection to a greater cause and meaningful impact within the organization and community. Improved autonomy is also crucial.

Interventions combining *emotional intelligence training, leadership skills,* and *self-care* techniques can mitigate burnout even with brief interventions: using a train-the-trainer approach and focusing on self-awareness, self-care, self-compassion, and boundary setting, a pilot study of a 2-day workshop to train program directors showed sustainable effects for the subsequent 9-month follow-up period (Ghossoub et al. 2018). Participants reported an improved ability to detect burnout, to improve their own work-life balance, and to better manage trainees' burnout as a result.

At Stanford University, the Golden Ticket Project was evaluated as a success (Gribben et al. 2018) as a tool for communicating appreciation and promoting a positive environment via building peer support and recognition for resident physicians. For Stanford faculty, the Academic Biomedical Career Customization initiative has been active for 2 years and focuses on mitigating work-life and work-work conflict (Fassiotto et al. 2018), also with success. *Work-life conflict,* simple to understand, revolves around meeting of family, spouse, and home demands and the requisites of personal self-care. *Work-work conflict,* on the other hand, consists of the conflicting demands of research, teaching, and clinical care in addition to those of service and administration. An innovative time-banking system allows credits to be assigned for activities deemed unpopular—such as mentoring or covering for colleagues on short notice—and exchanged or redeemed for support services at home (e.g., housecleaning, laundry, meal delivery, errand outsourcing, car service) or work (e.g., grant writing, manuscript editing, speech coaching, lab management services, website design, graphics for presentations, office organizing). Stanford University is also the first university to assign a chief wellness officer dedicated to promoting organizational wellness.

Psychiatrists and other medical professionals are part of the fabric of healthcare systems, and recent evidence highlights the importance of *civility* in the workplace and the price of incivility for workplace retention of healthcare workers (Pattani et al. 2018). Ostracism, harassment, and bullying fall along the same spectrum of incivility. The end product, a toxic work environment, has a negative impact on productivity and employee retention (Anjum et al. 2018). So what is a healthcare system to do? The first step is to curtail overtly negative behaviors, but this has to be followed by positively shaping workplace culture and promoting engagement with that positive culture (Pattani et al. 2018). This is most difficult in larger systems (Shortell et al. 1995). At Baylor College of Medicine, a pilot institutional effort, "Professionalism and Engagement Elevating Physician and Scientist Satisfaction," that focused on building ties among staff members across disciplines and across medical and nonmedical staff showed sustained positive results over 18 months (E. Friedman, personal communication, December 13, 2018). The program focused on reducing isolation, enhancing the sense of community, and validating the challenges staff were experiencing in the work setting. To achieve this goal, the program matched individuals from clinical and nonclinical departments at various levels of seniority and facilitated regularly scheduled casual, social-like meetings, in addition to education and support regarding burnout prevention. This undertaking was complemented by the "Threads Among Us" project, consisting of a video as well as a facilitator's handbook for a 60-minute workshop to be used across departments and by other institutions. The intended audience included staff physicians, nonphysician providers, medical trainees, nurses, and other allied healthcare professionals.

Systemic Approaches for Decreasing Burnout in Large and Small Healthcare Systems

Both large and small healthcare systems face challenges in promoting well-being. As emphasized in the introduction to the chapter, there is no one-size-fits-all solution; however, keeping in mind the aim of maintaining compassion and delivering humane and standard-compliant treatments, every system has strengths and weaknesses. Antiburnout and wellness efforts center on detection and treatment of burnout. The best-designed solutions are customized to career phase, physician specialty, and practice setting. System size affects ability to detect or treat burnout or both.

As a system grows, an impersonal quality typically becomes dominant, with lessened communication between individuals who do not have direct collaborative relationships, a lessened sense of community, decreasing communication between clinical and nonclinical departments, and potentially decreased access to leadership. Conscious organizational efforts are needed to contain those factors that can undermine well-being and productivity.

Those efforts may coincide with efforts needed to promote an organization's image in the community or to advertise an organization to patients. However, the well-being of physicians has become a target of institutional efforts only very recently (Shanafelt et al. 2017). System growth occurs better with staff believing that this growth will benefit them or their community, whether morally or financially, and this includes the feeling of participating in a meaningful operation. So, in large institutions where individualized burnout detection may suffer because of institution size, comprehensive wellness programs endowed with regular standardized assessment tools can facilitate detection.

Small systems, on the other hand, do not have to contend with this impersonal quality, and closer interpersonal ties among physicians, staff, and consultants may exist. However, this may also translate into heavier schedules and less support. For smaller systems, this may also mean that fewer resources are dedicated to community efforts, wellness efforts, or personalized wellness assessments combined with customized achievement plans, which are rapidly becoming standard in the field of antiburnout efforts. Smaller systems may also have less effective electronic health records and fewer trainees to shoulder the burden of night and emergency calls. Thus, detection of burnout signs, including irritability, increased absenteeism, substance use problems, and medical errors may be faster and more personalized. Conversely, mitigation and treatment could be a luxury in a small system that cannot afford absences, coverage, and so on. Evidence points to the fact that shorter shifts and sometimes shorter rotations correlate with better well-being (West et al. 2014).

Transformational leadership is an asset regardless of system size and characteristic because leadership can promote design and implementation of measures and policies that are well suited to the system at hand.

Burnout Among Psychiatrists

The role and image of the psychiatrist has been in flux for the past few decades, just as the burnout concept has evolved, keeping pace with the revolution in healthcare. Rates of burnout in psychiatrists are estimated to be around 40%, based on a meta-analysis of more than 9,000 psychiatrists (O'Connor et al. 2018), with the most prevalent symptom being emotional exhaustion. The specific pattern that seems to emerge for psychiatrists is high emotional exhaustion but moderate scores on cynicism and loss of meaning and depersonalization. Increasing age is associated with an improved sense of achievement but also an increased risk of depersonalization. Lack of role clarity was mentioned by a majority of mental health professionals as a risk factor for burnout, whereas supervision is considered a protective factor. In a survey of psychiatrists at the Department of Veterans Affairs hospitals, perceived unfair treatment by supervisors and feeling that inadequate resources are being allocated to one's practice mediate cynicism and emotional exhaustion (Villarosa-Hurlocker et al. 2019). This finding highlighted a direct link between organizational factors and burnout dimensions in psychiatrists. It is noteworthy that psychiatrists (probably because of training) do not display levels of depersonalization as high as other specialties, but they may transition to a diminished sense of meaning associated with practice (Weilenmann et al. 2018). Psychiatrists and primary care physicians show different levels of emotional engagement with emotional patient disclosures (Davidsen and Fosgerau 2014). Higher rates or increased vulnerability for burnout for psychiatrists working on community mental health programs and certain types of outreach efforts such as assertive community treatment (ACT) programs (Rosen et al. 2007) are a classic example of how the high frequency of difficult cases with no foreseeable improvement or resolution, as discussed earlier, leads to higher burnout symptomatology.

Factors that affect psychiatry are not limited to the demands and challenges of electronic health record use, detailed in Chapter 8, "Electronic Health Records and Physician Burnout," but also include the changing landscape with medication management versus psychotherapy in psychiatric practice. Over the past two decades, the percentage of patients receiving psychotherapy has decreased (Marcus and Olfson 2010). The percentage of patients receiving psychotropics for symptomatic treatment *without* a mental health diagnosis has increased significantly as well (Maust et al. 2017), with particular increases in sedative-hypnotic use in older adults and antidepressants in patients with pain diagnoses. The percentage of psychiatrists providing *psychotherapy* (regardless of the type), defined as providing a service of more than 30 minutes, in office, declined sharply to about 10% of all psychiatrists by 2005 (Mojtabai and Olfson 2008).

Picture an individual with insomnia and subacute to chronic pain who is receiving psychotropic medications. That patient may never receive psychotherapy, may experience discontinuation symptoms when the antidepressant is stopped, and may finally arrive in a psychiatrist's office in a crowded schedule and possibly experience the stigma of being labeled as mentally ill. Treating this kind of patient may epitomize the lack of role clarity mentioned earlier, which is a driving factor in the burnout epidemic for psychiatrists specifically.

Strengths pertaining to psychiatry training include a presumed better ability for emotional regulation, through sheer practice and extensive supervision that is a required part of psychiatric training. Such supervision is not part of other residency trainings. One of the first interventions for burnout focused on Balint training, which indeed lowers burnout rates (Clough et al. 2017; Stojanovic-Tasic et al. 2018); Balint groups, named after the psychoanalyst Michael Balint, have clinicians meet regularly to present and discuss clinical cases. They bear some similarities to the supervision that psychiatry residents get.

Better emotional regulation is associated with better well-being and quality of life measures. This serves as the basis for many of the mindfulness interventions that have been found to be successful in mitigating burnout because these interventions promote acceptance of unpleasant emotional states, better emotional control, and more thoughtful management of one's feelings. Unsurprisingly, models promoting proper managing of emotions, emotional regulation, and empathy-based processes show promise in preventing burnout and improving well-being (Weilenmann et al. 2018). Even though, as mentioned, the percentage of psychiatrists providing therapy has declined, psychotherapy training remains a cornerstone of psychiatric training, placing psychiatrists in a unique position to combat burnout given the right workplace setting.

Weaknesses in psychiatric training may include resistance to change when in a burned-out state. In a study of acute mental health wards in the United Kingdom, higher levels of burnout in psychiatric staff were related to less self-confidence for initiating change and more resistance to change (Laker et al. 2019). Thus, burnout may be self-perpetuating by embroiling the individual in a web of perseverating negative or maladaptive coping patterns. Additionally, because psychiatrists-in-training get exposed to more violence than other specialties (except emergency medicine), they also may have a somewhat higher propensity to use substances or self-medicate with sedative or anxiolytic medications, according to the BOURBON national survey of French interns (Fond et al. 2018).

The interplay of psychiatric training and institutional efforts to prevent and treat burnout can potentially be a match made in heaven: flexible supervision adapted to the load difficulty of psychiatrists' cases, reward schedule adapted to productivity (clinical and nonclinical), and encouragement of the practice of applicable useful psychotherapy modalities on departmental levels can mesh well with institution-level humanist efforts and programs highlighting the importance of physician-patient relationships.

Technological Innovation in Burnout Assessment and Intervention

The power of organizational interventions resides in their scope and ability to enforce implementation. Technological advances can be used to improve detection and management of burnout manifestations, but they have not yet matured to the point of systemwide utilization. Ideally, technological advances, once fully validated and proven, can be offered at institutions alongside other health benefits, such as wellness programs, smoking cessation programs, or weight management curricula.

The elements of technology that are pertinent to burnout assessment and treatment fall into the areas of biomonitoring and biobehavioral sensing. *Biomonitoring* simply relates to measuring biological parameters in relationship to burnout, such as cortisol in burned-out individuals versus control subjects. Biobehavioral sensing is the ultimate frontier in the collaboration between psychiatry and engineering. *Biobehavioral sensing* is the art and science of using sensors to measure biological parameters and then linking them to behavioral parameters, for example, linking fluctuations in heart rate or sleep or steps taken during the day to mood/anxiety, wellness, burnout ratings, or even specific outcomes, such as certain behaviors including self-harm or substance use. Smartphones, ubiquitous as they are, can be instrumental in advancing the field of burnout detection. Smartphones have several sensors including motion, temperature, infrared sensors, and, with some modifications, the ability to measure vital signs via video recordings or even skin perfusion (linking to anxiety, mild flushing) (Kumar et al. 2016).

The first step to using technology in detecting and treating burnout is to appreciate the physiological manifestations of this condition. Burnout is a stressful state to the human organism and affects cortisol secretion and inflammatory markers as well as heart rate variability, among others. Biomonitoring via measurements of midday cortisol secretions can be helpful in tracking burnout levels (Pilger et al. 2018), and lowered heart rate variability correlates with levels of burnout as well. Higher levels of burnout link to lower heart rate variability (Kanthak et al. 2017), especially cynicism (Viljoen and Claassen 2017). In addition, high levels of burnout are considered a risk factor for coronary events (Zhang et al. 2018). The Dresden study, currently under way, aims to examine biological correlates of burnout over 10 years (Penz et al. 2018).

Some useful and successful interventions have employed smartphone apps to deliver mindfulness interventions without employing biobehavioral sensing. Mobile or audio delivery of mindfulness applications for 10–20 minutes daily for 30 days contributed to decreased stress levels in medical student cohorts (Yang et al. 2018), and mindfulness-based resilience training delivered via an app had better effects than in-person training (Mistretta et al. 2018). In terms of interventions, smartphone and wearable device–based applications can provide ongoing monitoring and personalized warnings or interventions when burnout levels or associated parameters exceed certain preset thresholds (such parameters could include vital signs, self-ratings, or activity or sleep changes). The concept is facilitated by evidence supporting the fact that single-item questions about burnout correlate well with emotional exhaustion and depersonalization scores (West et al. 2009), bypassing the need for extensive questionnaires.

We have piloted a brief smartphone-based application for trainees in psychiatry that consisted of a set of two to five statements about well-being and work stressors three times per week, for which the participant was asked to rate approval on an analog scale. Participants were also asked to rate one's own perceived burnout level. The 6-week intervention showed positive effect in decreasing self-rated burnout levels with minimal time involvement and showed that self-rated burnout on a visual analog scale correlated well with the emotional exhaustion on the Maslach Burnout Inventory (Maslach and Jackson 1981).

The field of biobehavioral sensing in burnout is not fully mature, but it is very promising, especially for institutions willing to make wellness a priority.

Innovations in Healthcare and Burnout Reduction

Innovations in psychiatric care and delivery may also contribute to mitigating burnout and impact well-being and job satisfaction. Bearing in mind the complexity and chronic nature of some mental illnesses, various innovative transformations in healthcare delivery could be critical in changing the psychiatry practice landscape.

Integrated care, an umbrella term referring to linking mental health/behavioral care to other specialties or primary care, represents a major *evolution* in the practice of psychiatry. It refers to multiple models that focus on improving general healthcare and that follow chronic disease management strategies (Joseph et al. 2017). Sometimes, psychiatry can be part of the patient-centered medical home. Different specialties can be physically colocated or have common care management plans. Collaborative care models have shown higher efficacy in treating nonpsychotic disorders such as anxiety and depression (Thota et al. 2012) and lead to better clinician engagement (Moise et al. 2018). Burnout in participating psychiatrists has not been formally studied, but a Swiss survey reported improved well-being and fewer burnout ratings with increased collaboration (Baumgardt et al. 2015).

ACT has been touted as one of the best means to deal with chronic severe mental illness and has success with outcomes such as treatment adherence and decreased rehospitalizations. However, analyses comparing ACT teams internationally show increased rates of burnout, specifically emotional exhaustion, in some teams (Harvey et al. 2011, 2012). We speculate that model fidelity adherence and team logistics play a bigger role than previously thought in safeguarding the staff's mental health and well-being. Often, inclusion of a wide range of interventions (besides medication adherence, e.g., vocational and substance use treatment) and other evidence-based interventions is vital to prevent team burnout (Rosen et al. 2007).

Training psychiatrists and psychiatric staff to deal with specific conditions that make patients "difficult" is instrumental. The difficult patient in psychiatry is, of course, different than those in other specialties. Patients with personality disorders and chronic severe mental illness (specifically psychosis) and those who have experienced long-term residential treatments are the patients most cited as difficult. Training arms psychiatric staff with tools for more effective treatment and the ability to navigate negative feelings stemming from difficult patient interactions. In an exploratory pilot study, training staff in cognitive-analytic therapy, an integrative and relational model of psychotherapy, helped reduce burnout scores and improve scores on measurements of engagement (Caruso et al. 2013). Using *intervention mapping,* a method for development, implementation, and evaluation of health interventions, Koekkoek et al. (2010) developed an interpersonal community psychiatric treatment model and identified three main areas to target for more effective psychiatric care delivery: 1) inconsistent, shifting symptoms that prevent the clinician from achieving a clear diagnosis (and then initiating treatment); 2) ambivalent or poorly adherent care seeking; and 3) social problems (e.g., homelessness, poverty, unemployment, legal issues) that patients expect their psychiatrists to solve.

Conclusion

We are living in an exciting era when maintaining wellness is finally being seen as a task above and beyond resilience in the individual physician. Institutions can play a major role in promoting and maintaining wellness. Training psychiatrists to deal with difficult patients and deliver more effective care is crucial to greater work engagement and less burnout.

KEY POINTS

- Wellness and burnout are considered to be the result of interplay between individual factors and organizational factors.

- Institutions can play a major role in implementing interventions to detect burnout, facilitate self-care, and provide system-level solutions to worsening burnout levels.

- Several institutional-level programs are already under way and have shown usefulness.

- Advances in technological detection of burnout can pave the way to systemwide smartphone and wearable device applications, allowing automated detection of physiological parameters of burnout.

- More collaborative models of care delivery, including assertive community treatment and integrated care, may be protective against burnout when adequately implemented.

References

Ahola K, Salminen S, Toppinen-Tanner S, et al: Occupational burnout and severe injuries: an eight-year prospective cohort study among Finnish forest industry workers. J Occup Health 55(6):450–457, 2013 24162145

American Board of Internal Medicine, American College of Physicians-American Society of Internal Medicine, European Federation of Internal Medicine, et al: Medical professionalism in the new millennium: a physician charter. Ann Intern Med 136(3):243–246, 2002 11827500

An PG, Manwell LB, Williams ES, et al: Does a higher frequency of difficult patient encounters lead to lower quality care? J Fam Pract 62(1):24–29, 2013 23326819

Anjum A, Ming X, Siddiqi AF, et al: An empirical study analyzing job productivity in toxic workplace environments. Int J Environ Res Public Health 15(5):E1035, 2018 29883424

Baumgardt J, Moock J, Rössler W, et al: Aspects of sustainability: cooperation, job satisfaction, and burnout among Swiss psychiatrists. Front Public Health 3:25, 2015 25717469

Boulet JR, Durning SJ: What we measure...and what we should measure in medical education. Med Educ 53(1):86–94, 2019 30216508

Brazeau CM, Shanafelt T, Durning SJ, et al: Distress among matriculating medical students relative to the general population. Acad Med 89(11):1520–1525, 2014 25250752

Cannarella Lorenzetti R, Jacques CH, Donovan C, et al: Managing difficult encounters: understanding physician, patient, and situational factors. Am Fam Physician 87(6):419–425, 2013 23547575

Caruso R, Biancosino B, Borghi C, et al: Working with the 'difficult' patient: the use of a contextual cognitive-analytic therapy based training in improving team function in a routine psychiatry service setting. Community Ment Health J 49(6):722–727, 2013 23292306

Chirico F: Job stress models for predicting burnout syndrome: a review. Ann Ist Super Sanita 52(3):443–456, 2016 27698304

Clark SA: The impact of the Hippocratic Oath in 2018: the conflict of the ideal of the physician, the knowledgeable humanitarian, versus the corporate medical allegiance to financial models contributes to burnout. Cureus 10(7):e3076, 2018 30280071

Clough BA, March S, Chan RJ, et al: Psychosocial interventions for managing occupational stress and burnout among medical doctors: a systematic review. Syst Rev 6(1):144, 2017 28716112

Davidsen AS, Fosgerau CF: General practitioners' and psychiatrists' responses to emotional disclosures in patients with depression. Patient Educ Couns 95(1):61–68, 2014 24492158

Demerouti E, Bakker AB, Nachreiner F, et al: The job demands-resources model of burnout. J Appl Psychol 86(3):499–512, 2001 11419809

Eren N: Psychometric properties of difficulties of working with patients with personality disorders and attitudes towards patients with personality disorders scales. Noro Psikiyatri Arsivi 51(4):318–327, 2014 28360649

Fassiotto M, Simard C, Sandborg C, et al: An integrated career coaching and time-banking system promoting flexibility, wellness, and success: a pilot program at Stanford University School of Medicine. Acad Med 93(6):881–887, 2018 29298183

Fernando AT 3rd, Consedine NS: Beyond compassion fatigue: the transactional model of physician compassion. J Pain Symptom Manage 48(2):289–298, 2014 24417804

Fond G, Bourbon A, Micoulaud-Franchi JA, et al: Psychiatry: a discipline at specific risk of mental health issues and addictive behavior? Results from the national BOURBON study. J Affect Disord 238:534–538, 2018 29936392

Ghossoub Z, Nadler R, El-Aswad N: Targeting physician burnout through emotional intelligence, self-care techniques, and leadership skills training: a qualitative study. Mayo Clin Proc Innov Qual Outcomes 2(1):78–79, 2018 30225436

Gribben V, Bogetz A, Bachrach L, et al: The Golden Ticket Project for peer recognition. Clin Teach 2018 29806729 [Epub ahead of print]

Harvey C, Killaspy H, Martino S, et al: A comparison of the implementation of assertive community treatment in Melbourne, Australia and London, England. Epidemiol Psychiatr Sci 20(2):151–161, 2011 21714362

Harvey C, Killaspy H, Martino S, et al: Implementation of assertive community treatment in Australia: model fidelity, patient characteristics and staff experiences. Community Ment Health J 48(5):652–661, 2012 22089145

Joseph R, Kester R, O'Brien C, et al: The evolving practice of psychiatry in the era of integrated care. Psychosomatics 58(5):466–473, 2017 28606419

Kanthak MK, Stalder T, Hill LK, et al: Autonomic dysregulation in burnout and depression: evidence for the central role of exhaustion. Scand J Work Environ Health 43(5):475–484, 2017 28514792

Koekkoek B, van Meijel B, Schene A, et al: Development of an intervention program to increase effective behaviours by patients and clinicians in psychiatric services: Intervention Mapping study. BMC Health Serv Res 10:293, 2010 20973985

Kumar M, Suliburk J, Veeraraghavan A, et al: PulseCam: high-resolution blood perfusion imaging using a camera and a pulse oximeter. Conf Proc IEEE Eng Med Biol Soc 2016:3904–3909, 2016 28269139

Laker C, Cella M, Callard F, et al: Why is change a challenge in acute mental health wards? A cross-sectional investigation of the relationships between burnout, occupational status and nurses' perceptions of barriers to change. Int J Ment Health Nurs 28(1):190–198, 2019 29993168

Mangione S, Chakraborti C, Staltari G, et al: Medical students' exposure to the humanities correlates with positive personal qualities and reduced burnout: a multi-institutional U.S. survey. J Gen Intern Med 33(5):628–634, 2018 29380213

Marcus SC, Olfson M: National trends in the treatment for depression from 1998 to 2007. Arch Gen Psychiatry 67(12):1265–1273, 2010 21135326

Maslach C, Jackson SE: The measurement of experienced burnout. Journal of Occupational Behaviour 2(2):99–113, 1981. Available at: https://onlinelibrary.wiley.com/doi/abs/10.1002/job.4030020205. Accessed June 2, 2019.

Maust DT, Blow FC, Wiechers IR, et al: National trends in antidepressant, benzodiazepine, and other sedative-hypnotic treatment of older adults in psychiatric and primary care. J Clin Psychiatry 78(4):e363–e371, 2017 28448697

McLellan MF: Images of physicians in literature: from quacks to heroes. Lancet 348(9025):458–460, 1996 8709790

Mistretta EG, Davis MC, Temkit M, et al: Resilience training for work-related stress among health care workers: results of a randomized clinical trial comparing in-person and smartphone-delivered interventions. J Occup Environ Med 60(6):559–568, 2018 29370014

Moise N, Shah RN, Essock S, et al: Sustainability of collaborative care management for depression in primary care settings with academic affiliations across New York State. Implement Sci 13(1):128, 2018 30314522

Mojtabai R, Olfson M: National trends in psychotherapy by office-based psychiatrists. Arch Gen Psychiatry 65(8):962–970, 2008 18678801

O'Connor K, Muller Neff D, Pitman S: Burnout in mental health professionals: a systematic review and meta-analysis of prevalence and determinants. Eur Psychiatry 53:74–99, 2018 29957371

Pattani R, Ginsburg S, Mascarenhas Johnson A, et al: Organizational factors contributing to incivility at an academic medical center and systems-based solutions: a qualitative study. Acad Med 93(10):1569–1575, 2018 29901655

Pellegrini VD Jr, Guzick DS, Wilson DE, et al: Governance of academic health centers and systems: a conceptual framework for analysis. Acad Med 94(1):12–16, 2019 30113361

Penz M, Wekenborg MK, Pieper L, et al: The Dresden Burnout Study: protocol of a prospective cohort study for the bio-psychological investigation of burnout. Int J Methods Psychiatr Res 27(2):e1613, 2018 29611872

Pilger A, Haslacher H, Meyer BM, et al: Midday and nadir salivary cortisol appear superior to cortisol awakening response in burnout assessment and monitoring. Sci Rep 8(1):9151, 2018 29904183

Rider EA, Kurtz S, Slade D, et al: The International Charter for Human Values in Healthcare: an interprofessional global collaboration to enhance values and communication in healthcare. Patient Educ Couns 96(3):273–280, 2014 25103181

Rider EA, Gilligan MC, Osterberg LG, et al: Healthcare at the crossroads: the need to shape an organizational culture of humanistic teaching and practice. J Gen Intern Med 33(7):1092–1099, 2018 29740787

Rosen A, Mueser KT, Teesson M: Assertive community treatment—issues from scientific and clinical literature with implications for practice. J Rehabil Res Dev 44(6):813–825, 2007 18075939

Santos SR, Cox K: Workplace adjustment and intergenerational differences between matures, boomers, and Xers. Nurs Econ 18(1):7–13, 2000 11029913

Shanafelt TD, Noseworthy JH: Executive leadership and physician well-being: nine organizational strategies to promote engagement and reduce burnout. Mayo Clin Proc 92(1):129–146, 2017 27871627

Shanafelt T, Goh J, Sinsky C: The business case for investing in physician well-being. JAMA Intern Med 177(12):1826–1832, 2017 28973070

Shortell SM, O'Brien JL, Carman JM, et al: Assessing the impact of continuous quality improvement/total quality management: concept versus implementation. Health Serv Res 30(2):377–401, 1995 7782222

Siegrist J, Li J: Work stress and altered biomarkers: a synthesis of findings based on the effort-reward imbalance model. Int J Environ Res Public Health 14(11):E1373, 2017 29125555

Sinsky CA, Dyrbye LN, West CP, et al: Professional satisfaction and the career plans of US physicians. Mayo Clin Proc 92(11):1625–1635, 2017 29101932

Stansfeld S, Candy B: Psychosocial work environment and mental health—a meta-analytic review. Scand J Work Environ Health 32(6):443–462, 2006 17173201

Stojanovic-Tasic M, Latas M, Milosevic N, et al: Is Balint training associated with the reduced burnout among primary health care doctors? Libyan J Med 13(1):1440123, 2018 29493438

Swensen S, Kabcenell A, Shanafelt T: Physician-organization collaboration reduces physician burnout and promotes engagement: the Mayo Clinic experience. J Healthc Manag 61(2):105–127, 2016 27111930

Thota AB, Sipe TA, Byard GJ, et al: Collaborative care to improve the management of depressive disorders: a community guide systematic review and meta-analysis. Am J Prev Med 42(5):525–538, 2012 22516495

Viljoen M, Claassen N: Cynicism as subscale of burnout. Work 56(4):499–503, 2017 28339417

Villarosa-Hurlocker MC, Cuccurullo LJ, Garcia HA, Finley EP: Professional burnout of psychiatrists in a Veterans Health Administration: exploring the role of the organizational treatment. Adm Policy Ment Health 46(1):1–9, 2019 29948427

Weilenmann S, Schnyder U, Parkinson B, et al: Emotion transfer, emotion regulation, and empathy-related processes in physician-patient interactions and their association with physician well-being: a theoretical model. Front Psychiatry 9:389, 2018 30210371

West CP, Dyrbye LN, Sloan JA, et al: Single item measures of emotional exhaustion and depersonalization are useful for assessing burnout in medical professionals. J Gen Intern Med 24(12):1318–1321, 2009 19802645

West CP, Dyrbye LN, Rabatin JT, et al: Intervention to promote physician well-being, job satisfaction, and professionalism: a randomized clinical trial. JAMA Intern Med 174(4):527–533, 2014 24515493

West CP, Dyrbye LN, Shanafelt TD: Physician burnout: contributors, consequences and solutions. J Intern Med 283(6):516–529, 2018 29505159

Yang E, Schamber E, Meyer RML, et al: Happier healers: randomized controlled trial of mobile mindfulness for stress management. J Altern Complement Med 24(5):505–513, 2018 29420050

Zhang M, Liu L, Shi Y, et al: Longitudinal associations of burnout with heart rate variability in patients following acute coronary syndrome: a one-year follow-up study. Gen Hosp Psychiatry 53:59–64, 2018 29859340

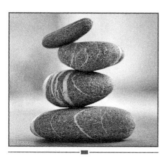

PART V

ETHICS AND BURNOUT

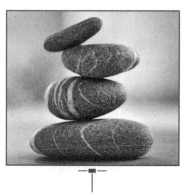

CHAPTER 14

ESTABLISHING AND MAINTAINING PROPORTIONAL AUTHORITY, RESPONSIBILITY, AND EXPERTISE TO PREVENT BURNOUT

Anthony L. Rostain, M.D., M.A.

David Pollack, M.D.

Howard Dichter, M.D.

Authority, responsibility, and expertise (ARE) are key dynamic forces affecting psychiatric roles in healthcare delivery. These elements often are out of balance or misaligned, leading to work stress, dissatisfaction, alienation, and eventual burnout. For many physicians, the loss of real or desired professional autonomy and the lack of sufficient authority are common complaints that arise from these imbalances. At the same time, significant changes in the health delivery system have resulted in team-based collaborative care as the predominant model in a wide range of clinical settings. How can we reconcile the profound changes in how mental health care is delivered with the need to support and help psychiatric providers to adapt to and feel good about their work with patients and other participants in the delivery of care? Key tasks in preventing burnout and restoring professional fulfillment include all of the following: examining career goals, expectations, and limits; evaluating the options for achieving an acceptable degree of ARE balance; understanding the types of imbalance that are operative in specific situations; and learning how to navigate these to work successfully within professional settings.

We view the intertwined and interdependent concepts of ARE as a salient starting point for considering the changes that have occurred in the roles psychiatrists[1] play in healthcare delivery. To begin with, ARE confers privileges, advantages, risks, and responsibilities routinely assumed by practitioners. Psychiatrists take on positions of leadership and control as physicians with the legal authority to conduct physical and mental examinations, diagnose, write prescriptions, provide somatic interventions (e.g., electroconvulsive therapy, transcranial magnetic stimulation), determine eligibility for entitlements, and, when necessary, recommend or authorize inpatient hospitalization. By completing general medical education, residency training, and state licensing procedures, psychiatrists are assigned a host of critical functions. Although other mental health professionals carry out many of these functions, society has deemed that psychiatrists have a unique role in patient care.

When properly balanced, ARE can buffer against burnout and can enhance professional autonomy and job satisfaction. Despite multiple clinical demands that psychiatrists may be asked to undertake, several factors mitigate against emotional exhaustion, compassion fatigue, depersonalization, and loss of fulfillment. These include a sense that one's clinical judgment and expertise are respected by patients, colleagues, and other team members; the perception that one's professional responsibilities are generally reasonable; and the delegation of appropriate authority to exercise one's professional duties in an ethical and compassionate fashion. As has been described in earlier chapters of this book (see Chapter 1, "The History of Burnout in Society, Medicine, and Psychiatry," and Chapter 2, "The Social Context of Physician Burnout"), there is no guarantee that the ARE of practicing psychiatrists is universally recognized—if anything, there is growing concern that the components of ARE are being eroded in the current healthcare environment. In addition to recog-

---

[1]Throughout this chapter, many times when we refer to psychiatrists, our commentary is generally applicable to all physicians and, in some cases, to all other health professionals.

nizing the widespread impact of systems changes on professional role status, we think it is worthwhile to identify the specific, concrete conditions in which psychiatrists are working to consider how to prevent burnout.

The roots of the current healthcare environment date back to two developments in the mid-1990s: the ascendance of managed care and the emergence of an organized community psychiatry movement (Breakey 1996; Committee on Psychiatry and the Community of the Group for the Advancement of Psychiatry 2001; Diamond et al. 1995; Goetz et al. 1998; Moffic 1997; Vacarro and Clark 1996). Economic incentives to contain healthcare costs and regulate the processes of care led to growing standardization of care delivery. In response to these changes, however, psychiatrists practicing in community settings asserted the importance of maintaining professional standards and ethical values in providing care to persons with chronic mental illnesses.

Psychiatry is increasingly practiced in group settings (hospitals, clinics, community mental health centers, private groups, emergency departments) within a framework of "team-based care." Team-based care is widely variable, depending on *context,* particularly with respect to the institution's or organization's mission, vision, goals, culture/ethos, priorities, policies, human and economic resources, and delivery models. Moreover, we believe there will always be conflicts whenever psychiatrists assert the need for balanced ARE in complex healthcare settings.

In the best of circumstances, these conflicts can be identified, discussed, and resolved in a straightforward manner. All too often, however, these issues remain unaddressed in the current healthcare environment. Health systems face profound challenges, including increasing financial pressures on the industry as a whole, the emphasis on "bottom-line" thinking of administrators, attempts to increase productivity, the introduction of electronic health records (EHRs), new threats to patient privacy, the growing impact of social media on patient expectations and the clinician-patient relationship, and the growing medicalization of mental health care. We need to ask two fundamental questions: 1) What is the meaning of ARE in a team-based healthcare delivery system? 2) How can the Quadruple Aim of the healthcare system—to provide care that is patient-centered, population-based, and at acceptable costs, *and* that considers the needs of the work force—be configured to enable psychiatrists to fulfill their roles in meaningful and effective ways (Bodenheimer and Sinsky 2014)?

Authority, Responsibility, and Expertise Profoundly Affect Physician Identity and Professional Autonomy

Physician training has varied widely in its effectiveness to prepare graduates to adapt to the range of clinical and administrative dilemmas they inevitably face. Physician culture in Western medicine also fosters an expectation that physicians should be primary leaders in clinical settings and that their orders and decisions should not be debated or overridden. To support this, they often cite the increased legal and financial liability they face compared with other clinicians or team members. The prolonged and intensive training psychiatrists must undertake, and the licensing requirements they must meet in order to practice, serve to perpetuate and reinforce this expectation. Moreover, popular culture often presents distorted images of psychiatrists as social control agents, mind readers, or "head shrinks" with mysterious powers. As a result, many psychiatrists are vulnerable and at risk for the emergence of disappointment, discouragement, conflict, confusion, and even despair.

Some physicians expect or demand to prevail in clinical care decisions and insist on maintaining a dominant position in relation to aspects of care. There are substantial data to support the notion that collaborative care relationships lead to better clinical and fiscal outcomes in most settings (Committee on Quality of Health Care in America and Institute of Medicine 2001; Interprofessional Education Collaborative 2011). These are settings and organizations in which there is some degree of shared, but clear designation of, authority. Changes can be pursued and prioritized by their relative urgency. The physician, although not necessarily the "leader" of the team, may provide important insights and guidance in a wide range of ways.

One way of taking care of oneself as a mental health clinician is to self-assess for types of imbalance of ARE, to evaluate work satisfaction, and to determine what problems can and should be addressed to restore or maintain a sense of professional job satisfaction. Proportionately *balanced* ARE form the basis of our fiduciary and ethical obligations to patients/families, to teams, and to the community. This assertion may fly in the face of some previously espoused views about the roles of physicians in healthcare settings, which have increasingly marginalized the influence of psychiatrists on the conditions affecting their workplaces.

In our opinion, if the dynamic factors leading to psychiatrist dissatisfaction, alienation, and burnout are properly identified and analyzed, it becomes more likely that these can be modified in ways that improve patient care and health outcomes as well as clinician well-being (see Table 14–1). It is important for clinicians to consider the factors that may be undermining their sense of professional satisfaction and sense of autonomy and to examine the ways in which ARE may be out of balance and lead to burnout. In the next subsections, we provide common examples of ARE imbalances.

Examples of Common Authority, Responsibility, and Expertise Imbalances

INSUFFICIENT AUTHORITY

A common dilemma that some psychiatric providers experience is feeling that the authority they have is not commensurate with the responsibilities

---

TABLE 14–1.   Dynamic factors leading to clinician burnout

Unrealistic expectations → toxic stress

　　Too many demands

　　Too many conflicting roles and ethical dilemmas

　　Excessive productivity demands

　　Time constraints

Conflicts with patients over the goals and methods of treatment

Conflicts with team members over decisions affecting patient care

Conflicts with institutional priorities/policies that compromise patient care

Conflicts with payers/insurers

Conflicts with regulatory bodies

Compassion fatigue

Vicarious (secondhand) traumatization

---

that their jobs entail. This may be related to the lack of autonomy in clinical decision making; risk of inappropriate or inadequate care carried out by other team members; personal, financial, or legal liability tied to the actions of others within the care setting; and limited resources preventing optimal care provision and outcomes.

VIGNETTE 1

The medical director for a behavioral health managed care organization (BHMCO) evaluates grievances regarding the denial of inpatient hospital days. Two psychiatrists are assigned to review grievances. One psychiatrist's evaluations include reviewing the medical record and the adjoining letter outlining the reason for the extended stay. The additional inpatient days are authorized if the clinical record or the letter support the need for continued stay. The other psychiatrist limits the evaluation to the adjoining letter without considering the clinical record. The BHMCO administrator prefers the evaluations by the second psychiatrist, who authorizes fewer inpatient days. The authority of the psychiatrist is compromised when clinical decision making is limited by administrative rules that are designed to maximize profit or promote organizational goals at the expense of patient well-being.

VIGNETTE 2

Psychiatrists working in a community setting are asked to share medical visits with a treatment team consisting of a variety of medical and social service professionals as well as peer specialists. Decisions are shared, and the psychiatrist is expected to refrain from talking or "thinking you know everything." The psychiatrist's expertise and authority are subordinated to the team. However, the psychiatrist's responsibilities are unchanged; she remains responsible for treatment decisions. No mechanism is available to reconcile differences, which occur when the psychiatrist's decisions vary from most of the team members. Burnout occurs when the psychiatrist is faced with the responsibility for decisions supported by the team but not by the psychiatrist herself. Conversely, the psychiatrist can overrule the expectation of team decisions and face the possibility of being viewed as controlling and uncooperative.

INSUFFICIENT RESPONSIBILITY

Issues of insufficient responsibility can arise when clinicians are expected to authorize practices or policies about which they have little or no information or direct involvement with in the clinical situation. When psychiatrists are reduced to being merely prescribers of medication, with limited or marginal input in the organization, their sense of responsibility integral to their skills and expertise is thwarted.

VIGNETTE 3

An outpatient clinic maximizes income with 6-minute psychiatric "med visits." During these visits, psychiatrists review a patient's clinical status, assess response to medication, and make decisions regarding adjusting medical regimens. These visits are used to facilitate ongoing treatment planning. Psychiatrists recognize that some patients require more time, but visit frequency and duration are conditions of employment, and the opportunity to extend the visit is limited. The physician's authority is diminished by the imposed work requirements. Time constraints compromise the psychiatrist's expertise because there can be insufficient time to collect adequate clinical information and discuss the risks and benefits of treatment options while maintaining a therapeutic relationship. The psychiatrist increases efficiency by narrowly focusing on symptoms and side effects. Responsibility is compromised with insufficient attention to dynamic and social variables, leading to a chronic feeling of clinical compromise and "burnout."

EXCESSIVE RESPONSIBILITY

Excessive responsibility—psychiatrists are asked to take on more than they should or can reasonably be expected to handle—is one of the primary drivers of burnout. This includes excessive workload, productivity demands, documentation requirements, long hours (including night call), and unrealistic deadlines for completing work. A glaring and commonly cited factor contributing to this issue is the EHR, which has placed a huge additional burden on physician work-life balance. The pressure to allow work to intrude on one's personal time and space undermines work-life balance, as has been considered in earlier chapters (see especially, Chapter 8, "Electronic Health Records and Physician Burnout") in this volume.

VIGNETTE 4

An attending psychiatrist assigned to a busy inpatient unit at a community hospital serving an inner-city population is asked to cover an additional inpatient unit for a colleague who is on maternity leave. The psychiatrist, already stressed by the demands of covering one service and maintaining an outpatient practice at the hospital's affiliated mental health center, is now facing the prospect of 3 months of increased responsibility for patient care. The hospital administration claims that it does not have the resources to hire a psychiatrist on a temporary basis to cover the service but agrees to reduce the attending's outpatient duties by 30%. The attending's contract does not have a clause that protects her from occasional increases in clinical duties, and she is not entitled to extra income for taking on these additional duties.

INSUFFICIENT EXPERTISE

Many providers experience another form of imbalance, especially during and in the first years after completing training but also during later career stages. This is the range of concerns that clinicians experience and express regarding the feeling that their perceived or real expertise is inadequate to address the challenges that they face in their work, whether it be clinical, administrative, teaching, or research. The well-known "imposter syndrome" is one of the outcomes of this imbalance. It can undermine self-confidence and contribute to a variety of negative consequences, such as depression, acting out that reflects impaired performance, burnout, or early cessation of one's career, all of which have been described in other chapters of this book. There are other instances in which the psychiatrist's expertise does match what is being requested in the clinical encounter (e.g., determining patient's suitability for work or for driving an automobile).

Given the myriad of skills and functions that psychiatrists are asked to implement and perform, it is not always clear that a practitioner possesses the requisite expertise to fulfill his or her job requirements. This may be a function of inexperience or lack of continuing medical education. It may also reflect limits on the science and art of contemporary psychiatry and medicine. Regardless of the context, when psychiatrists are asked to perform assessments of dangerousness, capacity to make medical decisions, and end-of-life requests, there is often an expectation that physicians (M.D.s) have the authority and responsibility but may not have the expertise to meet the demands assigned to them.

Some clinicians do not effectively keep up with the emerging literature or clinical practice guidance developed within their practice areas. Others do not maintain sufficient documentation skills. Other manifestations of the lack of skill, knowledge, or appropriate therapeutic attitude (as described by Caplan and Caplan [1970]), including a tendency to fall prey to "theme interference" or other losses of objectivity, are at least partially related to this type of imbalance. In brief, *theme interference* is a form of countertransference, usually the loss of objectivity that occurs when a clinician occasionally or consistently jumps to illogical conclusions about a patient based on subjective judgments related to extraneous or marginal characteristics of the patient (e.g., race, body size, gender, sexual orientation, social class, diagnosis), resulting in inaccurate and unhelpful projections of likely outcomes for such patients. Additionally, severe lack of resources or support is often associated with people getting burned out.

VIGNETTE 5

A psychiatrist tends to see all persons with schizophrenic disorders as being unable to have long-term relationships and unable to work, often discouraging his patients from taking the risks of entering into such experiences. He is surprised, discouraged, and defensive when others provide feedback to him about how poorly his patients are doing in their efforts to achieve some meaningful level of recovery.

Ethical Dimensions (Dignity, Respect, Ability to Do What One Believes Is Necessary)

Psychiatrists have an ethical responsibility to promote health and prevent suffering (American Psychiatric Association 2013). "Person-first perspectives" that insist patients' wishes should be of primary concern, although effective overall, can occasionally lead to treatment approaches that are not viewed as optimal by the psychiatrist. All too often, the consequence of a harm reduction approach is the relinquishment of decision-making authority to the patient, which can, in turn, inadvertently lead to serious health consequences.

Trade-offs between treatment efficacy and potential harm are prominent when psychiatrists work with patients who have both mental illness and a history of substance misuse. The psychiatric illness can be treated with psychotropic medication. However, the addition of medication in conjunction with illicit drug use can be dangerous. Patients may not reliably report the type and amount of substance misuse. In addition, information about the efficacy and risks associated with combining drug misuse and psychotropic medication is limited, further increasing safety risks. Medications to treat some conditions may be abused, contribute to overdoses, or be diverted by the patient.

VIGNETTE 6

Persons with opioid use disorder frequently have comorbid posttraumatic stress disorder and panic disorder. These patients often prefer benzodiazepines and report alternative medications as ineffective. The psychiatrist can choose to prescribe the requested medication, which can decrease anxiety while increasing the risk of overdose and diversion, or the psychiatrist can refuse to prescribe, which disrupts the treatment alliance. The conflict between the patient's desired treatment and a duty to prevent harm can lead to burnout. The psychiatrist can create treatment guidelines with administration and clinical staff for co-occurring opioid use disorder and anxiety disorders. These guidelines include the use of nonaddicting medications and psychotherapeutic strategies. Tapering strategies are recommended for patients with preexisting comorbid benzodiazepine use disorders. Burnout is thus mitigated through the incorporation of support, modified culture, and expanded treatment options.

Psychiatrists working in community settings often face resource limits, which interfere with health and contribute to suffering. Burnout often can occur from the psychiatrist's exposure to the suffering associated with an under-resourced setting or with the suffering resulting from widespread social determinants and economic inequities.

VIGNETTE 7

A psychiatrist consults at a small community unit that houses 16 persons with chronic mental illnesses who resided long term in a former inpatient hospital unit that had been designed for acute stays and had insufficient space for the long-term residents. The limited space contributed to recurrent acts of aggression among the residents. Many of the residents had histories of trauma, which were exacerbated when they were victims of aggression, witnessed the aggression, or feared harm. The psychiatrist recognizes the problem but does not have the authority or access to resources to initiate changes. However, the psychiatrist is able to work with recreational staff to increase off-unit activities. In addition, discharge criteria are modified to allow the discharge of some patients to less-stimulating community settings. Although the physical facility remains largely unchanged, these modifications reduce the level of conflict on the unit and help to mitigate burnout.

Working with highly vulnerable patients who require social and housing services as well as income support or education is difficult enough in optimal settings. This becomes especially hard when patients receive only minimal social supports. Clinicians are limited in the extent to which they can influence the social/environmental determinants of their patients' health and welfare. The rising rates of mental illness in the U.S. population mean that psychiatrists will be mandated to take on more duties than before, with ever more likelihood of experiencing secondary stress/distress.

Finally, profit motives can impinge on clinical and fiduciary responsibilities and undermine the ethical integrity of psychiatric practice, especially when these motives influence decisions that are not in patients' best interests.

VIGNETTE 8

The administrator of an inpatient unit seeks to increase revenues by maximizing the census. On occasion, patients are authorized by their payer organization for more days than is clinically required. Both the psychiatrist and the patient agree to an earlier discharge than the maximum allowable stay. The administrator disagrees with the psychiatrist's treatment recommendation to release the

patient before the maximum number of authorized days and threatens to sanc-
tion or fire the psychiatrist. In this example, the administrator expects that the
psychiatrist's clinical decision should maximize revenue to the detriment of the
treatment goals and the patient's best interests, contravening the treatment
plan mutually agreed on by the psychiatrist and the patient. This compromises
the psychiatrist's ARE. Working in an environment where patients' best interests are subordinate to revenue generation may lead to burnout.

In the best of circumstances, psychiatrists are empowered to practice
within an ethical framework that includes respect for patient autonomy, beneficence, nonmaleficence ("do no harm"), veracity, and social equity. When
institutions impinge on these principles, they foster professional dissatisfaction, alienation, burnout, and staff turnover. Obviously, workforce development strategies with long-term goals and measurable outcomes are critically
important at the system level to address some of these concerns.

Collaboration in Relationships With Patients and Colleagues

Veach (1972) and later Emanuel and Emanuel (1992) described the types of
relationships that can manifest between physicians and patients. The *priestly*
or *paternal model*, in which the physician took control of the care and treated
the patient more as an illness than a person, dominated healthcare from the
Hippocratic beginnings of medicine until the latter part of the twentieth century. At that time, more physicians began to adopt the *engineering* or *infor-
mative model*, in which the physician, like a technician or scientific expert,
would provide information in a relatively neutral way and expect the patient
to decide what action to take. In more recent years, two models emerged;
these models represent forms of collaboration between the physician and patient. They have been described and refined most clearly by Emanuel and
Emanuel (1992). The *interpretive model* posits that the physician elicits and
interprets the patient's values and goals and collaborates with the patient to
arrive at clinical decisions that are consistent with the patient's wishes. The
deliberative model involves a more active role in which the physician helps
to clarify, shape, or refine the patient's values/goals by using the physician's
own medical knowledge and understanding of the patient but leaves the decision making to the patient.

All four models may still be applicable to different clinical situations and settings, but the shift to more collaborative-type (interpretive and deliberative)
models has clearly become more dominant than the first two models. It is unclear whether the type of relationship model is correlated with greater or less
risk of burnout in physicians, but there is general agreement that many patients
prefer and benefit from a more collaborative relationship with their providers.

Clearly, we have moved beyond the age of paternalism, although the image of the doctor as being autonomous and in charge of patient care contin-

ues for many physicians to be linked to self-image. For them, the loss of desired autonomy is a major blow to self-esteem. It is still essential for physicians to have the right amount of credibility, influence, and respect in the settings in which they work. Healthy adaptation to the new realities of how care is delivered is necessary for physicians to not suffer needlessly, while it is also critical for all participants in the delivery of care to have input into the ways to improve organizational culture, policies, and processes. The perceived loss of control that many physicians experience can be addressed at individual, team, and higher levels, but opportunities for physicians to participate in the leadership and improvement of the systems in which they work must be included. The recommendations in this book on improving workplace environment and transforming institutional culture provide clear guidance for achieving better ARE balance.

Life Span Developmental Considerations— Authority, Responsibility, and Expertise Changes Over the Professional Life Span

The development of a psychiatrist's ARE proceeds along a time continuum beginning with training (i.e., residency and fellowship) and extending through the various stages of one's career. Unquestionably, the balance among these dimensions of professionalism changes with context, experience, and personal growth. This section highlights key stress points that emerge at different stages.

During residency and fellowship, the greatest sources of stress and burnout are linked to several key factors including lack of knowledge, inexperience, subordinate status, role insecurity, availability of supervision, clinical acuity of patients, and the cognitive dissonance between one's sense of one's abilities and the demanding characteristics of the workplace. Traditionally, these stressors were mediated by the structure of training (with its emphasis on direct supervision) and the close relationships that developed among trainees and faculty. Recently, however, these protective factors have been eroded by social, technological, and economic forces (Thomas et al. 2016). Among these forces are the following:

1. Regulatory factors (such as Accreditation Council for Graduate Medical Education program requirements) that place a greater burden on program faculty
2. Economic factors that have led to increased productivity requirements and to decreased teaching time for faculty
3. Changes in the clinical learning environment dictated by new rules for hospital and ambulatory care reimbursement requiring attending physicians to oversee or provide a greater portion of patient care activities

4. Social factors, including stigma regarding mental illness, the increasing diversity of the U.S. population, and the relative insufficiency of psychiatry curricula in nonpsychiatric training programs
5. Information technology factors (e.g., EHR, portable devices) that provide increased access to information and knowledge, although these factors also reduce time for doctor-patient encounters, team-based discussions, and direct supervision of patient care

We conclude that to address the challenges facing modern psychiatric education and training, closer attention needs to be paid to "factors that influence teacher-learner interactions and clinical care team dynamics. In preparing trainees to work in more integrated care environments with colleagues from other specialties and professions, psychiatric educators must model quality collaborative care in their institutions" (Thomas et al. 2016, p. 868). Moreover, more resources and energy need to be directed to reducing burnout and promoting wellness and resilience for learners at all levels of training.

An editorial in *Academic Psychiatry* (Beresin et al. 2016) pointed to the development and dissemination of well-being curricula in medical schools and residency training programs. These include activities such as participating in small, process-oriented reflective seminars; teaching methods for developing reflective practices (including mindfulness and narrative medicine); introducing curricula that specifically address sources of stress and burnout and that assist students and trainees to develop strategies to better deal with these; and promoting opportunities for learners to participate in relationship-building and community-building events. The key to success for these strategies is to invite or even require all faculty members to participate in the process of promoting wellness in both professional and personal spheres.

What about the stages following training? Little attention has been given to differences in stress and burnout across the professional life span of psychiatrists, especially when it comes to ARE. We can surmise that early-career psychiatrists are concerned about their expertise in assuming patient care duties without direct supervision by a senior clinician. They may also be (di)stressed by taking on too many different responsibilities with which they are not yet comfortable or efficient (e.g., patient care, administrative duties, teaching/supervision). It is not uncommon for younger practitioners to be asked to take the most undesirable work shifts and vacation schedules, thereby adding to an imbalance between work and personal life. One important coping resource for young practitioners is to identify mentors and clinical supervisors who can provide instrumental assistance as well as social support, especially during the transition from training into early-career status.

With respect to mid-career psychiatrists, there appear to be gender-based and other demographic differences in sources of stress and burnout. For women who are parents, especially single parents, the conflicting role demands of parenting and clinical psychiatry can easily lead to inordinate stress, especially when children are young. The constant juggling of responsibilities to family and to patients becomes particularly difficult when the demands of either domain make it impossible to meet the demands of the other domain. Fortunately, in recognition of the needs of physician-mothers, many health-care institutions are providing increased access to childcare (including childcare when children are sick), modified work schedules, and peer support groups to reduce the sense of isolation and exhaustion. For physician-fathers who want to participate in parenting, there remain significant institutional barriers to modifying work schedules and providing peer support.

Senior clinicians face the challenges of staying current with advances in clinical neuroscience and psychiatry, of managing the new technology that has come to dominate healthcare delivery, of meeting excessive productivity requirements in a timely fashion, and of facing the diminished energy level and concentration that may come with aging. The wisdom that derives from clinical experience often conflicts with the growing reliance on algorithm-driven practices, leaving older practitioners to wonder if their opinions are "out of sync" with modern psychiatry. The expectation that clinicians participate in continuing medical education and maintenance of certification is designed to ensure that the latest treatment advances are incorporated into patient care. Moreover, it may be valuable to give senior psychiatrists the opportunity to reduce their clinical load and productivity demands while taking advantage of their accumulated clinical reasoning and consultative skills when feasible.

Rebalancing Authority, Responsibility, and Expertise

As we have asserted throughout this chapter, professional dissatisfaction and burnout are highly associated with a perceived loss of control and autonomy. Psychiatrists need to exert more influence on local and national health policy (including health reform) and must ensure that their voices are heard and their opinions respected. The American Psychiatric Association Work Group on Psychiatrist Well-being and Burnout was created in 2017 to provide informational tools and online resources that psychiatrists can use to improve conditions. The chair of the work group, Richard F. Summers, asserts that burnout is

> caused by stress from the workplace overwhelming the doctor's ability to manage. It's addressed through a combination of better self-care and really importantly, changes in the workplace. To prevent burnout, doctors need some degree of autonomy, a sense of community, a reasonable workflow, leadership and management they can communicate with, and a sense of purpose in their organizations. (American Psychiatric Association 2018)

The emphasis is on the need to address specific *environmental* causes of stress, distress, and burnout as well as strategies promoting individual resilience.

The American Psychiatric Association (2018) Well-Being Ambassador Tool Kit offers a framework of interventions to help guide psychiatrists' efforts at institutional change (see Figure 14–1). Component 4 is aimed at building community, which entails creating social events, developing shared resources, providing peer-to-peer coaching and mentoring, and holding team-building activities devoted to improving communication and problem solving among professionals and staff members. Component 6 focuses on improving the workplace environment by updating the health information technology with guidance from the users, redesigning the physical environment to create shared spaces that foster teamwork, enabling personnel to work at the top of their licenses (i.e., working to the full extent of education and training) through task shifting, and providing sufficient autonomy for physicians to spend at least 20% of their workday in meaningful activities. Optimally, administrative and clinical leaders would support these types of initiatives, would welcome input into the strategic planning regarding operations, and would provide needed resources to facilitate professional well-being in the workplace.

At the institutional level, adequate organizational and administrative support for well-being initiatives is imperative for any positive changes to occur. One of the biggest challenges for physicians is to recognize the "system-driven" realities they face in practice and to minimize maladaptive or disruptive behaviors that may emerge in response to these. To effectively adapt to such situations does not mean to simply accept all aspects of the current reality. Adaptation includes conducting an effective assessment of the elements affecting the balance of ARE and selecting appropriate and significant actions to modify some aspects of the imbalance while accepting those aspects that may be resistant to change. The American Medical Association (2015) has advanced a framework to prevent burnout in organizational settings. It emphasizes the importance of establishing wellness as a quality indicator, distributing annual wellness surveys, developing a strategy for addressing key concerns, implementing changes, and gathering data to evaluate the effectiveness of these change efforts.

The interplay between individual and systems factors should be clarified to fully address the multiple sources of burnout that result from challenges to psychiatrists' ARE. The organizational interventions need to address issues of professionalism, leadership, and clinical decision making by using a multidisciplinary, collaborative framework. Beyond individual professional competencies and common competencies across all professions, there are *interprofessional* collaborative competencies that demand a different way of thinking, practicing, and acting in team-based collaborative care delivery (Interprofessional Education Collaborative 2011). The core competencies of collaborative care require that *all* participants in the team be aligned in relation to the following:

• Shared values and ethics
• Awareness of their respective roles and responsibilities, including understandings of how and when roles overlap or are distinct

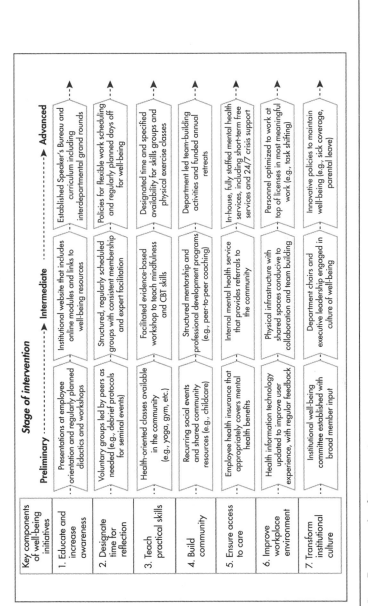

FIGURE 14–1. Framework of interventions.

CBT = cognitive-behavioral therapy.

- Good interpersonal communication skills
- Understanding of teams and teamwork

It is apparent to us that these interprofessional competencies rely on interprofessional education, most of which is not currently provided in professional schools and training programs. In view of this, we propose that healthcare delivery settings should provide ongoing continuing education to all providers on the fundamentals of interprofessionality (D'Amour and Oandasan 2005), which is defined by the following:

> The process by which professionals reflect on and develop ways of practicing that provides an integrated and cohesive answer to the needs of the client/family/population…. [It] involves continuous interaction and knowledge sharing between professionals, organized to solve or explore a variety of education and care issues all while seeking to optimize the patient's participation…. Interprofessionality requires a paradigm shift, since interprofessional practice has unique characteristics in terms of values, codes of conduct, and ways of working. These characteristics must be elucidated. (p. 8)

In addition to adopting these collaborative competencies, every team member must understand, accept, and honor the ARE of psychiatrists. In turn, psychiatrists must understand, accept, and honor other team members' ARE. Everyone in the team needs to gain a broader view of one's professional role and to insist one is respected and valued appropriately within one's work context. Mutual respect and recognition can only be achieved through open communication, dialog, shared problem solving, and openness to feedback. This is not easy to accomplish in any workplace setting, but it is especially difficult in clinical settings.

Inevitably, it is up to each individual to take charge of one's own professional development, to identify the threats or challenges to ARE that one is facing in the current work environment, to consider ways to reduce the imbalances that exist in the setting, and to mindfully take steps to enhance one's ARE, both to restore one's sense of professional well-being as well as to promote better patient care delivery processes and outcomes (i.e., team-based care). At some level, this may require redefining one's vision of doctoring to fit in with the realities of the modern healthcare environment. It can be helpful to understand and take stock of the "big picture" (i.e., systemic, macro/micro influences on mental health practice) and to avoid personalizing or internalizing system failures or limitations that could be interfering with the balance of one's perceived ARE. At another level, this means accepting limits on ARE that are present in the workplace but, at the same time, working toward reasonable goals to make things better for everyone. Of course, if the setting itself is too overwhelming, alienating, unsupportive, or incompatible with one's sense of professional identity, it might be time to make a job change.

Steps Forward

We propose a series of questions to assist psychiatrists in assessing how well one's professional identity, authority, responsibility, and expertise are being supported by one's current practice setting. The key question to raise is simple: Are my authority, responsibility, and expertise in balance, and if not, why not?

The following questions are offered to assist the reader in taking stock of the situation:

- How would I assess the proportional balance between the ARE that I have in the different roles/jobs that I have?
- Is my situation one in which I am pushed beyond my capacity or tolerance? If so, what seems to be contributing to this imbalance?
- Do I feel that my voice is heard? Do I have sufficient input to the organizational operations, the clinical processes, etc.?
- Is my professional-personal life balance acceptable? Do I have enough time, energy, and interest to play and enjoy various aspects of my life/family/friendships?
- How do my sense of my work, the proportion/balance of ARE, and self-perceived capabilities fit in relation to the stage of my career?
- Do I get enough variety and stimulation from my work?
- Do I find myself doing work that, in effect, is patching up problems that are derived from upstream factors that were they addressed more effectively would not be presenting as often or as severely?
- Am I working the right amount of time for my needs? Too much? Not enough?
- Is there adequate time for me and my colleagues/teammates to address the processes of care, the ethical dilemmas, the non-revenue-generating tasks (e.g., prior authorizations, obtaining information from collateral informants), without having to extend our work time beyond the expected duration of our workday/workweek?

Moving from these questions, it may be helpful to develop a broader framework from which to tackle the challenges to ARE one is facing and to construct a road map for restoring the most essential aspects of one's professional fulfillment. For instance, one needs to step back from the immediate situation and ask oneself "what really matters most" about one's current practice and one's career journey. A deeper look at the meaning of work in one's life can be a liberating step in generating alternative paths. More to the point, developing and nurturing mindfulness practices can promote well-being by keeping one focused on the bigger picture, empathizing with one's current stress/suffering, and coming to a deeper realization that one is the creator of one's experience and the author of one's narrative. This requires a process of "mentalization" through which one gains better insight into the underlying psychic sources of stress, alienation, and burnout. Using the

tools of self-reflection and communication with trusted others, it is possible
to arrive at a new understanding of the approach to one's career. This per-
mits us to set appropriate limits on the demands we place on ourselves and
those that others place on us.

By maintaining an appropriate distance between ourselves and the work-
based imbalances that threaten us, it becomes possible to imagine new solutions to the professional challenges we face. For some, it suggests learning to
say "no" to unrealistic job demands; for others, it means stepping away from
an intolerable position to pursue alternative work opportunities.

VIGNETTE 9

A junior attending on the consultation-liaison service returns from her first
maternity leave to find that there have been major changes in the clinical duties to which she is assigned. To begin with, the hospital's psychiatry residents
have been reassigned to work exclusively with the newly hired chief of the consultation-liaison psychiatry service, leaving the attending psychiatrist with
minimal teaching duties, a role from which she previously derived a great deal
of professional satisfaction. In addition, her work assignment is changed in
such a manner that she is required to provide emergency department consults
for 60% of her time—a job that she finds particularly stressful and unreward-
ing. Finally, her request for a modified schedule that would enable her to leave
work in time to pick up her baby from childcare is denied by the service chief.
After many discussions and much agonizing and soul searching, the attending
resigns from her position to pursue private practice—an option she deems will
be more conducive to her personal and professional life goals.

Beyond the individual perspective, it is imperative to address the relational dimensions of ARE in the multidisciplinary work setting. This requires
analyzing organizational issues, exploring team dynamics, and charting a
path toward greater mutual respect among everyone on the healthcare team.
The Stanford Tripartite Model of Physician Fulfillment is an effective way of
conceptualizing this process (see Figure 14–2). The three areas to consider
when examining one's work setting include the efficiency of practice, the culture of wellness, and one's personal resilience. We encourage psychiatrists to
engage in the following steps:

1. Develop creative "ubiquitous" leadership skills—multiple perspectives—
   collaboration frame.
2. Negotiate conflicts in a constructive manner.
3. Redefine roles when they are unclear, unrealistic, or imbalanced.
4. Create a sustainable work setting where team members can raise and address issues of concern.
5. Identify and discuss issues of ARE imbalances whenever they occur.

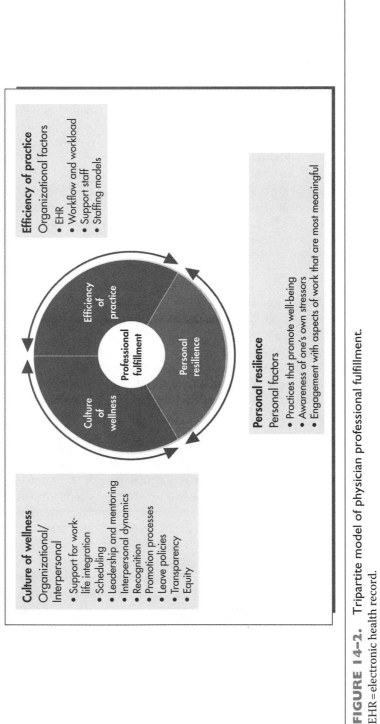

FIGURE 14–2. Tripartite model of physician professional fulfillment.

EHR = electronic health record.

Pie chart from Stanford Model for Physician Well-Being. Reprinted from Bohman B, Dyrbye L, Sinsky CA: "Physician Well-Being: The Reciprocity of Practice Efficiency, Culture of Wellness, and Personal Resilience." NEJM Catalyst, August 7, 2017. Property of Stanford University, Stanford, California. Copyright © 2016. Used with permission.

Conclusion

The "Triple Aim" of healthcare innovation (Berwick et al. 2008) includes improving the experience of care, improving the health of populations, and reducing per capita costs of healthcare. More recently, in response to the growing recognition of clinician burnout as a serious concern for healthcare delivery, Bodenheimer and Sinsky (2014) added a fourth aim, namely, improving the work-life balance of healthcare providers, including clinicians and staff. One of the most challenging aspects of this objective is to find ways to achieve it without undermining the other three aims. Healthcare systems are now being challenged to make changes to accommodate this fourth aim. Bodenheimer and Sinsky proposed several practical steps that healthcare organizations should take to improve conditions for primary care physicians, many of which are also applicable to psychiatric practice settings. These include team documentation, previsit planning, expanded roles for collaborative staff, prescription refill standardization, and reengineering roles, all of which are applicable to mental health care delivery. Beyond these steps, we propose that individual physicians and their organizations can best address the well-being and burnout of healthcare professional staff by advocating and promoting collaborative team-based care practices while simultaneously working to rebalance their respective ARE. This should be possible to achieve without compromising the other three aims, provided adequate financial and human resources are applied to this effort.

Southwick and Southwick (2018) suggest that "resilience research" offers helpful insights into the critical impact of a *loss of a sense of control* as a major contributor to physician burnout. As we suggest throughout this chapter, this loss is especially apparent for practitioners working in large healthcare systems in which individual autonomy is diminished by work conditions and organizational priorities. Southwick and Southwick (2018, p. 666) cite findings from resilience research to endorse the adoption of proactive coping mechanisms and to recommend "that health care organizations adopt a distributive leadership model that encourages physicians to actively participate in governing and improving the systems in which they work." This serves as a good starting point for initiating workplace discussions aimed at improving organizational and interpersonal factors that contribute to burnout. By actively participating in the redesign of mental health care delivery at the institutional level, psychiatrists can play a critical role in rebalancing and realigning ARE to preserve their autonomy and restore their sense of professional fulfillment.

KEY POINTS

————————■————————

- Authority, responsibility, and expertise (ARE) are key dynamic forces affecting psychiatric roles in healthcare delivery. These elements often are out of balance or misaligned, leading to work stress, dissatisfaction, alienation, and eventual burnout.

- For many clinicians, the loss of real or preferred professional autonomy and the lack of enough authority are common complaints that arise from these ARE imbalances.

- Key tasks in preventing burnout and restoring professional fulfillment include the following: examining career goals, expectations, and limits; evaluating the options for achieving an acceptable degree of ARE balance; understanding the types of imbalance that are operative in specific situations; and learning how to navigate these situations to work successfully within professional settings.

————————■————————

References

American Medical Association: 7 steps to prevent burnout in your practice. AMA Wire, Aug 11, 2015. Available at: https://wire.ama-assn.org/practice-management/7-steps-prevent-burnout-your-practice. Accessed November 4, 2018.

American Psychiatric Association: The Principles of Medical Ethics With Annotations Especially Applicable to Psychiatry, 3rd Edition. Arlington, VA, American Psychiatric Association 2013

American Psychiatric Association: Well-Being Resources (web page). Washington, DC, American Psychiatric Association, 2018. Available at: https://www.psychiatry.org/psychiatrists/practice/well-being-and-burnout/well-being-resources. Accessed November 4, 2018.

Beresin EV, Milligan TA, Balon R, et al: Physician wellbeing: a critical deficiency in resilience education and training. Acad Psychiatry 40(1):9–12, 2016 26691141

Berwick DM, Nolan TW, Whittington J: The triple aim: care, health, and cost. Health Aff (Millwood) 27(3):759–769, 2008 18474969

Bodenheimer T, Sinsky C: From triple to quadruple aim: care of the patient requires care of the provider. Ann Fam Med 12(6):573–576, 2014 25384822

Breakey WR (ed): Integrated Mental Health Services: Modern Community Psychiatry. New York, Oxford University Press, 1996

Caplan G, Caplan RB: The Theory and Practice of Mental Health Consultation. New York, Basic Books, 1970

Committee on Psychiatry and the Community of the Group for the Advancement of Psychiatry: Can the public sector survive managed care? Psychiatr Serv 52(7):867, 2001 11433099

Committee on Quality of Health Care in America, Institute of Medicine: Crossing the Quality Chasm: A New Health System for the 21st Century. Washington, DC, National Academies Press, 2001

D'Amour D, Oandasan I: Interprofessionality as the field of interprofessional practice and interprofessional education: an emerging concept. J Interprof Care 19 (suppl 1):8–20, 2005 16096142

Diamond RJ, Goldfinger SM, Pollack D, et al: The role of psychiatrists in community mental health centers: a survey of job descriptions. Community Ment Health J 31(6):571–577, discussion 579–581, 1995 8608701

Emanuel EJ, Emanuel LL: Four models of the physician-patient relationship. JAMA 267(16):2221–2226, 1992 1556799

Goetz R, Cutler D, Pollack D, et al: A three-decade perspective on community and public psychiatry training in Oregon: 25 years of evolution and adaptation. Psychiatr Serv 49(9):1208–1211, 1998 9735964

Interprofessional Education Collaborative: Core Competencies for Interprofessional Collaborative Practice: Report of an Expert Panel, May 2011. Washington, DC, Interprofessional Education Collaborative, 2011. Available at: https://members.aamc.org/eweb/upload/Core%20Competencies%20for%20Interprofessional%20Collaborative%20Practice_Revised.pdf. Accessed July 28, 2018.

Moffic HS: The Ethical Way: Challenges and Solutions for Managed Behavioral Healthcare. San Francisco, CA, Jossey Bass Publishers, 1997

Southwick FS, Southwick SM: The loss of a sense of control as a major contributor to physician burnout: a neuropsychiatric pathway to prevention and recovery. JAMA Psychiatry 75(7):665–666, 2018 29799941

Thomas CR, Rostain AL, Beresin EV: Modern trends: the impact of social, technological, and economic forces on psychiatric education and training. Acad Psychiatry 40(6):863–868, 2016 27761880

Vacarro J, Clark GH (eds): Practicing Psychiatry in the Community: A Manual. Washington, DC, American Psychiatric Press, 1996

Veach R: Models for ethical medicine in a revolutionary age. What physician-patient roles foster the most ethical relationship? Hastings Cent Rep 2(3):5–7, 1972 4679693

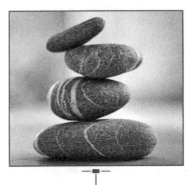

CHAPTER 15

WELL-BEING, PROFESSIONALISM, AND THE ETHICS OF RESILIENCE

Joan M. Anzia, M.D.

One of the central tenets of this volume is that the diagnosis and healing of patients rests firmly on the well-being of a very precious resource: the physicians who provide care and lead the healthcare team. When we are sick, we want a physician who is alert and attuned to us, who can carefully elicit symptoms, who can perceive subtle and nuanced signs, and who can think clearly and treat with skill and compassion. The set of values and ethical principles for the practice of medicine with regard to the physician's self-care is described in detail by the American Medical Association (AMA) *Journal of Ethics*:

To preserve the quality of their performance, physicians have a responsibility to maintain their health and wellness, construed broadly as preventing or treating acute or chronic diseases, including mental illness, disabilities, and occupational stress. When health or wellness is compromised, so may the safety and effectiveness of the medical care provided. When failing physical or mental health reaches the point of interfering with a physician's ability to engage safely in professional activities, the physician is said to be impaired.

In addition to maintaining healthy lifestyle habits, every physician should have a personal physician whose objectivity is not compromised. Physicians whose health or wellness is compromised should take measures to mitigate the problem, seek appropriate help as necessary, and engage in an honest self-assessment of their ability to continue practicing. (American Medical Association 2011, p. 700)

In addition to providing ethical principles regarding self-care, the AMA also details a much broader responsibility of physicians to the health and well-being of colleagues, asserting that medical professionals must be mindful of the following obligations: "promoting health and wellness among physicians; supporting peers in identifying physicians in need of help; intervening promptly when the health or wellness of a colleague appears to have become compromised" and states that physicians should ensure that impaired physicians refrain from practicing—and report those who do not (American Medical Association 2011, p. 700).

In Roberts and Dyer's (2004) *Concise Guide to Ethics in Mental Health Care,* the authors describe some of the ethical dilemmas that may face clinicians who attempt to assist peers, such as balancing confidentiality and privacy while ensuring the safety of both the clinician and patients. When considering current rates of burnout in physicians and trainees in the United States, it is clear that the ethical principles of self-care and care of colleagues have not been in the forefront of medicine until more recent research has amplified concerns (Shanafelt et al. 2012).

This chapter includes six major sections, discussing 1) ethical principles that are integral to physician well-being; 2) the implicit values of medicine and their impact on physician well-being, 3) the relationship between burnout, well-being, and professionalism; 4) life and career transitions that may be particularly challenging for physicians in maintaining well-being and resilience; 5) ethics and physician resilience; and 6) some suggestions for promoting well-being in medicine through medical education, practice, and leadership.

Ethical Principles in Physician Well-Being

Traditional principles of medical ethics can be applied to physician well-being by referencing the current body of literature in this area. Expanding these traditional principles to encompass physician self-care can help provide a foundation for initiatives to support 1) the individual physician's capacity to sustain a lifetime of caring for patients, 2) the creation of a system of medical education that promotes wellness in physicians, and 3) healthcare institutions that consider physician wellness a top priority. Roberts and Dyer (2004) highlight five ethical issues that are central in physician health:

1. The ethical obligation to maintain personal health in order to care for others
2. The ethical obligation to intervene in situations of impaired professionals and to assist colleagues under duress
3. Ethical dilemmas in providing care for medical colleagues
4. The ethical obligation to address the negative aspects of the culture of medicine
5. The ethical responsibility to ensure that our trainees are not exploited but, in fact, are taught to maintain their health and well-being

The ethical principles of beneficence, practice within the limits of competence, hope and optimism, nonmaleficence, justice, veracity, and fidelity all have implications for self-care, for addressing the negative aspects of the culture of medicine, and for ensuring that our trainees and students are not exploited. *Beneficence* is defined as the principle of doing good for others, but we now have abundant evidence that demonstrates that physicians do not exhibit optimal care for others when they are chronically fatigued, demoralized, and experiencing burnout and depression. In fact, we know that patients suffer from reduced quality of care and more medical errors when their physicians are burned out, and thus patients are less satisfied with their care (Shanafelt and Noseworthy 2017). A remodeled definition of beneficence might include the principle that physicians must take great care of their bodies, minds, and spirits—and those of their colleagues and trainees— in order to do good for others. To *practice within the limits of competence* could be expanded to assert that physicians must develop a sensitive awareness of and compassion for their own well-being in order to practice medicine in a competent manner. Recognition of fatigue, demoralization, cynicism, and isolation—and knowledge of how to mitigate the corrosive effects of those conditions—will be crucial for the capacity of physicians to adhere to this principle. Although there are robust current efforts to improve physicians' awareness of their own fatigue, isolation, and symptoms of burnout, these initiatives are relatively new in medicine and sometimes run counter to long-standing culture. *Hope* and *optimism* have traditionally been interpreted as for the patient. However, how can a hopeless, pessimistic, and cynical physician convey positive values to a patient? We know that even in the short years of residency training, young physicians become more pessimistic, more cynical, and less compassionate than when they began training (Dyrbye et al. 2010). If the medical profession highlighted the value of fostering and maintaining hope and optimism within physicians throughout medical training and practice, there would likely be considerable benefits for patients and healthcare teams. Physician leaders also need to develop and promulgate hope, optimism, and beneficence for colleagues who are struggling with burnout, depression, addiction, and maladaptive behaviors, such as disruptive communications, that are linked to burnout. *Disruptive communications* or *disruptive behaviors* in physicians are defined by the AMA and most hospitals' codes of conduct as behaviors that demean, disparage, or harm others (peers, healthcare team members, trainees, or patients). These behaviors include egregious behaviors (e.g., a surgeon throwing an instrument at a resident or nurse, the use of foul or obscene language, angry outbursts in the workplace, ethnic/racial/homophobic slurs). However, the AMA also lists passive behaviors—such as not returning pages, not responding to team members during a procedure, rolling the eyes, or smirking—as disruptive behaviors. The culture of medicine promotes a sense of perfectionism such that the discovery of any of these difficulties is met with shame and denial by both the suffering physician and often by physician leadership (Chew-Graham et al. 2003; Gold et al. 2015). We need to see these problems as common, multidetermined difficulties or illnesses in the course of a physician's life, and treatment must not be punitive or shameful. Instead of stigmatizing our fellow physicians, we need to assist them by providing the necessary care to restore their well-being.

The *principle of nonmaleficence* (first do no harm) needs to be extended not only to patients but to our colleagues and ourselves. Nonmaleficence operates not only at the level of the individual physician's self-care but also at the leadership level in healthcare institutions. Physician leadership must speak out and inform others about the impact of workplace and systems decisions on the life and work of physicians. The *principle of justice* speaks to the importance of providing physicians with the supports that they need to do their work well, in concordance with their clinical values. In the current healthcare environment, for example, this will mean providing adequate resources and assistance so that physicians stay healthy and safe while practicing at the top of their licenses (i.e., working to the full extent of education and training). For example, providing individual electronic health record (EHR) coaching so that physicians can avoid extra hours of charting at home would be an intervention that incorporates the principle of justice. The *principle of veracity* supports the importance of speaking honestly and assertively about needed changes in our work as physicians as well as in medical education and training. We need to be forthright in speaking to peers and trainees when they are not taking care of themselves and to leaders when they are neglecting the well-being of their physician staff. The *principle of fidelity* affirms that a physician must be a whole human being in order to be a physician—that is, fidelity to medicine also means faithfulness to one's whole self. All physicians struggle to a greater or lesser degree to balance different and conflicting values and ideals that underlie choices about how they live, work, and make meaning in their lives. The difficulty of that struggle, and the need for change, is evident in the numbers of physicians who are unhappy, unfulfilled, and experiencing burnout and depression.

Implicit Values in Medicine and Their Impact on Physician Well-Being

MORAL STRESS

Many investigators have described the multivariate drivers of burnout and career dissatisfaction among physicians (West et al. 2018), including work compression, the challenges of the EHR, loss of autonomy, loss of community, and isolation. Research on burnout has also highlighted conflicting values as a driver (Maslach and Leiter 1997). When physicians experience overwhelming work demands and conflicting values or threats to their professional values, they are subject to increased stress and reduced coping resources (Gabel 2011). In the current *high throughput* (emphasis on volume of patients seen over time) era of medicine (Ludmerer 2015), in which compensation may be based on relative value units (RVUs) and clinical schedules may be created by nonphysician managers, physicians can feel unable to deliver the quality of clinical care that meets their clinical standards and professional values. This incongruence of values (Gabel 2011) and moral strain—the inability to work according to one's conscience and moral values (Glasberg et al. 2007)—may be a less-studied contributor to burnout. The physician's values of beneficence and justice may be entirely different from the goals and strategies of healthcare systems. For example, when physicians perceive that they must discharge patients too soon from the hospital, must spend hours on the phone advocating with insurance representatives for patients to receive optimal medications, or are pressured not to admit patients with insufficient insurance to the hospital, they may feel demoralized, frustrated, and angry that they are not able to live and practice within their professional values. In a study of Canadian physicians, investigators found that among contributors to burnout (including excessive workload), only *values incongruence* (the disparity between a physician's clinical moral values and those of the healthcare system) predicted the perception of professional inefficacy (Leiter et al. 2009).

THE FAULT LINE

The term *fault line* usually refers to a geographic vulnerability in the Earth's crust to earthquakes; I have used it here to describe some of the personality characteristics and values of physicians that can render them more vulnerable to burnout. Another dimension of the core values of medicine, a second set of values, may contribute to burnout: the values of altruism, striving for excellence and perfection, compassion, hard work, and self-sacrifice. These values are at the center of medical education and practice, the formation of professional identity, and the beliefs and attitudes that flow from those values. These values inform how physicians live and work; they are often not explicit but deeply implicit. There have always been potential vulnerabilities, or areas of weakness, in this set of values—much like fine cracks in a vase or sculpture or geological faults—that have led to distorted beliefs that a physician must be invulnerable, perfect, self-reliant, tireless, and totally dedicated to medicine at the expense of self. When a physician perceives that he or she has failed to live up to these unrealistic standards, the result can be overwhelming shame and self-imposed isolation. Medical schools recruit students who demonstrate defined qualities and characteristics consistent with those values (Myers and Gabbard 2008):

- Perfectionism/compulsiveness
- Need for control: "If I just push myself harder, get more disciplined…"
- Strong need for achievement
- Exaggerated sense of responsibility
- Need to please everyone: "How do I say no?"
- Difficulty asking for help: "I'm self-sufficient and have always managed on my own before."
- Excessive, unrealistic guilt
- Suppression of feelings
- Difficulty taking time for oneself

These fault lines in our system of values have always had the potential to lead to human tragedy: physicians who lose marriages; are strangers to their children and families; struggle with compassion fatigue, burnout, chronic depression, a loss of zest and meaning in life; develop addiction; and die by suicide. In past decades, however, there were some protective factors in medicine that provided buffers for physicians: more autonomy and authority over one's work, many built-in opportunities for communities of peers and colleagues, and the ability to provide patient care in concordance with one's clinical values. In the current era of the "business" of medicine (Ludmerer 2015), of corporatization of healthcare systems, many of those supportive elements have been minimized or lost. In these systems, physicians often are seen as "providers"—rather than healers of the sick—who produce RVUs.

In addition, the qualities of perfectionism and of difficulty in asking for help are likely factors in the low percentage of physicians who have their own personal physicians (Gross et al. 2000). Even medical students are reluctant to reach out for help when in distress, especially for assistance with mental health concerns (Gold et al. 2015). Some of the resistance to help seeking is due to concerns about privacy, confidentiality, and potential negative impact on careers (e.g., licensure), but the amount of shame that many physicians, residents, and students express when they finally do reach out for care indicates that stigma about needing help is prominent.

TABLE 15–1.   Implicit values in the culture of medicine

Culture of medicine	Culture of well-being
I can do without sleep.	Adequate sleep is crucial for me to do my job.
I don't have time to exercise.	Some exercise is better than none.
I must eat and drink when I can, what I can.	I should try to stay hydrated and eat well to sustain energy.
I can always do more; I can get it done.	I'm probably not going to be able to do everything, but I can do most of the important and essential things.
I have to do it perfectly or it's a personal failure.	I'm going to do my absolute best, but I'm human, and perfection, even in medicine, is impossible.
I can't tell anyone if and when I have doubts or vulnerabilities.	It's not good for me to be isolated from my peers and suffer alone.
If I ask for help, my colleagues won't trust or respect me.	It's good to ask for help or advice when I feel I need it—good for me and my patients.
If I just work even harder and keep everything under control, it'll be OK. I can't say "no."	Trying to have everything under rigid control isn't good for me, my patients, my colleagues, or my family.

Let me briefly list some common implicit beliefs in medicine and medical education and compare them with corresponding assertions that would support physician well-being (see Table 15–1).

These are only a few examples of the implicit values of medicine and medical training that we encounter several times daily. A version of these values nearly always underlies the maladaptive beliefs of physicians in distress—and indeed, their peers, supervisors, and leaders. The following vignette helps demonstrate the extent to which leaders in medicine can perpetuate values of control, perfectionism, and invulnerability:

VIGNETTE 1: THE WELL-MEANING LEADER

A chairperson is concerned about one of her faculty members who is in his mid fifties, a much-beloved fellowship director and esteemed clinician-educator. The chair feels that something is clearly amiss with the faculty member because the latter had asked to step down from directing the fellowship and was talking about possibly retiring early. The chair requests that the medical staff health liaison officer proceed with a fitness-for-duty examination. The officer knows that the faculty member in question never said "no" to a referral or request to teach, so he asks the chair if she had thought about first discussing a reduction of workload and providing more tangible work support for the faculty member. Her response is that "It was so wonderful that the faculty member had always exceeded his RVU targets" and that "Everyone loves his accessibility."

It is clear that the chairperson failed to grasp the possibility that the faculty member's "accessibility" and high workload might be problematic, and that in her role as a leader she might first focus on the overall workplace well-being of her talented faculty member and not necessarily assume that there was "something wrong" *with him*—in effect, that he was insufficiently resilient or ill. This is an example of the kind of disconnection that can occur between a leader's more superficial awareness of the problem of burnout and the reality that it can be driven by environmental factors—and a long-standing implicit assumption that physicians will be able to manage ever-increasing workloads.

THE FAULT LINE AND ADVERSE CLINICAL EVENTS

The adverse event is often a nodal point in which a physician's implicit beliefs and values are challenged—oftentimes like a devastating hurricane. One of the long-standing, little-appreciated issues within medicine is the profound effect that adverse clinical events can have on physicians (Shapiro and Galowitz 2016). In many cases, physicians are shocked, stunned, grief-stricken, and feel deeply guilty and ashamed. They review the event repeatedly in the days afterward, looking for points of possible error or misjudgment. Many have difficulty sleeping for several days and feel anxious returning to the workplace the next day. Their confidence is undermined; many consider eliminating procedures from their work, changing specialties, or even leaving medicine altogether. An adverse event is not uncommonly the "last straw" for a physician who is already struggling with symptoms of burnout; some can develop clinical depression in the aftermath. Physicians believe they are to blame if the outcome is not good, that they are to blame if there is an error or less-than-perfect outcome even when they reasonably know that they performed in a competent manner. In the latter instance, physicians wonder what it means about the profession of medicine and their training that "everything can go right" and yet a patient can die. This is an experience that can be profoundly disturbing to many physicians. The default response of physicians following an adverse event is to isolate themselves from colleagues and staff and suffer in silence. Peer support systems for physicians in healthcare settings are a manifestation of the ethical principle of beneficent care for self and colleagues, one tool that can begin to ameliorate the distress and begin to change behaviors and culture around these events (Shapiro and Galowitz 2016).

Burnout, Well-Being, and Professionalism

CONTRIBUTION OF LIFE AND WORK STRESSORS TO BURNOUT AND UNPROFESSIONAL BEHAVIORS

Research on the relationships between physician burnout and deficits in ethical behaviors and professionalism in medicine is in the early stages; however, there is adequate evidence that individual well-being factors (including personal wellness and work-life stressors), healthcare team factors, and institutional factors can contribute to lapses in professionalism in physicians (Shanafelt and Noseworthy 2017). Impairment from fatigue, overwork, or the stress of a family illness or an adverse clinical event can compromise a physician's resources. Physicians often work as team leaders in critical, high-stakes situations and are exposed repeatedly to human loss and tragedy. Unexpected work and life events can sometimes overwhelm a physician's coping capacity and lead to deficits in professionalism. My personal observation is that many nonphysicians who work in healthcare settings are unaware of how personally stressed physicians feel throughout their workdays and how a seemingly minor event such as an email message about a decrease in patient satisfaction scores or a complaint from nursing staff can be the last straw that overburdens the physician's ability to cope. In a study of U.S. medical students that investigated the relationship between symptoms of burnout and instances of unprofessional behavior, the investigators found that students with burnout (but not with depression) were more likely to engage in unprofessional clinical behaviors and to fail to endorse values of altruism (Dyrbye et al. 2010).

A vignette drawn from my experience as a physician health liaison for a large academic medical center is helpful in illustrating how various life and work events can compromise both physician well-being and professionalism.

VIGNETTE 2: THE PERFECT STORM

An early-career faculty member in an internal medicine subspecialty has been identified as a future leader in his division. He is married to a physician in another specialty. He is serving for 4 months as team leader on a critical care service when one of the two other attending physicians falls ill and needs emergency surgery. There is no backup system, so this faculty member and the other attending are on phone call every other night and must cover on weekends. He takes this in stride and delays a planned vacation with his wife. He realizes he is somewhat sleep deprived but is confident that he can manage. He receives a call from his parents, who live in another city. His father has been diagnosed with colon cancer, and they have many questions for him. He feels guilty and anxious but explains that he cannot take time off to visit.

This physician arrives home one evening and his wife announces that she has decided to leave the marriage; he is shocked and devastated by this news. He cannot sleep that night, and in the following week, he obtains only 2–3 hours of sleep per night and loses 5 pounds because he cannot eat. He goes to work every day, and he tells no one about these events. By the beginning of the second week, he notices that he is having trouble concentrating at work, making mistakes in his documentation, and responding with irritation to the medical students and residents on his service. The nursing manager tells him that he failed to respond to three pages. In the middle of the second week, he explodes with an obscenity when a resident reports that he forgot to check some lab results. He feels overwhelmed, profoundly ashamed, and demoralized. He knows that he needs help but is unaware of resources that would be timely, confidential, and convenient. He contemplates drinking alcohol at night to help him sleep or self-prescribing a benzodiazepine medication but realizes that these would only worsen his situation.

In this vignette, a combination of a work event such as a significant staff shortage on a critical care unit plus a family illness and relationship loss, with resulting sleep deprivation and bereavement, has overtaxed the capacity of a very competent and resilient physician to maintain professional behaviors. Some aspects of the culture of medicine play a role in the physician's response to his dilemmas: his choice to remain silent about his life stressors, his decision to continue to work despite inadequate sleep, and his reticence and anxiety about seeking help.

Sleep deprivation and inadequate hydration and food are deficits of baseline physiological needs outlined in Maslow's (1943) hierarchy, and they can contribute to both deficiencies in well-being and professionalism.

VIGNETTE 3: BURNOUT AND SUBSTANCE USE

A single, midcareer surgical specialist works in a high-intensity hospital environment. Over a period of several years, he has taken on increasing clinical and administrative responsibilities without delegating or reducing any of his duties. His subspecialty division is small and has no service redundancy to accommodate team member illness or family needs; he usually ends up covering for others. He recognizes that he has exhibited the full spectrum of burnout signs and symptoms for over a year and frequently wonders if he should change jobs. Since his midthirties, he realized that two or three beers at night will help him relax and be able to initiate sleep, but over the past 5 years he has escalated his alcohol intake to nearly a fifth of vodka before going to sleep. He tries to time his alcohol intake so that his blood alcohol level will be negative by the time he goes to work in the morning.

This surgeon's chairperson meets with him to discuss unprofessional behaviors that he has exhibited over the past 6 months: chronic lateness to clinic, going to the wrong operating room, and complaints from nursing staff about some angry outbursts in the clinic and operating room.

This vignette is a frequent narrative heard by professionals who treat physicians with substance use disorders. Although substance use in physicians is driven by many factors besides burnout, especially genetic factors, physicians who struggle with symptoms of burnout may start or increase substance use as a form of self-treatment. Because physicians are often quite skilled at hiding their use of substances from others, the first manifestations in the work setting are often failures in the realm of professional behaviors. Physician burnout is more often correlated with increased use of alcohol compared with other substances (Oreskovich et al. 2012). In turn, excessive alcohol use can increase the likelihood of numerous unprofessional behaviors: tardiness, work absenteeism, failure to complete documentation, erratic team and patient interactions, and disruptive behaviors such as verbal and physical mistreatment of staff. In addition, excessive alcohol use can contribute to a decline in the quality of clinical work and an increase in medical errors.

BURNOUT IN DYSFUNCTIONAL CLINICAL TEAMS

As a physician health liaison, I am frequently asked by departmental leadership to evaluate individual physicians for unprofessional behaviors, and sometimes while investigating the context of these behaviors, I find that the physician has been identified as the "problem person" in a team whose culture is highly disruptive, negative, and interpersonally toxic. The phenomenon of negative teams is common, and it is crucial to be able to distinguish between physicians who are true instigators of a negative culture and those who begin to engage in disruptive behaviors as a *result* of destructive and demoralizing team function. If a physician is the main instigator of team dysfunction, he or she must be evaluated for substance use, depression, other mental illness (including personality disorders), medical illness, life stressors, and many other factors. However, in the situation of dysfunctional teams, a systems approach is indicated; communication, implicit team values and conflicts, team structure, and lines of authority must all be examined. Bullying, intimidation, shaming, harassment, and passive aggression are all manifestations of unprofessional behaviors that can flourish in maladaptive healthcare teams and that can have a profound negative impact on clinicians as well as quality of patient care.

IDENTIFYING AND CARING FOR THE PHYSICIAN WITH BURNOUT AND UNPROFESSIONAL BEHAVIORS

There are some aspects of implicit attitudes and culture about caring for struggling colleagues that should be mentioned as part of expanding the principle of beneficence. The highest priority must always be given to patient care and patient safety, but these highest values are always aligned with those that also support the well-being of the physician. Physicians who care for other physicians know that the initial response to a mandate that he or she enter addiction treatment, undergo neuropsychological testing, or have a course of behavioral coaching is usually one of great shame, embarrassment, and resistance. In addition, department heads and other physician leaders often identify with the shame and stigma experienced by the physician in question and avoid cup-of-coffee interventions and other crucial conversations that are necessary both to protect patient care and to help the clinician. This dimension of medicine—protecting patient care along with the health of our physicians—must undergo considerable growth in order to moderate the values of extreme perfectionism and autonomy and promote the values of humanistic self-care and care for our colleagues.

Life and Career Transitions That May Challenge Well-Being

Sometimes a physician's life transitions, such as new parenthood, combined with work stressors can trigger a series of events that result in burnout and sometimes deficits in professional behaviors. Some of the life events that occur during training and early attending years include finding a life partner, acknowledging one's sexual orientation, marriage, relationship breakups or divorce, purchasing a home, pregnancy and childbirth, personal illness, and family or partner illness or death.

VIGNETTE 4: THE NEW PARENT

A junior attending in a busy academic department of psychiatry is 2 years out of residency and has enjoyed her work and her colleagues in her workplace. She and her husband welcome their first child; she returns to work 6 weeks after a vaginal delivery because that is what her hospital's maternity leave policy allows. Like most first-time mothers, she finds the task of caring for a newborn challenging, and when she returns to work, she struggles with fatigue and anxiety about how her infant is doing in daycare. In addition, she finds that she is unable to adequately pump her breast milk during the 20-minute breaks that are built into the outpatient clinic schedule. She feels hesitant about asking to alter her clinic schedule because she does not want to appear as if she is asking for special favors, so she tries to adhere to the schedule, with the result that she runs behind in documentation. She begins writing her clinic notes at night from home but finds this very challenging because she and her husband are also caring for the baby in addition to doing increased household chores. Two months after her return to work, this physician is behind in her chart documentation for the first time in her career. She feels emotionally and physically exhausted, anxious, and ashamed and that she is "just going through the motions" in her clinical work. She notices that she has been abrupt and irritable with her clinic staff, and when her chair meets with her to discuss her delinquent charts as a "professionalism concern," she begins to think about leaving her job.

Very often residents and early-career attending physicians have had little, if any, guidance about questions such as how much time they should take off to care for a sick child, attend a family funeral, or grieve the loss of a significant other. Early-career physicians are also commonly burdened with repaying large student loans at the same time that they are beginning their careers, which can add considerable financial stress. Most residents and young physicians must find a way to manage these events on their own or with the advice of peers; there are few uniform built-in programs to provide coaching, support, and guidance. Physicians may choose not to seek help from nonphysician resources such as hospital employee assistance programs; they frequently feel that nonphysicians will not understand their situations. There are few medical school and residency curricula that focus explicitly on this crucial area: how to be a physician while navigating both planned and unplanned life events.

Another career transition that can prove challenging for physicians is preparation for reducing practice or approaching retirement. The average age of practicing physicians in the United States is rising (Dellinger et al. 2017), and many healthcare institutions are grappling with issues of senior physicians who wish to continue to practice, questions about mild cognitive impairment in physicians, and patient safety. Many U.S. physicians have had little to no guidance about when and how to "step back" and plan for a rewarding and meaningful retirement.

Ethics and Physician Resilience

Medicine has promoted a culture in which perfection is not only a goal but an expectation in our very human endeavors, and anything less than perfect is a failure. Physicians believe that they can and will always move on to the next case, the next patient, no matter what clinical loss or tragedy they have just experienced; that they should not get sick, and when they are sick, they can always continue to work. Improving physician well-being cannot be addressed by urging physicians to "take better care of themselves" so they can be "more resilient." The majority of physicians are very resilient people, and they find it insulting and demoralizing to be told that if they only practiced better self-care, they would be able to be more productive, meet their RVU targets, and complete their documentation in a timely manner. Many trainees have stated that they feel that they now have yet another set of obligations: to log their duty hours regularly, religiously monitor their sleep and hydration, and make sure that they "don't look too tired." It is well known in residency program circles that duty hours monitoring has led to some falsification of work hour reports in some specialties, and the expectation of obfuscating data about one's work hours during training can set up an ongoing moral conundrum for our physicians-in-training. Physicians are acutely sensitive to a mandate that they pay lip service to self-care when the major drivers in burnout—that is, work compression, documentation demands, and lack of resources and support to provide quality patient care—are ignored. There is evidence that some physician-directed interventions aimed at reducing burnout can produce small effects, but organization-directed interventions have been shown to have more robust impact in reducing physician burnout (Panagioti et al. 2017).

The role of advocating for a healthier and more supportive work environment is uncomfortable for most physicians, who have been trained to be uncomplaining under any stressors. Often, physician "resilience" is interpreted as the ability to suffer silently, without complaint, throughout busy workdays with lack of adequate resources such as water, access to healthy food, or a place to sleep when in the hospital overnight. A change in our view of the ethics of resilience is in order: a view of resilience that supports self-advocacy and negotiation for resources to ensure well-being of the physician and the healthcare team.

Promoting Well-Being in Medicine

SCHOLARSHIP

We need scholarship on how to reconfigure the values of medical education and physicianhood to develop values and ethical norms that clearly state that the maintenance of our core of altruism, compassion, and striving for excellence depend absolutely on the value of the quality of our own lives—our health in every aspect of our being and of our community of healers. We have to be able to demonstrate to our students and residents, through the way we live our lives as physicians and in how we guide them through training, clear ethical principles that will help them make choices that will promote and sustain long, meaningful, and fulfilling careers.

PHYSICIAN LEADERSHIP

Making positive changes for physician well-being will entail addressing multiple domains of our profession, especially deeply embedded cultural beliefs and values. Strategies that are implemented ad hoc, without solid grounding in an understanding of ethics, culture, and history, will be less likely to be successful. The process of positive change will require prolonged and steady effort; expanding and articulating ethical principles and explicitly and implicitly endorsing values is essential. For this reason, healthcare systems must include a physician leadership group whose purpose is to speak for the values of physician well-being in every major system decision and initiative. Physician leaders will need to advocate for their unique roles and for making changes in the structure and content of physicians' work. This advocacy in itself will involve a major cultural shift—physicians are far more comfortable advocating for their patients than for themselves—the residue of the cultural values of self-sacrifice and stoicism.

Expert physician well-being leaders must be trained in a number of aspects of physician well-being, including detailed knowledge of the lifelong development of physicians, quality improvement methodology, peer support, crucial conversations, and collaboration with healthcare teams. Leaders must develop secondary prevention systems for identifying physicians at risk for burnout and exhibiting signs of burnout and must develop programs and policies that provide early effective interventions in a supportive and humanistic environment.

MEDICAL EDUCATION

Medical education has a central role in promoting change with regard to physician well-being. Medical students identify with the implicit values of medicine within their first few years. They observe how their role models live their lives and engage in practice while caring for self and others.

As students enter their residency years, they are usually at the start of adulthood, with numerous life tasks ahead of them. It is challenging for young men and women at this age to devote the majority of their energies (physical and emotional) to developing the skills, knowledge, and identities of physicians while negotiating major life changes at the same time. Program directors and core faculty must take an active, involved role in assisting the trainee to manage these life events during residency and model healthy decisions for trainees. Faculty must be able to articulate the basic principles and values that come into play in a life in medicine. Many educators in graduate medical education have come to see their central roles, in addition to teaching skills and knowledge, as teaching residents to use values- and morals-based decision making about work-life integration in the formative training years.

Conclusion

The traditional principles of medical ethics can be expanded to provide a foundation of values that guide and support positive changes in physician well-being in the practice of medicine. The long-standing culture of medicine has fostered some implicit beliefs that can contribute to burnout and present obstacles to recognizing distress and seeking help. Burnout can be a significant causal factor in professionalism deficits, such as disruptive behaviors and substance use disorders; individual physicians, healthcare teams, medical educators, and healthcare leadership must learn early identification of symptoms of burnout and depression. Expectable life and work transitions can be challenging for physicians, and formal guidance and coaching may reduce some of the stress associated with transitions and promote resilience. Efforts to improve physician well-being must include initiatives in scholarship, medical education, training of physician leaders, and advocacy.

KEY POINTS

---■---

- Traditional principles of medical ethics support the importance of physician health and wellness, and new research demonstrates that physician well-being and quality patient care are intrinsically aligned.

- Some interpretations of the implicit cultural values of medicine, such as altruism, self-sacrifice, and perfectionism, have at times served to compromise physician well-being.

- Adverse clinical events cause significant distress for most physicians and are often a "last straw" occurrence in the development of burnout and withdrawal from medicine.

- Deficits in professional behaviors, including substance use disorders, are correlated with higher rates of burnout in physicians.

- Physicians would benefit from support and coaching to prepare for expectable life and work transitions and stages such as new parenthood, becoming an attending physician, and retirement.

- For adequate change in physician well-being to occur, physician leaders with knowledge and expertise in physician well-being must be included "at the table" in healthcare institutions.

---■---

References

American Medical Association: AMA code of medical ethics' opinions on physicians' health and conduct. AMA Journal of Ethics 13(10):700–702, 2011

Chew-Graham CA, Rogers A, Yassin N: 'I wouldn't want it on my CV or their records': medical students' experiences of help-seeking for mental health problems. Med Educ 37(10):873–880, 2003 12974841

Dellinger EP, Pellegrini CA, Gallagher TH: The aging physician and the medical profession: a review. JAMA Surg 152(10):967–971, 2017 28724142

Dyrbye LN, Massie FS Jr, Eacker A, et al: Relationship between burnout and professional conduct and attitudes among US medical students. JAMA 304(11):1173–1180, 2010 20841530

Gabel S: Ethics and values in clinical practice: whom do they help? Mayo Clin Proc 86(5):421–424, 2011 21531885

Glasberg AL, Eriksson S, Norberg A: Burnout and 'stress of conscience' among healthcare personnel. J Adv Nurs 57(4):392–403, 2007 17291203

Gold JA, Johnson B, Leydon G, et al: Mental health self-care in medical students: a comprehensive look at help-seeking. Acad Psychiatry 39(1):37–46, 2015 25082721

Gross CP, Mead LA, Ford DE, et al: Physician, heal thyself? Regular source of care and use of preventive health services among physicians. Arch Intern Med 160(21):3209–3214, 2000 11088080

Leiter MP, Frank E, Matheson TJ: Demands, values, and burnout: relevance for physicians. Can Fam Physician 55(12):1224–1225, 1225.e1–1225.e6, 2009 20008605

Ludmerer K: Let Me Heal: The Opportunity to Preserve Excellence in American Medicine. New York, Oxford University Press, 2015

Maslach C, Leiter MP: The Truth About Burnout. Hoboken, NJ, John Wiley and Sons, 1997

Maslow AH: A theory of human motivation. Psychol Rev 50(4):370–396, 1943

Myers MF, Gabbard GO: The Physician as Patient. Washington, DC, American Psychiatric Publishing, 2008

Oreskovich MR, Kaups KL, Balch CM, et al: Prevalence of alcohol use disorders among American surgeons. Arch Surg 147(2):168–174, 2012 22351913

Panagioti M, Panagopoulou E, Bower P, et al: Controlled interventions to reduce burnout in physicians: a systematic review and meta-analysis. JAMA Intern Med 177(2):195–205, 2017 27918798

Roberts LW, Dyer AR (eds): Ethics in Mental Health Care (Concise Guides Series, Hales RE, series ed). Arlington, VA, American Psychiatric Publishing, 2004

Shanafelt TD, Noseworthy JH: Executive leadership and physician well-being: nine organizational strategies to promote engagement and reduce burnout. Mayo Clin Proc 92(1):129–146, 2017 27871627

Shanafelt TD, Boone S, Tan L, et al: Burnout and satisfaction with work-life balance among US physicians relative to the general US population. Arch Intern Med 172(18):1377–1385, 2012 22911330

Shapiro J, Galowitz P: Peer support for clinicians: a programmatic approach. Acad Med 91(9):1200–1204, 2016 27355784

West CP, Dyrbye LN, Shanafelt TD: Physician burnout: contributors, consequences and solutions. J Intern Med 283(6):516–529, 2018 29505159

Index

Page numbers printed in **boldface** type refer to tables and figures.

Vignettes (*continued*)
  of residency choice, 181
  of resilient psychiatry resident, 96
  of senior physician, 187–188
  of support for ARE, 288
  of well-meaning leader, 299–300
  of work stressors, 301–302

Well-being, 137. *See also* Physicians;
    Self-care; Work-life balance
  awareness of, 40
  culture of, **299**
  metaphor for, 212–229
  model for maintaining well-being
      and preventing burnout for
      psychiatrists, 211–232
    phone applications of, 230
    problems with solutions, 217–219,
        220–221, 222–224, 225–226
    tactics for, 229
    tips for maintaining, 226–227
    triage tool for obligations, **219**
    vignettes, 212–213
  physician, xvi, 293–309
    adverse clinical events, 300
    burnout in dysfunctional clinical
        teams, 303
    caring for physician with
        burnout and unprofessional
        behaviors, 303–304
    contribution of life and work
        stressors to burnout and
        unprofessional behaviors,
        301–303
      vignettes of, 301–303
    ethical principles in, 294–297
    ethics and physician resilience,
        305–306
    life and career transitions that
        challenge well-being,
        304–305
      vignette of new parent, 304
    values in medicine and impact
        on, 297–300, **299**
      moral stress, 297

physician's fault line, 297–300
      vignette, 299–300
  promoting in medicine, 306–307
    medical education, 307
    physician leadership, 306–307
    scholarship, 306
Well-Being Index, 55–56, 256
Wellness. *See also* Work-life balance
  ACEP's focus on, 14
  among medical students/residents,
      201
  occupation-related, xv
  programs, 11–12
  of psychiatrists, 15–16
"Wellness booth," 13
"Wellness day," 114–115
WHO. *See* World Health Organization
Women
  burnout rates for, 178
  career progress for, 132
  childbirth and, 131
  leadership in medicine, 132
  prevalence of female physicians, 130
  suicide among female psychiatrists,
      109
Women Physicians' Health Study, 107
Workaholism, 135
Work-life balance, 46, 72, 92–93,
      127–147, 228, 256. *See also* Well-
      being; Wellness
  conflict and burnout, 134–136
  definition of, 128
  effects of conflict on the physician,
      130–134
    career choices, 131–133
      academic physicians, 132–133
      career changes and reduction
          in hours, 131–132
      career progress for women,
          132
      childbirth, 131
    home life, 130–131
    medical marriages, 133–134
    psychological factors, 134
    work life, 130